# Respiratory Medicine

**First and second edition authors**
Angus Jeffries
Andrew Turley
Pippa McGowan

**Third edition authors**
Harish Patel
Catherine Gwilt

**Fourth edition authors**
Sarah Hickin
James Renshaw

**Fifth edition authors**
Hannah Lawrence
Thomas Moore

## 6th Edition
# CRASH COURSE

SERIES EDITOR
## Philip Xiu
MA (Cantab), MB BChir, MRCP, MRCGP, MScClinEd, FHEA, MAcadMEd, RCPathME
Honorary Senior Lecturer
Leeds University School of Medicine
Medical Examiner
Leeds Teaching Hospital Trust
Leeds, United Kingdom

FACULTY ADVISOR
## Swapna Mandal
BSc (Hons), FRCP (UK), PhD
Associate Professor, University College London
Consultant in Respiratory Medicine
Royal Free London NHS Foundation Trust

# Respiratory Medicine

## Amar Shah
BSc Haematology (Hons) (UK), MBBS (UK), MRCP (UK)
Consultant in Sleep and Ventilation and Respiratory Medicine
Royal Free Hospital
London, United Kingdom

## Anita Saigal
BM Medicine (UK), BSc Biomedical Sciences (UK), MRCP (UK)
Consultant in Sleep and Ventilation and Respiratory Medicine
Royal Free Hospital
London, United Kingdom

## Natasha Patel
MBBS (UK), BSc Medical Studies With Management (Hons) (UK)
Post-Foundation Year 2 Doctor
Barnet Hospital
London, United Kingdom

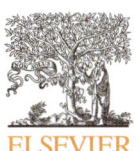

ELSEVIER

Elsevier

© 2026 Elsevier Limited. All rights are reserved, including those for text and data mining, AI training, and similar technologies.

Publisher's note: Elsevier takes a neutral position with respect to territorial disputes or jurisdictional claims in its published content, including in maps and institutional affiliations.

First edition 1999

Second edition 2003

Third edition 2008

Fourth edition 2013

Updated Fourth edition 2015

Fifth edition 2019

Sixth edition 2025

---

**Notices**

---

**ISBN:** 978-0-443-24984-6

*Content Strategist:* Trinity Hutton; Jennifer Dooley

*Content Development Specialist:* Ayan Dhar

*Project Manager:* Ayan Dhar

*Design:* Miles Hitchen

*Marketing Manager:* Deborah Watkins

Printed in India

Last digit is the print number: 9 8 7 6 5 4 3 2 1

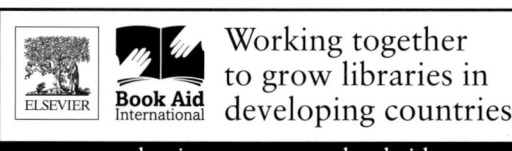

# Series editor's foreword

With great honour and pride, we present the latest edition of the *Crash Course* series. This series has traversed a journey of nearly a quarter-century, stemming from the vision of Dr Dan Horton-Szar, and his legacy continues to walk with us on this pathway of knowledge.

The series has been popular with students worldwide, selling over **1 million copies** and being translated into more than **eight languages**, reinforcing our commitment to global learning.

We remain extremely grateful for your unwavering trust. The series has once again been refreshed and fully upgraded in accordance with the rapidly changing medical guidelines, ensuring the content is comprehensive, accurate and fully up-to-date.

This latest series continues our tradition of integrating clinical practice with basic medical sciences, tailored meticulously for today's medical undergraduate curriculum. A central highlight of this instalment is our emphasis on high-yield exam content designed specifically for the MLA curriculum.

The addition of the **Rapid MLA Index** at the beginning of the book enhances this offering, serving as a valuable aid to students to track their exam preparation efficiently. We have also revised all self-assessment questions to align with the single best answer format in line with the latest MLA examination style. We have also added ***High-Yield Association Tables***. These are essential tools designed to aid students in recognizing clinical patterns and acing vignette-style exam questions. By condensing complex medical scenarios into digestible, manageable insights, these tables ensure efficient learning. They connect symptoms, diagnosis and treatment, bolstering understanding and confidence in tackling the rigorous MLA exams. This comprehensive approach makes these tables an indispensable asset in your exam preparations.

Utilizing student feedback, we have strived to maintain the core principles of this series: delivering precise and readable text that brings together depth and clarity. The authors are experienced junior doctors who successfully navigated these exams recently, ensuring practical and tested guidance. A team of expert faculty advisors from across the United Kingdom ensures the content's accuracy, making it resilient and reliable.

As we turn a new chapter with the latest edition, we honour the past, cherish the present and embrace the promise of the future. We wish you every success in your journey of learning and growth and hope that this series adds value to your life, both as students and as future medical professionals.

**Philip Xiu**

# Preface

## Authors

Being able to work in a field such as Respiratory Medicine allows us to combine key symptoms, physiological data and clinical signs with the relevant diagnoses. Respiratory Medicine encompasses acute admissions and chronic conditions, and it is important to recognize and optimize the underlying condition when treating these patients.

This textbook aims to provide a comprehensive and up-to-date exploration of respiratory medicine, catering to medical students. In this book, we cover the anatomy of the lungs, mechanisms of gas exchange and reasons for respiratory failure, as well as explore the diagnosis, treatment and management of a variety of respiratory disorders. This textbook integrates the latest clinical guidelines and clinical practices in turn.

In keeping with the latest MLA examination style, we have removed the extended matching questions and expanded the single best answer question bank, as well as linking chapters to the relevant MLA curriculum.

We hope this volume will be a valuable resource and potentially support others hoping to pursue a career in Respiratory Medicine.

**Amar Shah, Anita Saigal and Natasha Patel**

## Faculty Advisor

It has been a privilege to work alongside a team of dedicated professionals committed to advancing medical education. This book represents a collaborative effort to provide a comprehensive and up-to-date resource for medical students and practitioners alike.

Respiratory Medicine is a dynamic field that requires a deep understanding of both acute and chronic conditions. Our goal with this textbook is to bridge the gap between theoretical knowledge and clinical practice, offering insights into the anatomy of the lungs, mechanisms of gas exchange, chronic respiratory disease and respiratory failure. We have meticulously integrated the latest clinical guidelines and practices to ensure that our readers are well-equipped to diagnose, treat, and manage a wide range of respiratory disorders.

I hope this volume serves as a valuable resource, it is my sincere belief that the knowledge contained within these pages will contribute to the betterment of patient care.

**Swapna Mandal**

# Acknowledgements

## Authors

I would very much like to thank Phil Xiu and the *Crash Course* team for the opportunity to contribute to this new edition. I am also grateful for the ongoing support of the faculty advisor, Dr Swapna Mandal. With a gratitude always to my partner and children for their continued patience and support.

**Amar Shah**

I would like to thank Phil, Amar and the *Crash Course* team for the opportunity to contribute to this new edition and for their support through this process. With a gratitude always to my partner, children and parents for their support.

**Anita Saigal**

I would like to thank Dr Amar Shah for giving me the fantastic opportunity of contributing to this book. As a junior doctor, it has enriched my own learning while also allowing me to develop content that I would have found useful as a medical student. In addition, I would like to thank Phil Xiu for all his dedication and support during this process. Finally, my contributions are dedicated to my parents, Shane and Mimasha Patel; my siblings, Avni, Sid and Pranay Patel and my partner Nimit Dodhia; without their ongoing encouragement, I would not be where I am today.

**Natasha Patel**

# Series editor's acknowledgement

We would like to express our sincere gratitude to those who have provided their support and expertise in preparing this sixth edition of the *Crash Course* series. Our junior doctor contributors' participation in crafting the manuscript has been indispensable. Their first-hand experience and current medical knowledge have infused realism and practicality into our content.

Our faculty editors deserve a special note of thanks. They have extensively validated the correctness of the information, ensuring that the content is not just accurate but also contemporaneous, credible and aligns with the latest medical standards.

We extend our heartfelt thanks to our publisher, Elsevier. Their staff have demonstrated an unwavering commitment to quality, maintaining the high standards set since the first edition. Their insights have routinely enriched the content and process alike.

Our Commissioning Editor, Jeremy Bowes, deserves a special mention for his consistent support and guiding hand throughout the development process. His directions and advice have bettered this edition and spurred us on our quest for excellence.

We are greatly indebted to Alex Mortimer for her wisdom, practical insights and valuable guidance. A big thank you to our Content Strategists, Jennifer Dooley, Trinity Hutton and Cloe Holland-Borosh, who need special acknowledgement for meticulously outlining the direction and scope of the content. They've managed to mix details with a strategic plan, keeping our readers in mind.

Lastly, much gratitude is owed to our Content Product Managers, Taranpreet Kaur, Ayan Dhar, Shivani Pal and Tapajyoti Chaudhuri, who have juggled the numerous day-to-day tasks with utmost dedication and perseverance. Despite the ever-approaching deadlines, they have shown remarkable patience and steadfast determination, ensuring that each step of the book's development was accomplished seamlessly.

In conclusion, we sincerely thank each of these wonderful people for their outstanding contributions and support, without which this work wouldn't have been achieved. Their passion, commitment and collaborative effort have helped us bring this edition together.

**Philip Xiu**

# Rapid MLA Index

The MLA Curriculum Conditions Priority levels have been based on the below:

Level 1: Conditions that a newly qualified doctor should have a good knowledge of and be able to recognize and manage.

Level 2: Conditions requiring knowledge for recognizing and confirming diagnosis and planning first-line management in straightforward cases.

Level 3: Conditions where recognition of clinical presentation and describing principles of management are important.

**Table 1** MLA Conditions and Where to Find Them

| Priority | MLA Conditions | Chapter | Page |
|---|---|---|---|
| 3 | Acid-base abnormality | Chapter 10: The respiratory patient: clinical investigations | 94–95 |
| 1 | Acute bronchitis | Chapter 8: Taking a respiratory history | 78–79 |
| 1 | Allergic disorder | Chapter 13: The upper respiratory tract | 125–127 |
| 1 | Anaemia | Chapter 23: Respiratory manifestations of systemic disease | 214–215 |
| 1 | Anaphylaxis | Chapter 13: The upper respiratory tract | 125 |
| 2 | Ankylosing spondylitis | Chapter 23: Respiratory manifestations of systemic disease | 216–217 |
| 2 | Asbestos-related lung disease | Chapter 16: Disorders of the interstitium<br>Chapter 20: Pleural disease | 161–162<br>198–199 |
| 1 | Asthma | Chapter 7: Basic pharmacology<br>Chapter 9: Examination of the respiratory system<br>Chapter 14: Asthma | 69–70<br>85–86, 89, 91<br>133–144 |
| 3 | Asthma COPD overlap syndrome | Chapter 14: Asthma<br>Chapter 15: Chronic obstructive pulmonary disease | 137<br>147 |
| 1 | Breast cancer | Chapter 20: Pleural disease | 192 |
| 2 | Bronchiectasis | Chapter 9: Examination of the respiratory system<br>Chapter 19: Bronchiectasis and cystic fibrosis | 85, 91<br>185–187 |
| 3 | Bronchiolitis | Chapter 19: Bronchiectasis and cystic fibrosis | 147 |
| 1 | Cardiac arrest | Chapter 20: Pleural disease | 198 |
| 1 | Chronic obstructive pulmonary disease | Chapter 7: Basic pharmacology<br>Chapter 14: Asthma<br>Chapter 15: Chronic obstructive pulmonary disease | 69–70<br>137<br>145–153 |
| 1 | COVID-19 | Chapter 8: Taking a respiratory history<br>Chapter 18: Respiratory infections | 79<br>181–182 |
| 1 | Cystic fibrosis | Chapter 19: Bronchiectasis and cystic fibrosis | 188–190 |
| 1 | Diabetic ketoacidosis | Chapter 9: Examination of the respiratory system | 83 |
| 3 | Disease prevention/screening | Chapter 7: Basic pharmacology | 69–70, 73 |
| 1 | Drug overdose | Chapter 9: Examination of the respiratory system | 86 |
| 1 | Epistaxis | Chapter 23: Respiratory manifestations of systemic disease | 215–216 |

*continued*

**Table 2** MLA Presentations and Where to Find Them

*continued*

# Contents

# Section 1

# BASIC SCIENCE AND PHYSIOLOGY

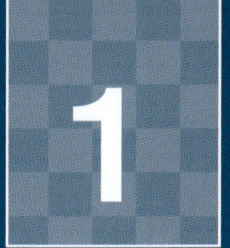

## INTRODUCTION TO RESPIRATORY MEDICINE

Understanding the respiratory system and the pathological processes that can affect it is a fundamental part of modern medicine. In the United Kingdom, approximately one in five people are diagnosed with asthma, chronic obstructive pulmonary disease (COPD) or another long-term respiratory condition during their lifetime. Unfortunately, a person dies from a respiratory disease every 5 minutes in the United Kingdom. Worldwide in 2019, four of the top ten causes of death were primary respiratory disorders (lower respiratory infections, COPD, lung cancers and tuberculosis), according to World Health Organization statistics.

There is significant morbidity associated with respiratory conditions, affecting millions of people across the world. In health, we hardly notice our breathing; however, when our breathing is compromised, we notice nothing else. In addition to morbidity, there are health economic consequences to respiratory disorders, with 8% of hospital admissions in the United Kingdom in 2011 due to respiratory disease. The implications of respiratory problems influence all medical and surgical specialities. An assessment of lung health is required before any surgery requiring general anaesthesia and informs the decision-making process prior to intensive care admission.

As a physician, understanding the respiratory system is vital in day-to-day practice. Having a firm grasp on normal physiology, control and response to insult is essential to recognizing, predicting and effectively managing illness. This book aims to outline the physiology, demonstrate how assessments are carried out and discuss the common conditions currently seen in respiratory medicine.

## OVERALL STRUCTURE AND FUNCTION

### Respiration

Respiration refers to the processes involved in oxygen transport from the atmosphere to the body tissues and the release and transportation of carbon dioxide produced in the tissues to the atmosphere.

Microorganisms rely on diffusion for the supply of oxygen to and removal of carbon dioxide from their environment. Humans, however, are unable to rely on diffusion because:

* Their surface area:volume ratio is too small.
* The diffusion distance from the surface of the body to the cells is too large and the process would be far too slow to be compatible with life.

Remember that diffusion time increases with the square of the distance, and, as a result, the human body has had to develop a specialized respiratory system to overcome this problem. This system has two components:

1. A gas-exchange system that provides a large surface area for the uptake of oxygen from, and the release of carbon dioxide to, the environment. This function is performed by the lungs.
2. A transport system that delivers oxygen to the tissues from the lungs and carbon dioxide to the lungs from the tissues. This function is carried out by the cardiovascular system.

### Structure

The respiratory system can be neatly divided into upper respiratory tract (nasal and oral cavities, pharynx, larynx and trachea) and lower respiratory tract (main bronchi and lungs) (Fig. 1.1).

### Upper respiratory tract

The upper respiratory tract has a large surface area and a rich blood supply, and its epithelium (respiratory epithelium) is covered by a mucus secretion. Within the nose, hairs are present, which act as a filter. The function of the upper respiratory tract is to warm, moisten and filter the air so that it is in a suitable condition for gaseous exchange in the distal part of the lower respiratory tract.

### Lower respiratory tract

The lower respiratory tract consists of the lower part of the trachea, the two primary bronchi and the lungs. These structures are contained within the thoracic cavity.

### Lungs

The lungs are the organs of gas exchange and act as both a conduit for air flow (the airway) and a surface for movement of oxygen into the blood and carbon dioxide out of the blood (the alveolar–capillary membrane).

The lungs consist of airways, blood vessels, nerves and lymphatics, supported by parenchymal tissue. Inside the lungs, the two main bronchi divide into smaller and smaller airways until the end respiratory unit (acinus) is reached (Fig. 1.2).

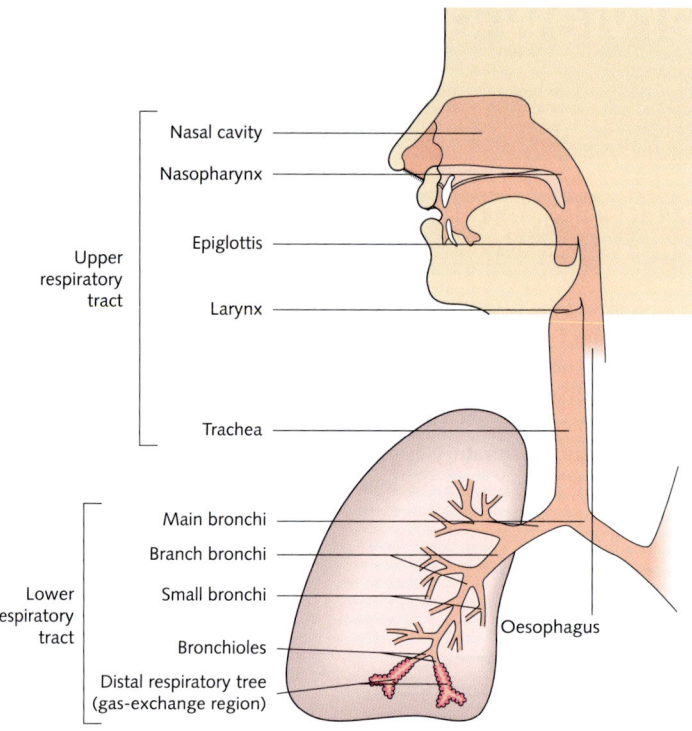

**Fig. 1.1** Schematic diagram of the respiratory tract.

## Acinus

The acinus is the part of the airway involved in gaseous exchange (i.e., the passage of oxygen from the lungs to the blood and carbon dioxide from the blood to the lungs). It begins with the respiratory bronchioles and includes subsequent divisions of the airway and alveoli.

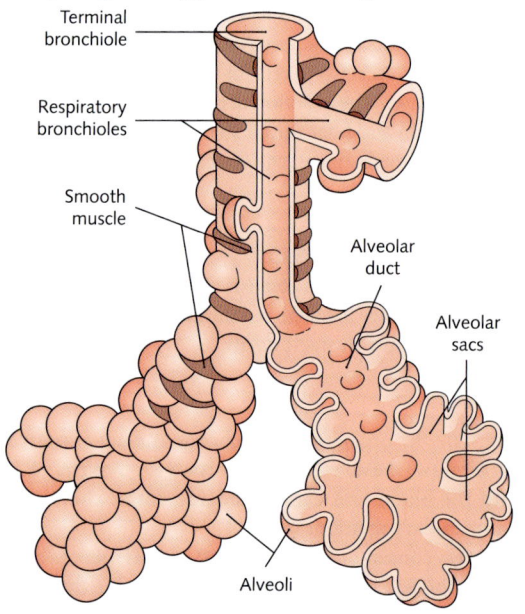

**Fig. 1.2** The acinus, or respiratory unit. This part of the airway is involved in gas exchange.

### Conducting airways

Conducting airways allow the transport of gases to and from the acinus but are themselves unable to partake in gas exchange. They include all divisions of the bronchi proximal to, but excluding, respiratory bronchioles.

### Pleurae

The lung, chest wall and mediastinum are covered by two continuous layers of epithelium known as the pleurae. The visceral pleura is the inner pleura covering the lung and the parietal pleura is the outer pleura covering the chest wall and mediastinum. These two pleurae are closely opposed and are separated by only a thin layer of liquid. The liquid acts as a lubricant and allows the two surfaces to slip over each other during breathing.

## BASIC CONCEPTS IN RESPIRATION

The supply of oxygen to body tissues is essential for life; after only a brief period without oxygen, cells undergo irreversible change and eventually die. The respiratory system plays an essential role in preventing tissue hypoxia by optimizing the oxygen content of

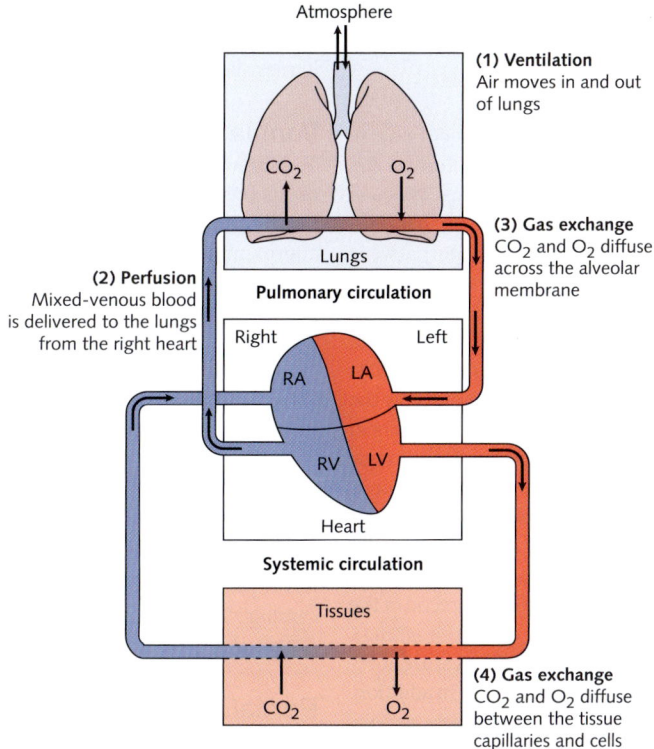

Atmosphere

**(1) Ventilation**
Air moves in and out
of lungs

$CO_2$    $O_2$

**(3) Gas exchange**
$CO_2$ and $O_2$ diffuse
across the alveolar
membrane

Lungs

**Pulmonary circulation**

**(2) Perfusion**
Mixed-venous blood
is delivered to the lungs
from the right heart

Right    Left

RA    LA

RV    LV

Heart

**Systemic circulation**

Tissues

**(4) Gas exchange**
$CO_2$ and $O_2$ diffuse
between the tissue
capillaries and cells

$CO_2$    $O_2$

**Fig. 1.3** Key steps in respiration. *LA,* Left atrium; *LV,* left ventricle; *RA,* right atrium; *RV,* right ventricle.

arterial blood through efficient gas exchange. The three key steps involved in gas exchange are:

1. Ventilation
2. Perfusion
3. Diffusion

Together these processes ensure that oxygen is available for transport to the body tissues and that carbon dioxide is eliminated (Fig. 1.3). If any of the three steps are compromised, e.g., through lung disease, then the oxygen content of the blood will fall below normal (hypoxaemia) and levels of carbon dioxide may rise (hypercapnia) (Table 1.1). In clinical practice, we do not directly test for tissue hypoxia but look for:

- Symptoms and signs of impaired gas exchange (e.g., breathlessness or central cyanosis).
- Abnormal results from arterial blood gas tests.

## Ventilation

Ventilation is the movement of air in and out of the respiratory system. It is determined by both:

- The respiratory rate (i.e., number of breaths per minute, normally 12–20).
- The volume of each breath, also known as the tidal volume.

**Table 1.1** Common respiratory terms

| Term | Definition |
|---|---|
| Hypocapnia | Decreased carbon dioxide tension in arterial blood ($P_aCO_2 < 4.6$ kPa or 35 mmHg) |
| Hypercapnia | Increased carbon dioxide tension in arterial blood ($P_aCO_2 > 6$ kPa or 45 mmHg) |
| Hypoxaemia | Deficient oxygenation of the arterial blood ($PaO_2 < 8$ kPa or 60 mmHg) |
| Hypoxia | Deficient oxygenation of the tissues |
| Hyperventilation | Ventilation that is in excess of metabolic requirements (results in hypocapnia) |
| Hypoventilation | Ventilation that is too low for metabolic requirements (results in hypercapnia) |

A change in ventilation in response to the metabolic needs of the body, can therefore be brought about by either:

- Altering the number of breaths per minute, or
- Adjusting the amount of air that enters the lungs with each breath.

In practice, the most common response to hypoxaemia is rapid, shallow breathing, which increases the elimination of carbon dioxide and often leads to hypocapnia. However, it should be noted that a raised respiratory rate, or tachypnoea, is not the same as hyperventilation. The term hyperventilation refers to a situation where ventilation is too great for the body's metabolic needs.

## The mechanisms of ventilation

The movement of air into and out of the lungs takes place because of pressure differences caused by changes in lung volumes. Air flows from a high-pressure area to a low-pressure area. We cannot change the local atmospheric pressure around us to a level higher than that inside our lungs; the only obvious alternative is to lower the pressure within the lungs. We achieve this pressure reduction by expanding the size of the chest.

The main muscle of inspiration is the diaphragm, upon which the two lungs sit. The diaphragm is dome shaped; contraction flattens the dome, increasing intrathoracic volume. This is aided by the external intercostal muscles, which raise the ribcage; this results in a lowered pressure within the thoracic cavity and hence the lungs, supplying the driving force for air flow into the lungs. Inspiration is responsible for most of the work of breathing; diseases of the lungs or chest wall may increase the workload so that accessory muscles are also required to maintain adequate ventilation.

Expiration is largely passive, being a result of elastic recoil of the lung tissue. However, in forced expiration (e.g., during coughing), the abdominal muscles increase the intraabdominal pressure, forcing the contents of the abdomen against the diaphragm. In addition, the internal intercostal muscles lower the ribcage. These actions greatly increase intrathoracic pressure and enhance expiration.

### Impaired ventilation

There are two main types of disorders that impair ventilation. These are:

1. Obstructive disorders:
   - Airways are narrowed and resistance to air flow is increased.
   - Mechanisms of airway narrowing include inflamed and thickened bronchial walls (e.g., asthma), airways filled with mucus (e.g., chronic bronchitis, asthma) and airway collapse (e.g., emphysema).
2. Restrictive disorders:
   - Lungs are less able to expand and so the volume of gas exchanged is reduced.
   - Mechanisms include stiffening of lung tissue (e.g., pulmonary fibrosis) or inadequacy of respiratory muscles (e.g., Duchenne muscular dystrophy).

Obstructive and restrictive disorders have characteristic patterns of lung function, measured by pulmonary function tests.

Ventilatory failure occurs if the work of breathing becomes excessive and muscles fail. In this situation, or to prevent it from occurring, mechanical ventilation is required.

## Perfusion

The walls of the alveoli contain a dense network of capillaries bringing mixed-venous blood from the right heart. The barrier separating blood in the capillaries and air in the alveoli is extremely thin. Perfusion of blood through these pulmonary capillaries allows diffusion, and therefore gas exchange, to take place.

## Ventilation:perfusion inequality

To achieve efficient gaseous exchange, it is essential that the flow of gas (ventilation: $V$) and the flow of blood (perfusion: $Q$) are closely matched. The $V/Q$ ratio in a normal, healthy lung is approximately one. Two extreme scenarios illustrate mismatching of ventilation and perfusion (Fig. 1.4). These are:

- Normal alveolar ventilation but no perfusion (e.g., owing to a blood clot obstructing flow).
- Normal perfusion but no air reaching the lung unit (e.g., owing to a mucus plug occluding an airway).

$V/Q$ inequality is the most common cause of hypoxaemia and underlies many respiratory diseases.

## Diffusion

At the gas-exchange surface, diffusion occurs across the alveolar–capillary membrane. Molecules of carbon dioxide and oxygen diffuse along their partial pressure gradients.

## Partial pressures

Air in the atmosphere, before it is inhaled and moistened, contains 21% oxygen. This means that:

- Twenty-one percent of the total molecules in air are oxygen molecules.
- Oxygen is responsible for 21% of the total air pressure; this is its partial pressure, measured in mmHg or kPa and abbreviated as $PO_2$ (Table 1.2).

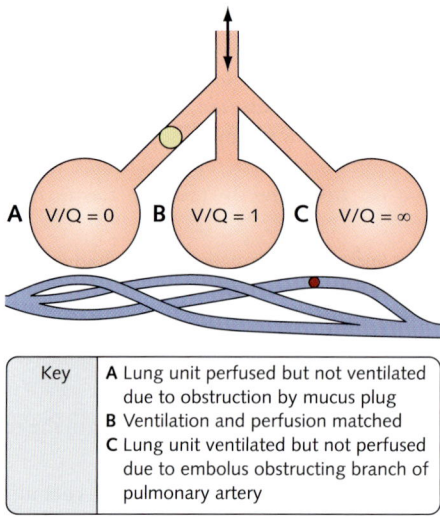

| Key | A Lung unit perfused but not ventilated due to obstruction by mucus plug |
|---|---|
|  | B Ventilation and perfusion matched |
|  | C Lung unit ventilated but not perfused due to embolus obstructing branch of pulmonary artery |

**Fig. 1.4** Ventilation:perfusion ($V/Q$) mismatching.

**Table 1.2** Abbreviations used in denoting partial pressures[a]

| Abbreviation | Definition |
| --- | --- |
| $PO_2$ | Oxygen tension in blood (either arterial or venous) |
| $P_aO_2$ | Arterial oxygen tension |
| $P_vO_2$ | Oxygen tension in mixed-venous blood |
| $P_AO_2$ | Alveolar oxygen tension |

[a]Carbon dioxide tensions follow the same format. ($PCO_2$, etc.)

Partial pressure also determines the gas content of liquids, but it is not the only factor. Gas enters the liquid as a solution, and the amount that enters depends on its solubility. The more soluble a gas, the more molecules will enter solution for a given partial pressure. The partial pressure of a gas in a liquid is sometimes referred to as its tension (i.e., arterial oxygen tension is the same as $P_aO_2$).

As blood perfusing the pulmonary capillaries is mixed-venous blood:

- Oxygen will diffuse from the higher $PO_2$ environment of the alveoli into the capillaries.
- Carbon dioxide will diffuse from the blood towards the alveoli, where $PCO_2$ is lower.

Blood and gas equilibrate as the partial pressures become the same in each and gas exchange then stops.

## Oxygen transport

Once oxygen has diffused into the capillaries, it must be transported to the body tissues. The solubility of oxygen in the blood is low and only a small percentage of the body's requirement can be carried in dissolved form. Therefore, most of the oxygen is combined with haemoglobin in red blood cells. Haemoglobin has four binding sites and the amount of oxygen carried by haemoglobin in the blood depends on how many of these sites are occupied. If they are all occupied by oxygen, the molecule is said to be saturated. The oxygen saturation ($S_aO_2$) tells us the relative percentage of the maximum possible sites that can be bound. Note that anaemia will not reduce $S_aO_2$; lower haemoglobin means there are fewer available sites but the relative percentage of possible sites that are saturated stays the same.

The relationship between the partial pressure of oxygen and percentage saturation of haemoglobin is represented by the oxygen dissociation curve.

## Diffusion defects

If the blood–gas barrier becomes thickened through disease, then the diffusion of oxygen and carbon dioxide will be impaired. Any impairment is particularly noticeable during exercise, when pulmonary flow increases and blood spends an even shorter time in the capillaries, exposed to alveolar oxygen. Impaired diffusion is, however, a much less common cause of hypoxaemia than $V{:}Q$ mismatching.

## CONTROL OF RESPIRATION

Respiration must respond to the metabolic demands of the body. This is achieved by a control system within the brainstem that receives information from various sources in the body where sensors monitor:

- Partial pressures of oxygen and carbon dioxide in the blood.
- pH of the extracellular fluid within the brain.
- Mechanical changes in the chest wall.

Based on the information they receive, the respiratory centres modify ventilation to ensure that oxygen supply and carbon dioxide removal from the tissues match their metabolic requirements. The actual mechanical change to ventilation is carried out by the respiratory muscles; these are known as the effectors of the control system.

### COMMON PITFALLS

It is easy to get confused about $P_aO_2$, $S_aO_2$ and oxygen content. $P_aO_2$ tells us the pressure of the oxygen molecules dissolved in plasma, not those bound to haemoglobin. It is not a measure of how much oxygen is in the arterial blood. $S_aO_2$ tells us how many of the possible haemoglobin binding sites are occupied by oxygen. To calculate the amount of oxygen, you would also need to know haemoglobin levels and how much oxygen is dissolved. Oxygen content ($C_aO_2$) is the only value that actually tells us how much oxygen is in the blood and, unlike $P_aO_2$ or $S_aO_2$, it is given in units that denote quantity (mL $O_2$/dL).

Respiration can also be modified by higher centres (e.g., during speech, anxiety, emotion).

## OTHER FUNCTIONS OF THE RESPIRATORY SYSTEM

Respiration is also concerned with a number of other functions, including metabolism, excretion, hormonal activity and, most importantly:

- The pH of body fluids.
- Regulation of body temperature.

### Acid–base regulation

Carbon dioxide forms carbonic acid in the blood, which dissociates to form hydrogen ions, lowering pH. By controlling the partial pressure of carbon dioxide, the respiratory system plays an important role in regulating the body's acid–base status;

lung disease can therefore lead to acid–base disturbance. In acute disease, it is important to test for blood pH and bicarbonate levels, and these are included in the standard arterial blood gas tests.

## Body temperature regulation

Body temperature is achieved mainly by insensible heat loss. Thus, by altering ventilation, body temperature may be regulated.

## Metabolism

The lungs have a huge vascular supply and thus a large number of endothelial cells. Hormones such as noradrenaline (norepinephrine), prostaglandins and 5-hydroxytryptamine are taken up by these cells and destroyed. Some exogenous compounds are also taken up by the lungs and destroyed (e.g., amphetamine and imipramine).

## Excretion

Carbon dioxide and some drugs (notably those administered through the lungs, e.g., general anaesthetics) are excreted by the lungs.

## Hormonal activity

Hormones (e.g., steroids) act on the lungs. Insulin enhances glucose utilization and protein synthesis. Angiotensin II is formed in the lungs from angiotensin I (by angiotensin-converting enzyme). Damage to the lung tissue causes the release of prostacyclin $PGI_2$, which prevents platelet aggregation.

---

### ● Chapter Summary

- Respiratory illness is a major cause of morbidity and mortality in the United Kingdom and worldwide. Knowledge of the respiratory system is important for doctors in all specialities.
- The main functions of the respiratory system are gas exchange and the transport of gases involved in respiration, the process in tissues responsible for production of energy.
- The three key steps involved in gas exchange are ventilation, perfusion and diffusion. Defects in these steps cause hypoxaemia.
- Ventilation is the movement of air into and out of the lungs. This movement takes place owing to pressure differences caused by changes in lung volumes. Air flows from a high-pressure area to a low-pressure area. Ventilation is determined by respiratory rate and the volume of each breath.
- Perfusion of blood through a dense network of capillaries brings mixed-venous blood from the right heart into contact with the extremely thin barrier separating the blood from the air in the alveoli.
- Diffusion occurs across the alveolar–capillary membrane. Molecules of $CO_2$ and $O_2$ diffuse along their partial pressure gradients.

## THE RESPIRATORY TRACT

The respiratory tract is the collective term for the anatomy relating to the process of respiration, from the nose down to the alveoli. It can be considered in two parts: that lying outside the thorax (upper tract) and that within the thorax (lower tract) (see Fig. 1.1). These will be considered in turn, detailing both macroscopic and microscopic structure.

## Macroscopic structure

### Upper respiratory tract

#### Nose and nasopharynx

The nose is the part of the respiratory tract superior to the hard palate. It consists of the external nose and the nasal cavities, which are separated by the nasal septum. The main functions of these structures are olfaction (which is not detailed in this book) and breathing.

The lateral wall of the nasal cavity consists of bony ridges called conchae or turbinates (Figs. 2.1 and 2.2), which provide a large surface area covered in highly vascularized mucous membrane to warm and humidify inspired air. Under each turbinate, there is a groove or meatus. The paranasal air sinuses (frontal, sphenoid, ethmoid and maxillary) drain into these meatuses via small ostia, or openings.

#### Nasal neurovascular supply and lymphatic drainage

The terminal branches of the internal and external carotid arteries provide a rich blood supply for the internal nose. The

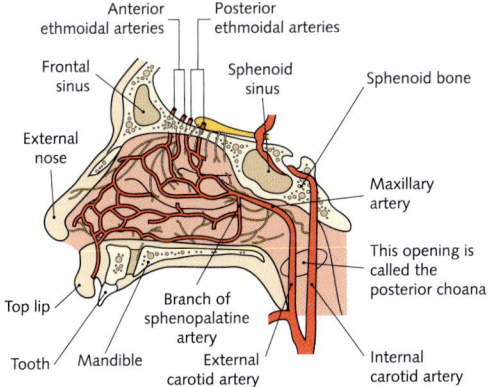

**Fig. 2.1** Lateral view of the nasal cavity showing the rich blood supply.

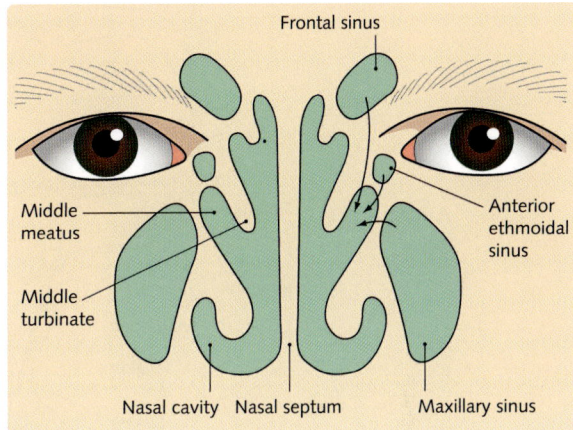

**Fig. 2.2** Frontal view of the nasal cavity drainage sites of the paranasal sinuses.

sphenopalatine artery (from the maxillary artery) and the anterior ethmoidal artery (from the ophthalmic) are the two most important branches. Sensation to the area is provided mainly by the maxillary branch of the trigeminal nerve. Lymphatic vessels drain into the submandibular node, then into deep cervical nodes.

#### Pharynx

The pharynx extends from the base of the skull to the inferior border of the cricoid cartilage, where it is continuous anteriorly with the trachea and posteriorly with the oesophagus. It is described as being divided into three parts: the nasopharynx, oropharynx and laryngopharynx, which open anteriorly into the nose, mouth and larynx, respectively (Fig. 2.3). The pharynx is part of both the respiratory and gastrointestinal systems.

The nasopharynx is situated above the soft palate and opens anteriorly into the nasal cavities at the choanae (posterior nares). During swallowing, the nasopharynx is cut off from the oropharynx by the soft palate. The nasopharynx contains the opening of the eustachian canal (pharyngotympanic or auditory tube) and the adenoids, which lie beneath the epithelium of its posterior wall.

#### Musculature, neurovascular supply and lymphatic drainage

The tube of the pharynx is enveloped by the superior, middle and inferior constrictor muscles, respectively. These receive arterial blood supply from the external carotid through the superior

9

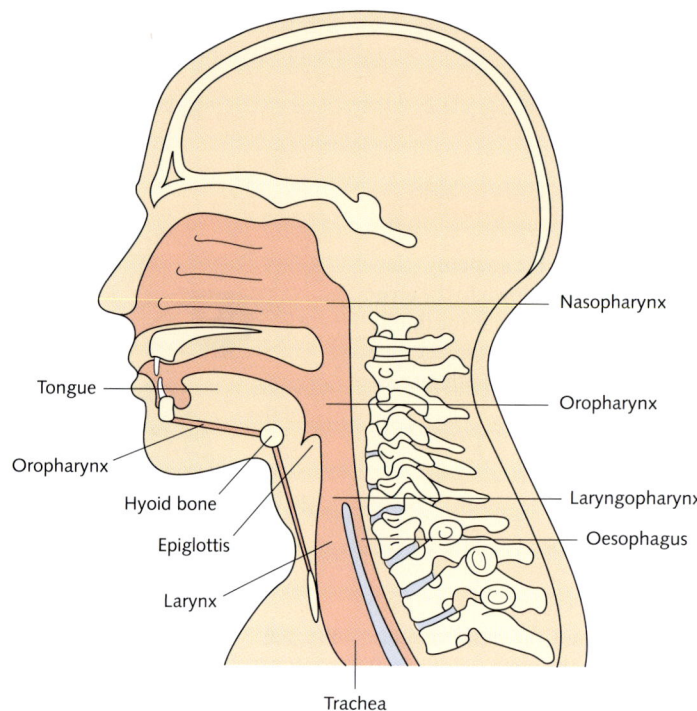

**Fig. 2.3** Schematic diagram showing midline structures of the head and neck.

thyroid, ascending pharyngeal, facial and lingual arteries. Venous drainage is by a plexus of veins on the outer surface of the pharynx to the internal jugular vein. Both sensory and motor nerve supplies are from the pharyngeal plexus (cranial nerves IX and X); the maxillary nerve (cranial nerve V) supplies the nasopharynx with sensory fibres. Lymphatic vessels drain directly into the deep cervical lymph nodes.

## Larynx

The larynx is continuous with the trachea at its inferior end. At its superior end, it is attached to the U-shaped hyoid bone and lies below the epiglottis of the tongue. The larynx consists of a cartilaginous skeleton linked by a number of membranes. This cartilaginous skeleton comprises the epiglottis, thyroid, arytenoid and cricoid cartilages (Fig. 2.4). The larynx has three main functions:

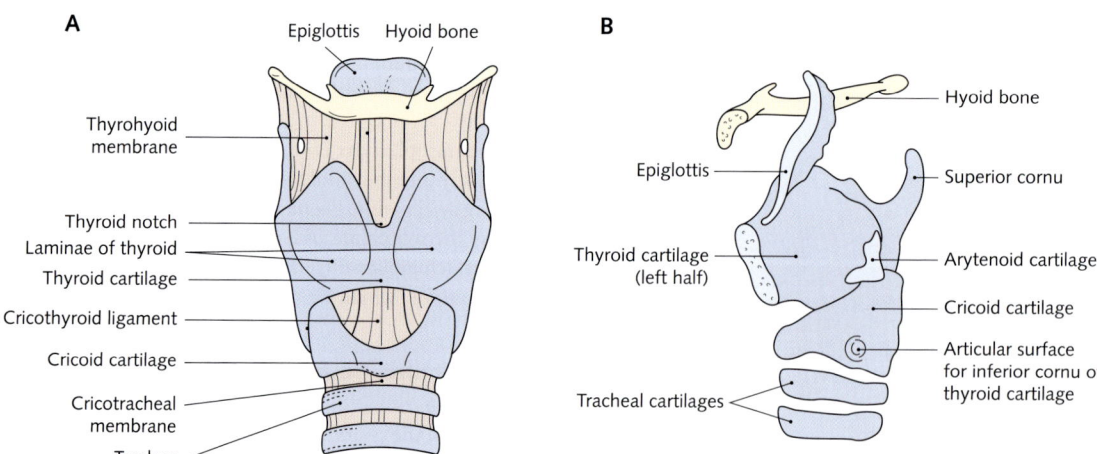

**Fig. 2.4** The larynx. (A) External view – anterior aspect. (B) Median section through the larynx, hyoid bone and trachea.

1. As an open valve, to allow air to pass when breathing.
2. Protection of the trachea and bronchi during swallowing. The vocal folds close, the epiglottis is pushed back covering the opening to the larynx, and the larynx is pulled upwards and forwards beneath the tongue.
3. Speech production (phonation).

## Musculature

There are external and internal muscles of the larynx. One external muscle, the cricothyroid, and numerous internal muscles attach to the thyroid membrane and cartilage. The internal muscles may change the shape of the larynx: they protect the lungs by a sphincter action and adjust the vocal folds in phonation.

## Blood and nerve supply and lymphatic drainage

The blood supply of the larynx is from the superior and inferior laryngeal arteries, which are accompanied by the superior and recurrent laryngeal branches of the vagus nerve (cranial nerve X). The internal branch of the superior laryngeal nerve supplies the mucosa of the larynx above the vocal cords, and the external branch supplies the cricothyroid muscle. The recurrent laryngeal nerve supplies the mucosa below the vocal cords and all the intrinsic muscles apart from the cricothyroid. Lymph vessels above the vocal cords drain into the upper deep cervical lymph nodes; below the vocal cords, lymphatic vessels drain into the lower cervical lymph nodes (Fig. 2.5 displays the lymphatic system).

## Trachea

The trachea is a cartilaginous and membranous tube of about 10 cm in length. It extends from the larynx to its bifurcation at the carina (at the level of the fourth or fifth thoracic vertebra). The trachea is approximately 2.5 cm in diameter and is supported by C-shaped rings of hyaline cartilage. The rings are completed

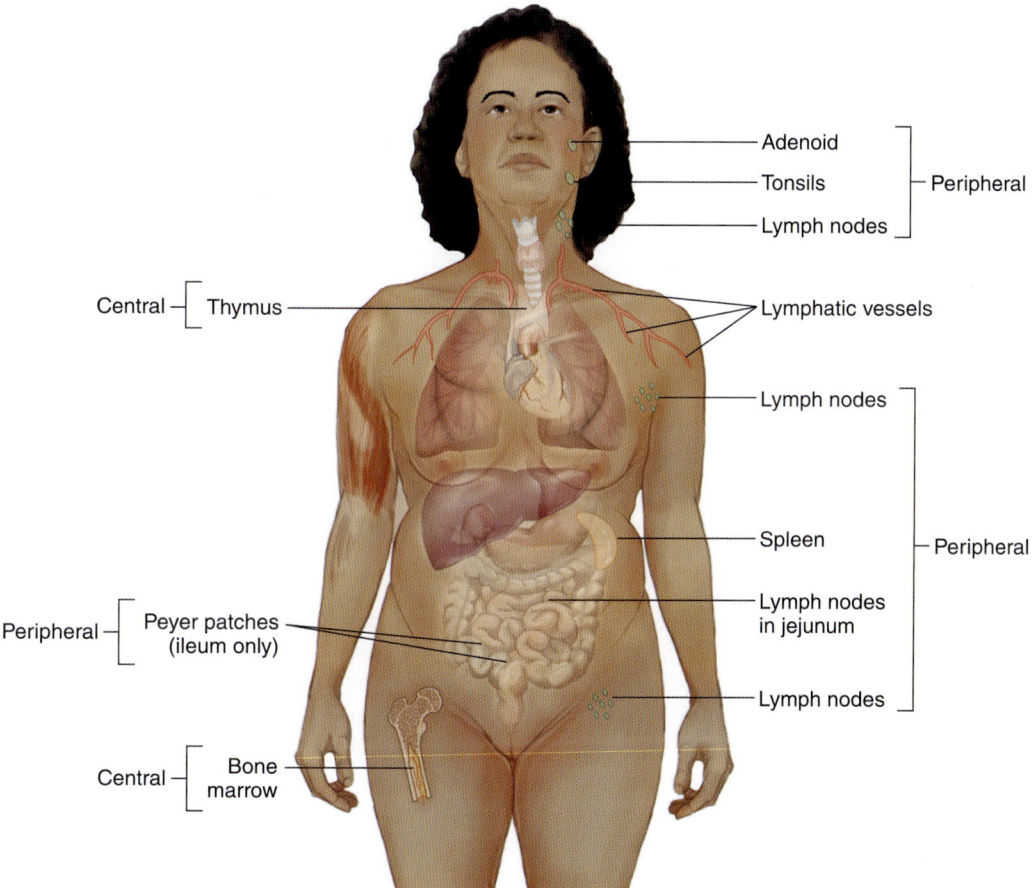

**Fig. 2.5** Diagram of lymphatic system. (Modified from McCance K, Huether S, Brashers V, Rote N. *Pathophysiology: The Biologic Basis for Disease in Adults and Children*. 8th ed. St. Louis: Elsevier; 2019.)

posteriorly by the trachealis muscle. Important relations of the trachea within the neck are:

1. The thyroid gland, which straddles the trachea, with its two lobes positioned laterally, and its isthmus anterior to the trachea with the inferior thyroid veins.
2. The common carotid arteries, which lie lateral to the trachea.
3. The oesophagus, which lies directly behind the trachea, and the recurrent laryngeal nerve, which lies between these two structures.

## Lower respiratory tract

The lower respiratory tract is that contained within the thorax, a cone-shaped cavity defined superiorly by the first rib and inferiorly by the diaphragm. The thorax has a narrow top (thoracic inlet) and a wide base (thoracic outlet). The thoracic wall is supported and protected by the bony thoracic cage, consisting of:

- Thoracic vertebrae
- Manubrium
- Sternum
- Twelve pairs of ribs with associated costal cartilages (Fig. 2.6).

Each rib makes an acute angle with the spine and articulates with the body and transverse process of its equivalent thoracic vertebra, and with the body of the vertebra above. The upper seven ribs (true ribs) also articulate anteriorly through their costal cartilages with the sternum. The 8th, 9th and 10th ribs (false ribs) articulate with the costal cartilages of the next rib above. The 11th and 12th ribs (floating ribs) are smaller and their tips are covered with a cap of cartilage.

The space between the ribs is known as the intercostal space. Lying obliquely between adjacent ribs are the internal and

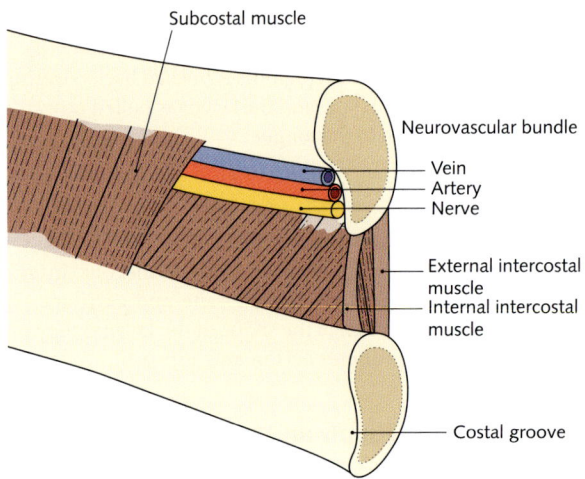

Fig. 2.7 Details of the subcostal neurovascular bundle.

external intercostal muscles. The intercostal muscles support the thoracic cage and their functions include:

- External intercostal muscles – raise the ribcage and increase intrathoracic volume.
- Internal intercostal muscles – lower the ribcage and reduce intrathoracic volume.

### CLINICAL NOTES

#### THE NEUROVASCULAR BUNDLE

Deep to the intercostal muscles and under cover of the costal groove lies a neurovascular bundle of vein, artery and nerve (Fig. 2.7). Knowledge of this anatomy is important during pleural procedures such as inserting a chest drain to remove fluid or air from the pleural space. Where possible the drain should be inserted above the rib to minimize damage to the neurovascular bundle during the procedure. More details on pleural procedures can be found in Chapter 20.

## Mediastinum

The mediastinum is situated in the midline and lies between the two lungs. It contains the:

- Heart and great vessels
- Trachea and oesophagus
- Phrenic and vagus nerves
- Lymph nodes.

## Pleurae and pleural cavities

The pleurae consist of a continuous serous membrane, which covers the external surface of the lung (parietal pleura) and is then reflected to cover the inner surface of the thoracic cavity

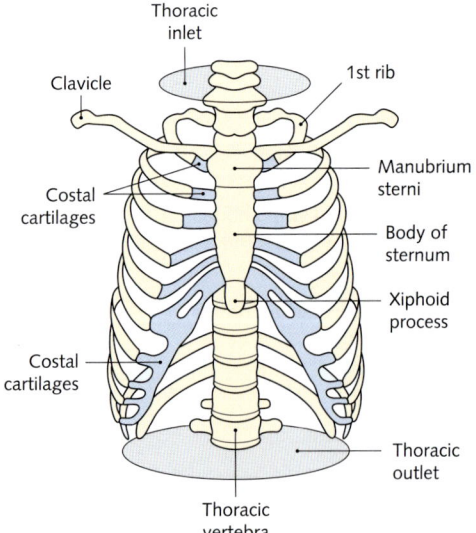

**Fig. 2.6** The thoracic cage.

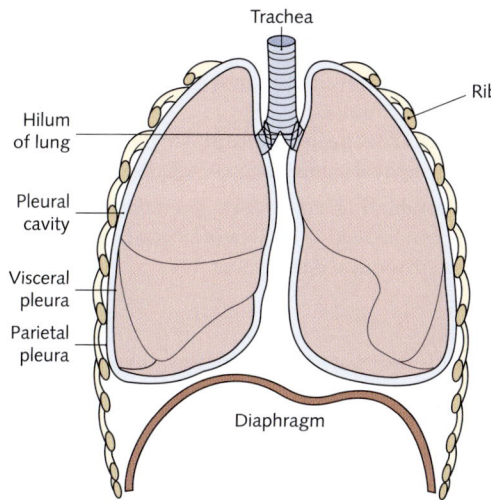

**Fig. 2.8** The two pleurae form a potential space called the pleural cavity.

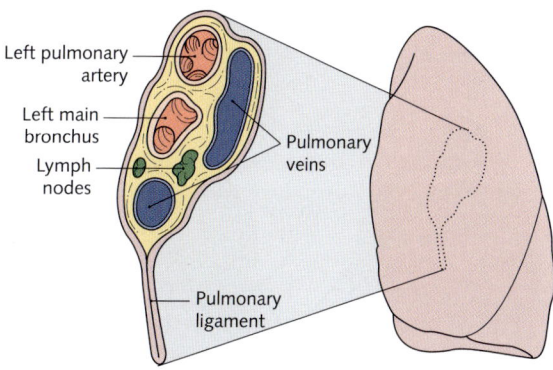

**Fig. 2.9** Contents of the hilum.

- Lymphatics and lymph nodes.
- Nerves.
- Supportive connective tissue (lung parenchyma), which has elastic qualities.

### Hilum of the lung
The hilum or root of the lung (Fig. 2.9) consists of:
- Bronchi
- Vessels: pulmonary artery and vein
- Nerves
- Lymph nodes and lymphatic vessels
- Pulmonary ligament.

### Bronchopulmonary segments
The trachea divides to form the left and right primary bronchi, which in turn divide to form lobar bronchi, supplying air to the lobes of each lung. The lobar bronchi divide again to give segmental bronchi, which supply air to regions of lung known as bronchopulmonary segments. The bronchopulmonary segment is both anatomically and functionally distinct. This is important because it means that a segment of diseased lung can be removed surgically (e.g., in tuberculosis).

### Surface anatomy
The surface anatomy of the lungs is shown in Figs 2.10–2.12.

## The respiratory tree and blood–air interface

### Respiratory tree
Inside the thorax, the trachea divides into the left and right primary bronchi at the carina. The right main bronchus is shorter and more vertical than the left (for this reason, inhaled foreign bodies are more likely to pass into the right lung). The primary bronchi within each lung divide into secondary or lobar bronchi. The lobar bronchi divide again into tertiary or segmental bronchi. The airways continue to divide, always splitting into two daughter airways

(visceral pleura) (Fig. 2.8), creating a potential space known as the pleural cavity. The visceral and parietal pleurae are so closely apposed that only a thin film of fluid is contained within the pleural cavity. This allows the pleurae to slip over each other during breathing, thus reducing friction. Normally, no cavity is actually present, although in pathological states, this potential space may expand, e.g., pneumothorax.

Where the pleura is reflected off the diaphragm and onto the thoracic wall, a small space is created which is not filled by the lung tissue; this space is known as the costodiaphragmatic recess. At the root of the lung (the hilum) in the mediastinum, the pleurae become continuous and form a double layer known as the pulmonary ligament.

The parietal pleura has a blood supply from intercostal arteries and branches of the internal thoracic artery. Venous and lymph drainage follow a return course similar to that of the arterial supply. Nerve supply is from the intercostal nerves and phrenic nerve; thus, inflammation of the pleurae may cause ipsilateral shoulder-tip pain. Conversely, the visceral pleura receives its blood supply from the bronchial arteries. Venous drainage is through the bronchial veins to the azygous and veins. Lymph vessels drain through the superficial plexus over the surface of the lung to bronchopulmonary nodes at the hilum. The visceral pleura has an autonomic nerve supply. It is not sensitive to pain but does have sensory fibres that detect stretch.

## Lungs
The two lungs are situated within the thoracic cavity on either side of the mediastinum and contain:
- Airways: bronchi, bronchioles, respiratory bronchioles, alveolar ducts, alveolar sacs and alveoli.
- Vessels: pulmonary artery and vein and bronchial artery and vein.

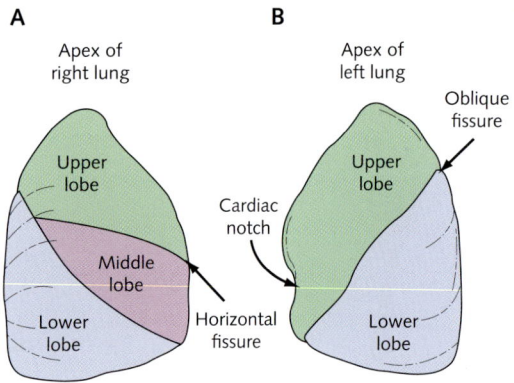

**Fig. 2.10** Lateral aspect of the lungs. The outer surfaces show impression of the ribs. (A) Right lung; (B) left lung.

of progressively smaller calibre until eventually forming bronchioles.

Table 2.1 outlines the structure of the respiratory tree. Each branch of the tracheobronchial tree can be classified by its number of divisions (called the generation number); the trachea is generation number zero. The trachea and bronchi contain cartilage in their walls for support and to prevent collapse of the airway. At about generation 10 or 11, the airways contain no cartilage in their walls and are known as bronchioles. Airways distal to the bronchi that contain no cartilage rely on lung parenchymal tissue for their support and are kept open by subatmospheric intrapleural pressure (radial traction).

Bronchioles continue dividing for up to 20 or more generations before reaching the terminal bronchiole. Terminal bronchioles are those which supply the end respiratory unit (the acinus).

The tracheobronchial tree can be classified into two zones:

1. The conducting zone (airways proximal to the respiratory bronchioles), involved in air movement by bulk flow to the end respiratory units.
2. The respiratory zone (airways distal to the terminal bronchiole), involved in gaseous exchange.

As the conducting zone does not take part in gaseous exchange, it can be seen as an area of 'wasted' ventilation and is described as anatomical dead space.

## Acinus

The acinus is the part of the airway involved in gaseous exchange (i.e., the passage of oxygen from the lungs to the blood and carbon dioxide from the blood to the lungs). The acinus consists of:

- Respiratory bronchioles, leading to the alveolar ducts.
- Alveolar ducts, opening into two or three alveolar sacs, which in turn open into several alveoli. Note: alveoli can also open directly into alveolar ducts and a few open directly into the respiratory bronchiole.

Multiple acini are grouped together and surrounded by parenchymal tissue, forming a lung lobule (Fig. 2.13). Lobules are separated by interlobular septa.

## The blood–air interface

The blood–air interface is a term that describes the site at which gaseous exchange takes place within the lung.

The alveoli are microscopic blind-ending air pouches forming the distal termination of the respiratory tract; there are 150–400 million in each normal lung. The alveoli open into alveolar sacs

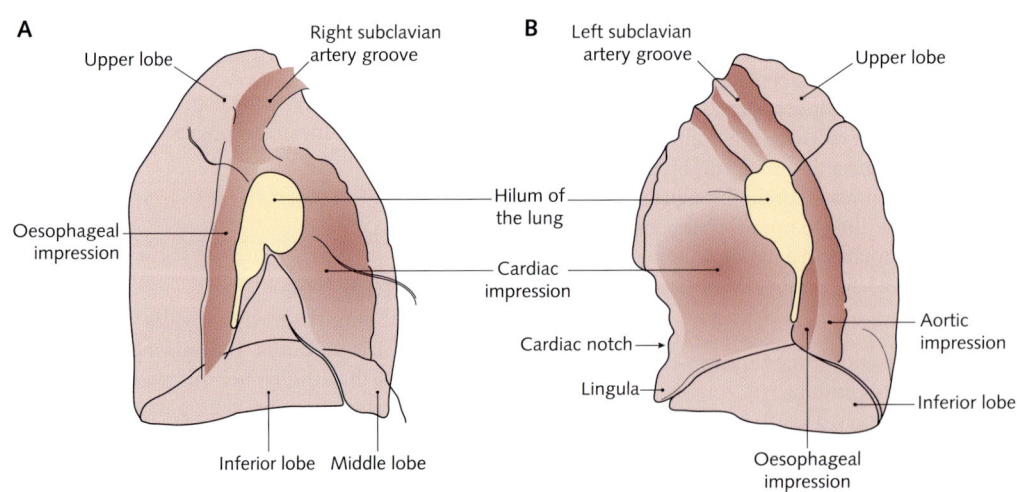

**Fig. 2.11** Relations of the lung. (A) Right lung; (B) left lung.

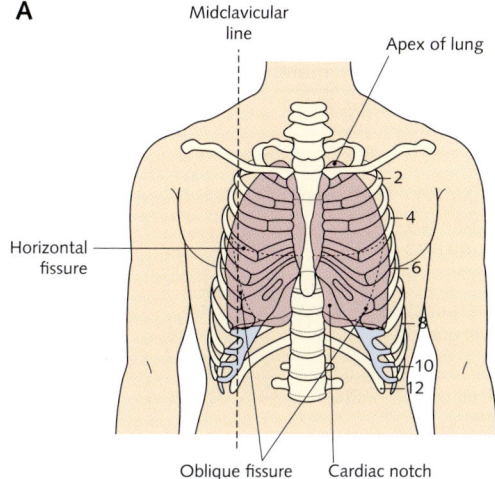

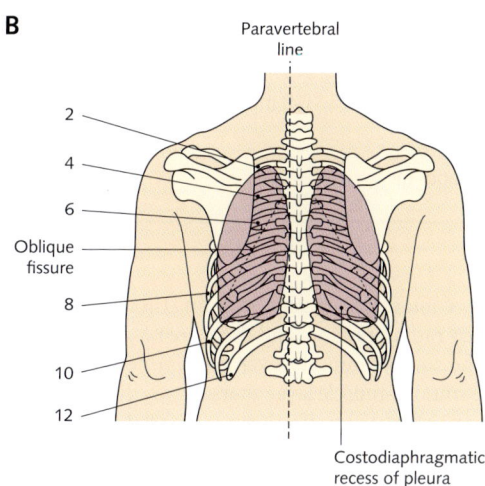

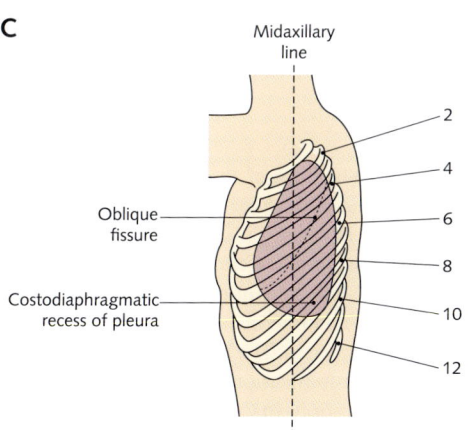

**Fig. 2.12** Surface anatomy of the lungs and pleura *(shaded area)*. (A) Anterior aspect; (B) posterior aspect; (C) lateral aspect. Numbering relates to relative rib position.

and then into alveolar ducts. The walls of the alveoli are extremely thin and are lined by a single layer of pneumocytes (types I and II) lying on a basement membrane. The alveolar surface is covered with alveolar lining fluid. The walls of the alveoli also contain capillaries (Fig. 2.14). It should be noted that:

- Average surface area of the alveolar–capillary membrane = 50–100 m$^2$.
- Average thickness of alveolar–capillary membrane = 0.4 mm.

This allows an enormous area for gaseous exchange and a very short diffusion distance.

## Microscopic structure

### Upper respiratory tract

#### Nose and nasopharynx
The upper one-third of the nasal cavity is the olfactory area and is covered in yellowish olfactory epithelium. The nasal sinuses and the nasopharynx (lower two-thirds of the nasal cavity) comprise the respiratory area, which is adapted to its main functions of filtering, warming and humidifying inspired air. These areas are lined with pseudostratified ciliated columnar epithelium (Fig. 2.15), also known as respiratory epithelium. With the exception of a few areas, this pattern of epithelium lines the whole of the respiratory tract down to the terminal bronchioles. Throughout these cells are numerous mucus-secreting goblet cells with microvilli on their luminal surface. Coordinated beating of the cilia propels mucus and entrapped particles to the pharynx, where it is swallowed, an important defence against infection.

#### Adenoids
The nasopharyngeal tonsil is a collection of mucosa-associated lymphoid tissue (MALT) that lies behind the epithelium of the roof and the posterior surface of the nasopharynx.

#### Oropharynx and laryngopharynx
The oropharynx and laryngopharynx have dual functions as parts of both the respiratory and alimentary tracts. They are lined with nonkeratinized stratified squamous (NKSS) epithelium several layers thick and are kept moist by numerous salivary glands.

#### Larynx and trachea
The epithelium of the larynx is made up of two types: NKSS epithelium and respiratory epithelium. NKSS epithelium covers the vocal folds, vestibular fold and larynx above this level. Below the level of the vestibular fold (with the exception of the vocal folds, which are lined with keratinized stratified squamous epithelium), the larynx and trachea are covered with respiratory epithelium.

### Lower respiratory tract
The basic structural components of the walls of the airways are shown in Fig. 2.16, although the proportions of these components vary in different regions of the tracheobronchial tree.

**Table 2.1** An overview of the respiratory tree and differences in structure of the airways

| Airway | Generation No. | Lining | Wall structure | Diameter | Function | Contractile |
|---|---|---|---|---|---|---|
| Trachea | 0 | Respiratory epithelium | Membranous tube supported by C-shaped rings of cartilage, loose submucosa and glands | 25 mm | Con | No |
| Bronchus | 1–11 | Respiratory epithelium | Fibromuscular tubes containing smooth muscle are reinforced by incomplete rings of cartilage and express B receptors | 1–10 mm | Con | Yes |
| Bronchiole | 12–16 | Simple ciliated cuboidal epithelium and Clara cells | Membranous and smooth muscle in the wall; no submucosal glands and no cartilage | 1.0 mm | Con | Yes |
| Respiratory bronchiole | 18+ | Simple ciliated cuboidal epithelium and Clara cells | Merging of cuboidal epithelium with flattened epithelial lining of alveolar ducts; membranous wall | 0.5 mm | Con/Gas | Yes |
| Alveolar duct | 20–23 | Flat nonciliated epithelium; no glands | Outer lining of spiral smooth muscle; walls of ducts contain many openings laterally into alveolar sacs | 0.5 mm | Gas | Yes |
| Alveolus | 24 | Pneumocytes types I and II | Types I and II pneumocytes lie on an alveolar basement membrane; capillaries lie on the outer surface of the wall and form the blood–air interface | 75–300 mm | Gas | No |

*Con, Conducting zone; Gas, gaseous exchange.*

## Trachea

The respiratory epithelium of the trachea is tall and sits on a thick basement membrane separating it from the lamina propria, which is loose and highly vascular, with a fibromuscular band of elastic tissue. Under the lamina propria lies a loose submucosa containing numerous glands that secrete mucinous and serous fluid. The C-shaped cartilage found within the trachea is hyaline in type and merges with the submucosa.

## Bronchi

The respiratory epithelium of the bronchi is shorter than the epithelium of the trachea and contains fewer goblet cells. The lamina propria is denser, with more elastic fibres, and it is separated from the submucosa by a discontinuous layer of smooth muscle. It also contains mast cells. The cartilage of the bronchi forms discontinuous flat plates and there are no C-shaped rings.

*Tertiary bronchi.* The epithelium in the tertiary bronchi is similar to that in the bronchi. The lamina propria of the tertiary bronchi is thin and elastic, being completely encompassed by smooth muscle. Submucosal glands are sparse and the submucosa merges with surrounding adventitia. MALT is present.

## Bronchioles

The epithelium here is ciliated and cuboidal but contains some Clara cells, which are nonciliated and secrete proteinaceous fluid.

Bronchioles contain no cartilage, meaning these airways must be kept open by radial traction, and there are no glands in the submucosa. The smooth-muscle layer is prominent. Adjusting the tone of the smooth-muscle layer alters airway diameter, enabling resistance to airflow to be effectively controlled.

*Respiratory bronchioles.* The respiratory bronchioles are lined by ciliated cuboidal epithelium, which is surrounded by smooth muscle. Clara cells are present within the walls of the respiratory bronchioles. Goblet cells are absent but there are a few alveoli in the walls; thus, the respiratory bronchiole is a site for gaseous exchange.

## Alveolar ducts

Alveolar ducts consist of rings of smooth muscle, collagen and elastic fibres. They open into two or three alveolar sacs, which in turn open into several alveoli.

*Alveoli.* An alveolus is a blind-ending terminal sac of respiratory tract (Fig. 2.17). Most gaseous exchange occurs in the alveoli. Because alveoli are so numerous, they provide the majority of lung volume and surface area. The majority of alveoli open into the alveolar sacs. Communication between adjacent alveoli is possible through perforations in the alveolar wall, called pores of Kohn. The alveoli are lined with type I and type II pneumocytes, which sit on a basement membrane. Type I pneumocytes are structural, whereas type II pneumocytes produce surfactant.

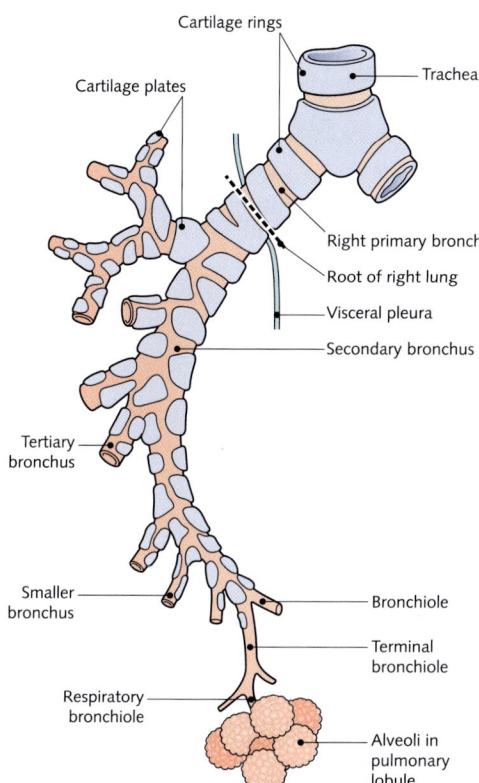

**Fig. 2.13** Visual representation of the bronchial tree.

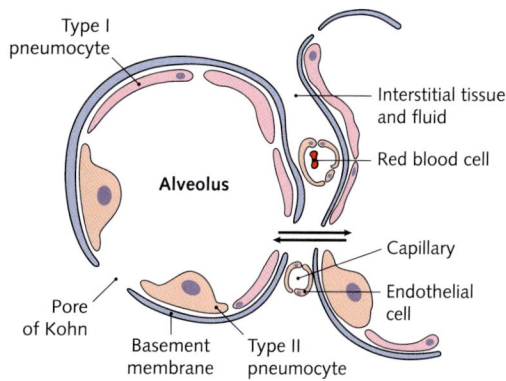

**Fig. 2.14** The alveolus.

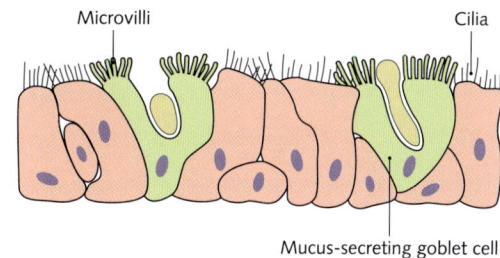

**Fig. 2.15** Respiratory epithelium.

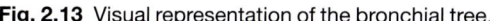

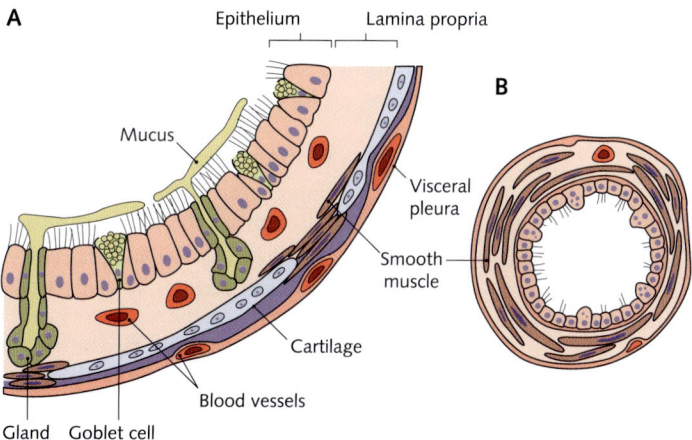

**Fig. 2.16** Structure of the airways: (A) bronchial structure; (B) bronchiolar structure. *Note there are no submucosal glands or cartilage in the bronchiole.*

**Type I pneumocytes.** To aid gaseous diffusion, type I pneumocytes are very thin; they contain flattened nuclei and few mitochondria. Type I pneumocytes make up 40% of the alveolar cell population and 90% of the surface lining of the alveolar wall. Cells are joined by tight junctions.

**Type II pneumocytes.** Type II pneumocytes are surfactant-producing cells containing rounded nuclei; their cytoplasm is rich in mitochondria and endoplasmic reticulum, and microvilli exist on their exposed surface. These cells make up 60% of the alveolar cell population, and 5%–10% of the surface lining of the alveolar wall.

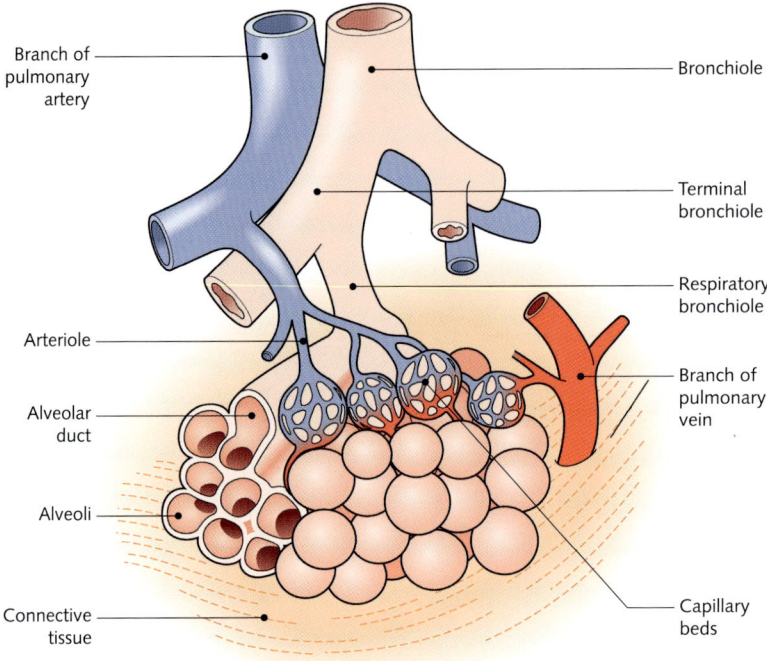

Branch of pulmonary artery

Bronchiole

Terminal bronchiole

Respiratory bronchiole

Arteriole

Branch of pulmonary vein

Alveolar duct

Alveoli

Connective tissue

Capillary beds

**Fig. 2.17** The relationship of the alveoli to the respiratory acinus.

## Alveolar macrophages

Alveolar macrophages are derived from circulating blood monocytes. They lie on an alveolar surface lining or on alveolar septal tissue. The alveolar macrophages phagocytose foreign material and bacteria; they are transported up the respiratory tract by mucociliary clearance. They are discussed later in this chapter.

## Mucosa-associated lymphoid tissue

MALT is noncapsulated lymphoid tissue located in the walls of the respiratory tract. It is also found in the gastrointestinal and urogenital tract. MALT is a specialized local system of concentrated lymphoid cells in the mucosa, and has a major role in the defence of the respiratory tract against pathogens.

## Pulmonary defence mechanisms

The lungs possess the largest surface area of the body in contact with the environment. They are therefore extremely susceptible to damage by foreign material and provide an excellent gateway for infection. The lungs are exposed to many foreign materials, e.g., bacteria and viruses, as well as dust, pollen and pollutants. Defence mechanisms to prevent infection and reduce the risk of damage by inhalation of foreign material are thus paramount (Fig. 2.18). There are three main mechanisms of defence:

1. Physical
2. Humoral
3. Cellular.

Physical defences are particularly important in the upper respiratory tract, while at the level of the alveoli, other defences, such as alveolar macrophages, predominate.

## Physical defences

Entry of particulates to the lower respiratory tract is restricted by the following three mechanisms:

1. Filtering at the nasopharynx – hairs within the nose act as a coarse filter for inhaled particles; sticky mucus lying on the surface of the respiratory epithelium traps particles, which are then transported by the wafting of cilia to the nasopharynx; the particles are then swallowed into the gastrointestinal tract.
2. Swallowing – during swallowing, the epiglottis folds back, the laryngeal muscles constrict the opening to the larynx and the larynx itself is lifted; this prevents aspiration of food particles.
3. Irritant C-fibre nerve endings – stimulation of irritant receptors within the bronchi by inhalation of chemicals, particles or infective material produces a vagal reflex contraction of bronchial smooth muscle; this reduces the diameter of airways and increases mucus secretion, thus limiting the penetration of the offending material.

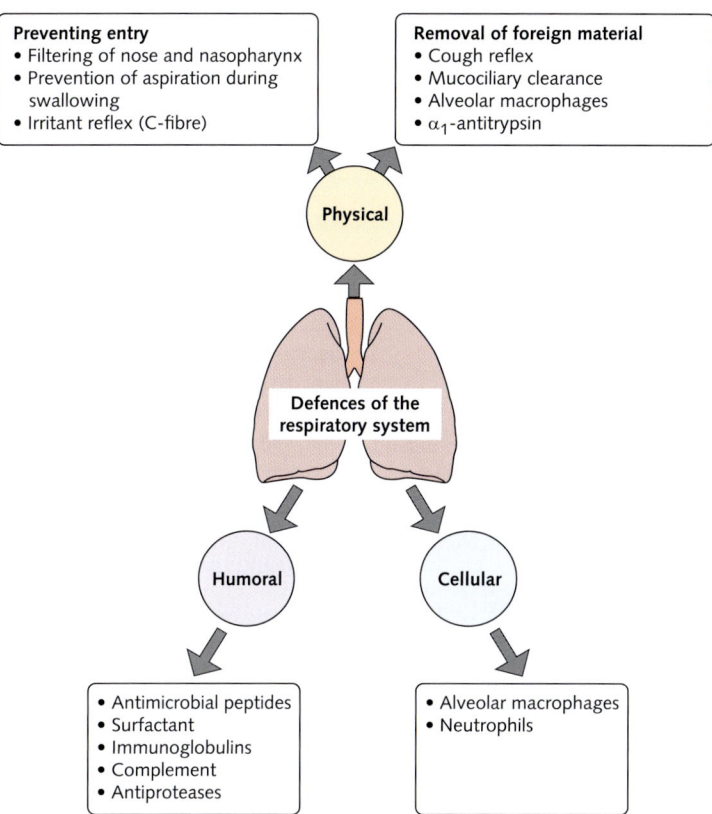

**Preventing entry**
- Filtering of nose and nasopharynx
- Prevention of aspiration during swallowing
- Irritant reflex (C-fibre)

**Removal of foreign material**
- Cough reflex
- Mucociliary clearance
- Alveolar macrophages
- $\alpha_1$-antitrypsin

Physical

Defences of the respiratory system

Humoral

Cellular

- Antimicrobial peptides
- Surfactant
- Immunoglobulins
- Complement
- Antiproteases

- Alveolar macrophages
- Neutrophils

**Fig. 2.18** Summary of defences of the respiratory system.

## Airway clearance
### Cough reflex
Inhaled material and material brought up the bronchopulmonary tree to the trachea and larynx by mucociliary clearance can trigger a cough reflex. This is achieved by a reflex deep inspiration that increases intrathoracic pressure while the larynx is closed. The larynx is suddenly opened, producing a high-velocity jet of air, which ejects unwanted material at high speed through the mouth.

### Mucociliary clearance
Mucociliary clearance deals with a lot of the large particles trapped in the bronchi and bronchioles and debris brought up by alveolar macrophages. Respiratory epithelium is covered by a layer of mucus secreted by goblet cells and submucosal glands. Approximately 10–100 mL of mucus is secreted by the lung daily. The mucus film is divided into two layers:

1. Periciliary fluid layer about 6 μm deep, immediately adjacent to the surface of the epithelium. The mucus here is hydrated by epithelial cells. This reduces its viscosity and allows movement of the cilia.

2. Superficial gel layer about 5–10 μm deep. This is a relatively viscous layer forming a sticky blanket, which traps particles.

The cilia beat synchronously at 1000–1500 strokes per minute. Coordinated movement causes the superficial gel layer, together with trapped particles, to be continually transported towards the mouth at 1–3 cm/min. The mucus and particles reach the trachea and larynx where they are swallowed or expectorated. Importantly, mucociliary clearance is inhibited by:

- Tobacco smoke
- Cold air
- Drugs (e.g., general anaesthetics and atropine)
- Sulphur oxides
- Nitrogen oxides.

The significance of mucociliary clearance is illustrated by cystic fibrosis (see Chapter 19), in which a defect in chloride channels throughout the body leads to hyperviscous secretions. In the lung, inadequate hydration causes excessive stickiness of the mucus lining the airways, preventing the action of the cilia in effecting mucociliary clearance.

## Humoral defences

Lung secretions contain a wide range of proteins which defend the lungs by various mechanisms. Humoral and cellular aspects of the immune system are considered only briefly here; for more information, see Vanbergen et al.[1]

### Antimicrobial peptides

A number of proteins in lung fluid have antibacterial properties. These are generally low-molecular-weight proteins such as defensins, lysozyme and lactoferrin.

### Surfactant

The alveoli are bathed in surfactant, which reduces surface tension and prevents the lungs from collapsing. Surfactant also contains proteins that play an important role in defence. Surfactant protein A (Sp-A) is the most abundant of these proteins and is hydrophilic. Sp-A has been shown to enhance the phagocytosis of microorganisms by alveolar macrophages. Sp-D, which is also hydrophilic, has a similar role to Sp-A in immune defence.

Sp-B and Sp-C, which are hydrophobic in nature, have a more structural role in that they are involved in maintaining the surfactant monolayer and further reducing the surface tension. Surfactant deficiency in preterm babies is a major contributor to infant respiratory distress syndrome.

### Immunoglobulins

Effector B lymphocytes (plasma cells) in the submucosa produce immunoglobulins. All classes of antibody are produced, but IgA production predominates. The immunoglobulins are contained within the mucus secretions in the respiratory tract and are directed against specific antigens.

### Complement

Complement proteins are found in lung secretions, in particularly high concentrations during inflammation, and they play an important role in propagating the inflammatory response. Complement components can be secreted by alveolar macrophages (see further in the chapter) and act as chemoattractants for the migration of cells such as neutrophils to the site of injury.

### Antiproteases

Lung secretions contain a number of enzymes (antiproteases) that break down the destructive proteases released from dead bacteria, macrophages and neutrophils. One of the most important of these antiproteases is $\alpha_1$-antitrypsin, produced in the liver. Its role is to oppose neutrophil elastase, which breaks down alveolar wall connective tissue in the lungs.

## Cellular defences

### Alveolar macrophages

Alveolar macrophages are differentiated monocytes, and are both phagocytic and mobile. They normally reside in the lining of the alveoli where they ingest bacteria and debris, before transporting them to the bronchioles to be removed from the lungs by mucociliary clearance. Alveolar macrophages can also initiate and amplify the inflammatory response by secreting proteins that recruit other cells. These proteins include:

- Complement components
- Cytokines (e.g., interleukin [IL]-1, IL-6) and chemokines
- Growth factors.

## Neutrophils

Neutrophils are the predominant cells recruited in the acute inflammatory response. Neutrophils emigrate from the intravascular space to the alveolar lumen, where intracellular killing of bacteria takes place by two mechanisms:

1. Oxidative – via reactive oxygen species
2. Nonoxidative – via proteases.

## Chapter Summary

- The respiratory tract is the collective term for the anatomy relating to the process of respiration, from the nose down to the alveoli. It is divided into the upper respiratory tract (outside the thorax) and the lower respiratory tract (within the thorax).
- The two lungs are situated within the thoracic cavity on either side of the mediastinum. The mediastinum contains the midline structures, including the heart, great vessels, trachea, oesophagus and phrenic and vagus nerves.
- The trachea is a cartilaginous and membranous tube of about 10 cm in length. It extends from the larynx to its bifurcation at the carina, where it divides into the left and right main bronchi. The right main bronchus is shorter and more vertical than the left.
- Bronchioles continue dividing for up to 20 or more generations before reaching the terminal bronchiole. Terminal bronchioles are those bronchioles which supply the end respiratory unit (the acinus).
- Different types of specialist epithelium line the respiratory tract at different stages, from respiratory epithelium lining the trachea through to pneumocytes lining the alveoli.
- Gas exchange takes place at the blood–air interface within the acinus.
- The three main defence mechanisms to prevent infection within the lungs are physical (e.g., airway clearance and mucociliary clearance), humoral (e.g., surfactant) and cellular (e.g., alveolar macrophages).

### MLA Conditions
Bronchiectasis

### Reference

1. Vanbergen O, Redhouse White G. *Crash Course: Haematology and Immunology*. Elsevier; 2019.

## INTRODUCTION

This chapter will provide an overview of the pulmonary circulation, exploring the important concepts and factors that influence lung perfusion. The pulmonary circulation is a highly specialized system that is adapted to accommodate the entire cardiac output both at rest and during exercise. The pulmonary circulation can do this because it is:

- A low-pressure, low-resistance system.
- Able to recruit more vessels with only a small increase in arterial pulmonary pressure.

Sufficient lung perfusion is only one factor that ensures blood is adequately oxygenated. The most important determinant is the way in which ventilation and perfusion are matched at the level of each individual alveolus. Mismatching of ventilation:perfusion is a common pathophysiological process in many common lung diseases.

## BLOOD SUPPLY TO THE LUNGS

The lungs have a dual blood supply from the pulmonary and bronchial circulations. The bronchial circulation is part of the systemic circulation.

## Pulmonary circulation

### Function
The primary function of the pulmonary circulation is to allow the exchange of oxygen and carbon dioxide between the air in the alveoli and the blood in the pulmonary capillaries. Oxygen is taken up into the blood whilst carbon dioxide is released from the blood into the alveoli.

### Anatomy
Mixed-venous blood is pumped from the right ventricle through the pulmonary arteries and then through the pulmonary capillary network. The pulmonary capillary network is in contact with the respiratory surface (Fig. 3.1) and provides a huge gas-exchange area, approximately 50–100 m$^2$. Gaseous exchange occurs (carbon dioxide given up by the blood, oxygen taken up by the blood) and the oxygenated blood returns through the pulmonary venules and veins to the left atrium.

## Bronchial circulation

The bronchial circulation is derived from the systemic circulation. The bronchial arteries (usually two left and one right

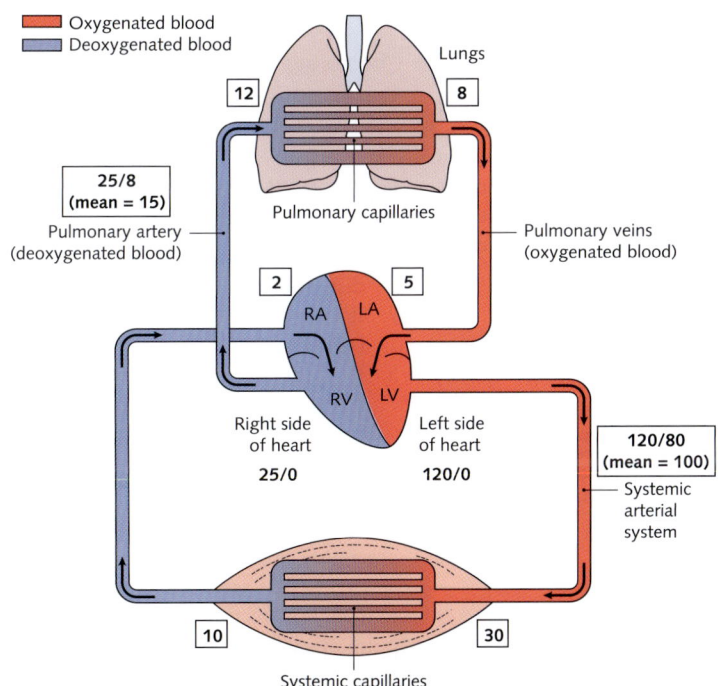

**Fig. 3.1** The pulmonary circulation. *LA*, Left atrium; *LV*, left ventricle; *RA*, right atrium; *RV*, right ventricle.

bronchial artery) are derived from the thoracic aorta. They form a broad network with pre- and postcapillary anastomoses to the pulmonary circulation.

## Function

The function of the bronchial circulation is to supply oxygen, water and nutrients to:

- Lung parenchyma
- Airways – smooth muscle, mucosa and glands
- Pulmonary arteries and veins
- Pleurae.

An additional function of the bronchial circulation is in the conditioning (warming) of inspired air.

## Venous drainage

Both the pulmonary and bronchial circulation in the lungs are drained by the pulmonary veins. These large veins carry oxygenated blood from the lungs into the left atrium of the heart.

## PULMONARY BLOOD FLOW

## Mechanics of the circulation

Flow through the pulmonary artery is considered to be equal to cardiac output. However, in real terms the blood flow through the pulmonary vasculature is slightly less than cardiac output. This is because a proportion of the coronary circulation from the aorta drains directly into the left ventricle and the bronchial circulation from the aorta drains into pulmonary veins, bypassing the lungs.

Pressures within the pulmonary circulation are much lower than in equivalent regions within the systemic circulation (Table 3.1). The volume of blood flowing through both circulations is approximately the same; therefore, the pulmonary circulation must offer lower resistance than the systemic circulation.

**Table 3.1** Pressures within the pulmonary circulation compared with the systemic circulation

| Site | Pulmonary circulation Mean pressure (mmHg) | Systemic circulation Mean pressure (mmHg) |
|---|---|---|
| Arterial pressure (systolic/diastolic) | 15 (25/8) | 100 (120/80) |
| Arteriole | 12 | 30 |
| Venule | 8 | 10 |
| Atrium | 5 | 2 |

Pulmonary capillaries and arterioles cause the main resistance to flow in the pulmonary circulation. Low resistance in the pulmonary circulation is achieved in two ways:

1. The large number of resistance vessels that exist are usually dilated; thus, the total area for flow is very large.
2. Small muscular arteries contain much less smooth muscle than equivalent arteries in the systemic circulation, meaning they are more easily distended.

Many other factors affect pulmonary blood flow and pulmonary vascular resistance. These are discussed later.

### CLINICAL NOTES

**PULMONARY HAEMORRHAGE AND INFARCTION FOLLOWING PULMONARY EMBOLISM**

A pulmonary embolism (PE) causes a blockage of the pulmonary circulation to an area of lung. The bronchial circulation continues to supply the capillaries in the affected area via capillary anastomoses. The bronchial circulation is at higher pressure than the pulmonary circulation. After a PE there is locally increased vascular permeability owing to tissue injury at the site. Red blood cells therefore move out of the vessels into the alveoli, causing haemorrhage. As blood flow is restored, the red cells will be reabsorbed. If, however, the pressure in the bronchial circulation is also decreased (e.g., in hypotension caused by shock), the area of lung may infarct. In both cases this may be represented by a wedge-shaped opacity at the periphery of the lung on a chest X-ray or computed tomography scan. This is a useful sign to look for in a patient with suspected PE.

## Hydrostatic pressure

Hydrostatic pressure has three effects.

1. It distends blood vessels: as hydrostatic pressure rises, distension of the vessel increases.
2. It is capable of opening previously closed capillaries (recruitment).
3. It causes flow to occur; in other words, a pressure difference ($\Delta P$) between the arterial and venous ends of a vessel provides the driving force for flow.

In situations where increased pulmonary flow is required (e.g., during exercise), the cardiac output is increased, which raises pulmonary vascular pressure. This causes recruitment of previously closed capillaries and distension of already open capillaries (Fig. 3.2), which reduces the pulmonary vascular resistance to flow. It is for this reason that resistance to flow through the pulmonary vasculature decreases with increasing pulmonary vascular pressure.

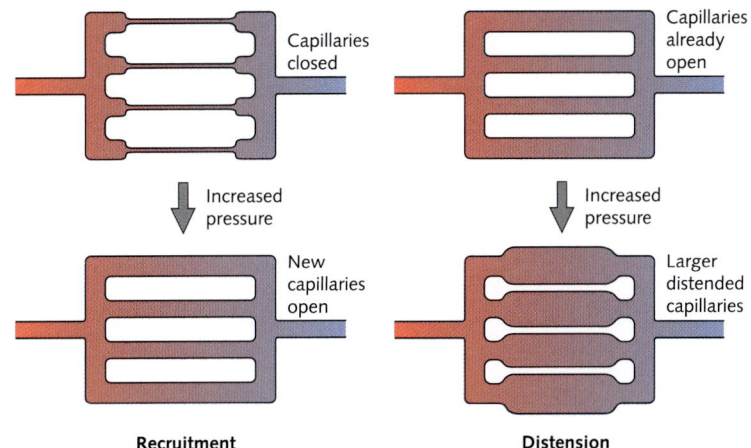

**Fig. 3.2** Effect of increased pressure on pulmonary vasculature. To minimize pulmonary vascular resistance when pulmonary arterial pressure increases, new vessels are recruited and vessels that are already open are distended.

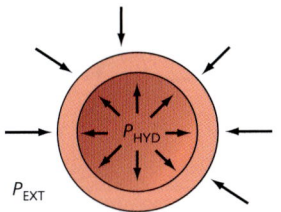

**Fig. 3.3** Transmural pressure in pulmonary capillary. $P_{EXT}$, External pressure; $P_{HYD}$, hydrostatic pressure.

## External pressure

Pressure outside a blood vessel will act to collapse the vessel if the pressure is positive, or aid distension of the vessel if the pressure is negative.

The tendency for a vessel to distend or collapse is also dependent on the pressure inside the lumen. Thus, it is the pressure difference across the wall (transmural pressure) that determines whether a vessel compresses or distends (Fig. 3.3).

Pulmonary vessels can be considered in two groups (Fig. 3.4): alveolar and extraalveolar vessels.

## Alveolar vessels

There is a dense network of capillaries in the alveolar wall; these are the alveolar vessels. The external pressure affecting these capillaries is alveolar pressure (normally atmospheric pressure). As the lungs expand, the capillaries are compressed. The diameter of the capillaries is dependent on the transmural pressure (i.e., the difference between hydrostatic pressure within the capillary lumen and pressure within the alveolus). If the alveolar pressure is greater than capillary hydrostatic pressure, the capillary will tend to collapse.

Vessels in the apex of the lung may collapse as the alveoli expand. This is more likely during diastole when venous (capillary) pressure falls below alveolar pressure.

## Extraalveolar vessels

Extraalveolar vessels are arteries and veins contained within the lung tissue. As the lungs expand, these vessels are distended by radial traction. The external pressure is similar to intrapleural pressure (subatmospheric, i.e., negative); therefore, transmural pressure tends to distend these vessels.

During inspiration, intrapleural pressure and thus the pressure outside the extraalveolar vessels becomes even more negative, causing these vessels to distend even further, reducing vascular resistance and increasing pulmonary blood flow. At large lung volumes, the effect of radial traction is greater and the extraalveolar vessels are distended more.

## Effects of lung volume on alveolar capillaries

Hydrostatic pressure within the capillaries is lowered during deep inspiration. This is caused by negative intrapleural pressure around the heart. This changes the transmural pressure and the capillaries tend to be compressed, increasing pulmonary vascular resistance (Fig. 3.5). At large lung volumes, the alveolar wall is stretched and becomes thinner, compressing the capillaries and increasing vascular resistance. This is a key mechanism in the development of pulmonary hypertension in patients with chronic obstructive pulmonary disease.

## Smooth muscle within the vascular wall

Smooth muscle in the walls of extraalveolar vessels causes vasoconstriction, thus opposing the forces caused by radial traction and hydrostatic pressure within the lumen that are trying to distend these vessels. Drugs that cause contraction of smooth muscle therefore increase pulmonary vascular resistance.

## Measurement of pulmonary blood flow

Pulmonary blood flow can be measured by three methods:

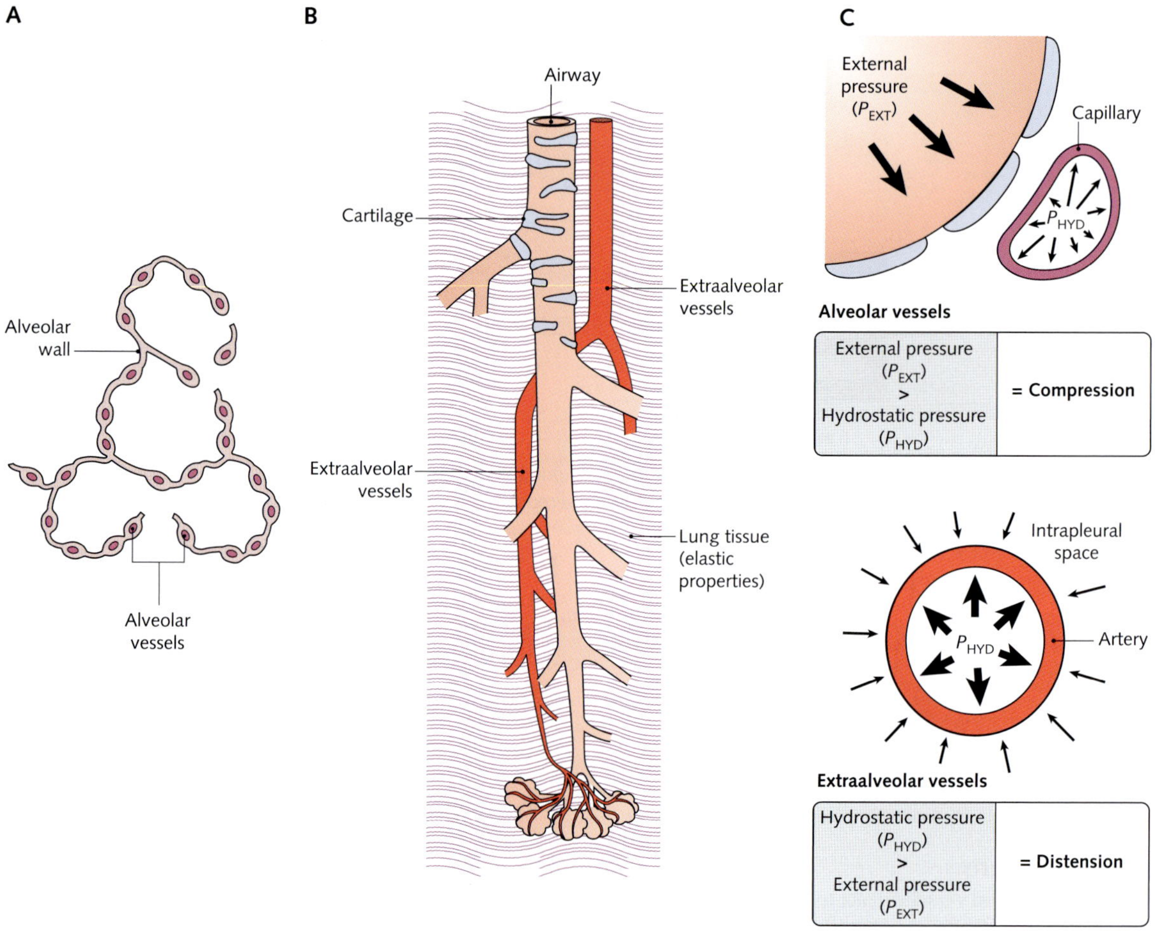

A

B

C

External pressure ($P_{EXT}$)

Airway

Capillary

Cartilage

$P_{HYD}$

Extraalveolar vessels

**Alveolar vessels**

| External pressure ($P_{EXT}$) > Hydrostatic pressure ($P_{HYD}$) | = Compression |
|---|---|

Alveolar wall

Extraalveolar vessels

Lung tissue (elastic properties)

Intrapleural space

Alveolar vessels

$P_{HYD}$

Artery

**Extraalveolar vessels**

| Hydrostatic pressure ($P_{HYD}$) > External pressure ($P_{EXT}$) | = Distension |
|---|---|

**Fig. 3.4** Alveolar and extraalveolar vessels. (A) Alveolar vessels. (B) Extraalveolar vessels. (C) Alveolar vessels tend to collapse on deep inspiration, whereas extraalveolar vessels distend by radial traction.

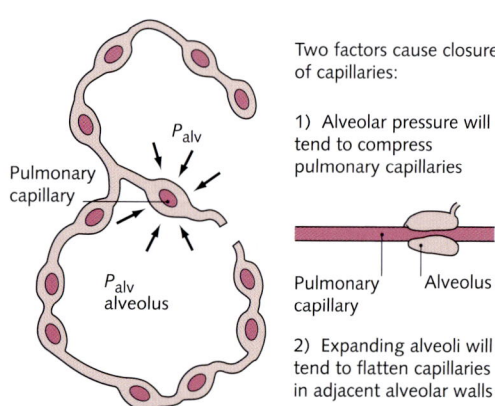

$P_{alv}$

Pulmonary capillary

$P_{alv}$
alveolus

Pulmonary capillary

Alveolus

Two factors cause closure of capillaries:

1) Alveolar pressure will tend to compress pulmonary capillaries

2) Expanding alveoli will tend to flatten capillaries in adjacent alveolar walls

**Fig. 3.5** Alveolar pressure and capillary compression.

1. Fick principle (Fig. 3.6).
2. Indicator dilution method: a known amount of dye is injected into venous blood and its arterial concentration is measured.
3. Uptake of inhaled soluble gas (e.g., $N_2O$, nitrous oxide): the gas is inhaled and arterial blood values are measured.

Both the first and second methods give average blood flow, whereas the third method measures instantaneous flow. The third method relies upon $N_2O$ transfer across the gas-exchange surface being perfusion-limited.

Fick theorized that, because of the laws of conservation of mass, the difference in oxygen concentration between mixed-venous blood returning to the pulmonary capillary bed $[O_2]_{pv}$ and arterial blood leaving the heart $[O_2]_{pa}$ must be caused by uptake of oxygen within the lungs. This uptake must be equal to the body's consumption of oxygen (see Fig. 3.6).

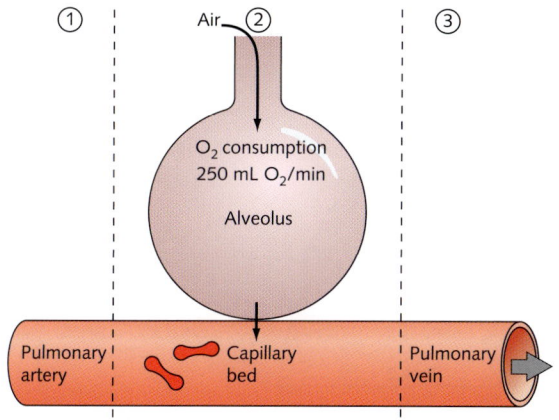

**Fig. 3.6** Fick principle for measuring pulmonary blood flow. Fick theorized that the difference in oxygen content between pulmonary venous blood and pulmonary arterial blood must be due to uptake of oxygen in the pulmonary capillaries, and therefore the pulmonary blood flow can be calculated.

## Distribution of blood within the lung

Blood flow within the normal (upright) lung is not uniform. Blood flow at the base of the lung is greater than at the apex, owing to the influence of gravity. Therefore, the pulmonary vessels at the lung base will have a greater hydrostatic pressure than vessels at the apex.

The hydrostatic pressure exerted by a vertical column of fluid is given by the relationship:

$$P = \rho g h$$

where $\rho$ = density of the fluid, h = height of the column and g = acceleration due to gravity. From the equation above, it can be seen that:

- Vessels at the lung base are subjected to a higher hydrostatic pressure.

- The increase in hydrostatic pressure will distend these vessels, lowering the resistance to blood flow. Thus, pulmonary blood flow in the bases will be greater than in the apices.

In diastole, the hydrostatic pressure in the pulmonary artery is 11 $cmH_2O$. The apex of each lung is approximately 15 cm above the right ventricle, and the hydrostatic pressure within these vessels is lowered or even zero. Vessels at the apex of the lung are therefore narrower or even collapse because of the lower hydrostatic pressure within them.

Ventilation also increases from apex to base, but is less affected than blood flow because the density of air is much less than that of blood.

## Pattern of blood flow

The distribution of blood flow within the lung can be described in three zones (Fig. 3.7).

### Zone 1 (at the apex of the lung)

In zone 1, arterial pressure is less than alveolar pressure: capillaries collapse and no flow occurs. Note that, under normal conditions, there is no zone 1 because there is sufficient pressure to perfuse the apices.

### Zone 2

In zone 2, arterial pressure is greater than alveolar pressure, which is greater than venous pressure. Postcapillary venules open and close depending on hydrostatic pressure (i.e., hydrostatic pressure difference in systole and diastole). Flow is determined by the arterial–alveolar pressure difference (transmural pressure).

### Zone 3 (at the base of the lung)

In zone 3, arterial pressure is greater than venous pressure, which is greater than alveolar pressure. Blood flow is determined by arteriovenous pressure difference as in the systemic circulation.

## Control of pulmonary blood flow

Pulmonary blood flow can be controlled by several local mechanisms in order to improve the efficiency of gaseous exchange, such as:

- Changes in hydrostatic pressure (as previously discussed).
- Local mediators (thromboxane, histamine and prostacyclin), as in systemic circulation.
- Contraction and relaxation of smooth muscle within walls of arteries and arterioles.
- Hypoxic vasoconstriction (this is an important mechanism in the pathophysiology of respiratory failure).

### Hypoxic vasoconstriction

The aim of breathing is to oxygenate the blood sufficiently. This is achieved by efficient gaseous exchange between the alveoli and the bloodstream. If an area of lung is poorly ventilated and the alveolar partial pressure of oxygen (alveolar oxygen tension) is low, perfusion of this area with blood would lead to inefficient gaseous

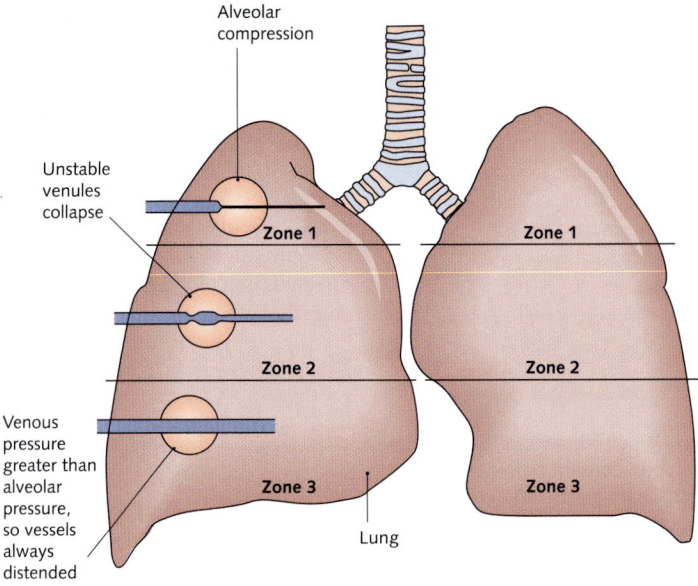

**Fig. 3.7** Zones of pulmonary blood flow.

exchange. It would be more beneficial to perfuse an area that is well ventilated. This is the basis of hypoxic vasoconstriction.

Small pulmonary arteries and arterioles which are in close proximity to the gas-exchange surface and alveolar capillaries are surrounded by alveolar gas. Oxygen passes through the alveolar walls into the smooth muscle of the blood vessel by diffusion. The high oxygen tension to which these smooth muscles are normally exposed acts to dilate the pulmonary vessels. In contrast, if the alveolar oxygen tension is low, pulmonary blood vessels are constricted, which leads to reduced blood flow in the area of lung that is poorly ventilated and diversion to other regions where alveolar oxygen tension is high.

It should be noted that it is the partial pressure of oxygen in the alveolus ($P_AO_2$) and not in the pulmonary artery ($P_aO_2$) that causes this response. The actual mechanism and the chemical mediators involved in hypoxic vasoconstriction are not known.

## ● Chapter Summary

The lungs have a dual blood supply from the pulmonary and bronchial circulations. The bronchial circulation derives from the systemic circulation.
- The primary function of the pulmonary circulation is to allow the exchange of oxygen and carbon dioxide between the blood in the capillaries and the air in the alveoli.
- Pressures with the pulmonary circulation are much lower than within equivalent regions of the systemic circulation.
- Pulmonary vascular resistance is low and falls with an increase in cardiac output owing to capillary recruitment and distension.
- Blood flow is not uniform throughout the lungs but is greater at the lung bases than the apices. This is owing to gravity and greater hydrostatic pressure in the vessels at the lung bases.
- Hypoxic vasoconstriction reduces inefficient gas exchange by decreasing blood flow to poorly ventilated area of the lung.

# Physiology, ventilation and gas exchange

# 4

## INTRODUCTION

This chapter will provide an overview of the important principles that govern ventilation and gas exchange in the lungs. Ventilation is the movement of air through the conducting passages of the respiratory system, from between the atmosphere to the lungs. The movement of air in and out of the lungs occurs due to a pressure gradient and the respiratory muscles create these pressure differences by creating changes in lung volume.

The process of inspiration is active and involves the contraction of the accessory muscles of breathing in addition to those used in quiet inspiration (the diaphragm and external intercostals). This increases the volume of the thoracic cavity and decreases the intraalveolar pressure, so air flows into the lungs (inhalation).

Conversely, during expiration, relaxation of the diaphragm and elastic recoil of the tissue decrease the volume of the thoracic cavity, which increases the intraalveolar pressure (pushing air out of the lungs – i.e., exhalation). The processes of inspiration and expiration are displayed in Fig. 4.1.

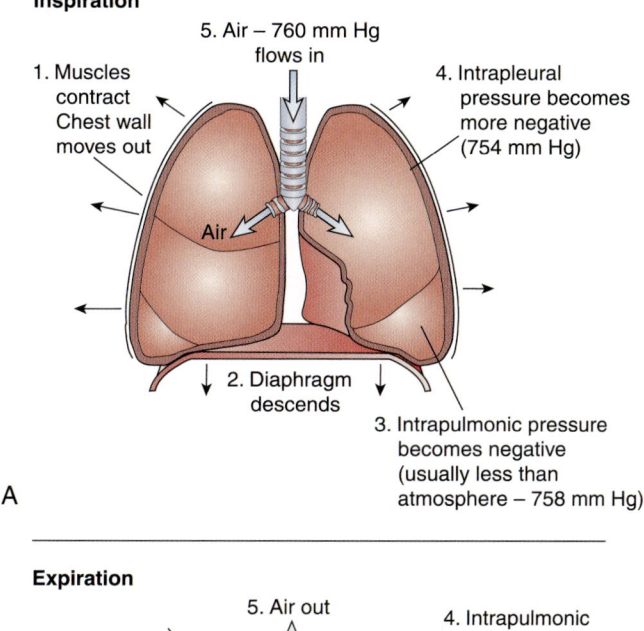

**Inspiration**

5. Air – 760 mm Hg flows in

1. Muscles contract Chest wall moves out

4. Intrapleural pressure becomes more negative (754 mm Hg)

Air

2. Diaphragm descends

3. Intrapulmonic pressure becomes negative (usually less than atmosphere – 758 mm Hg)

A

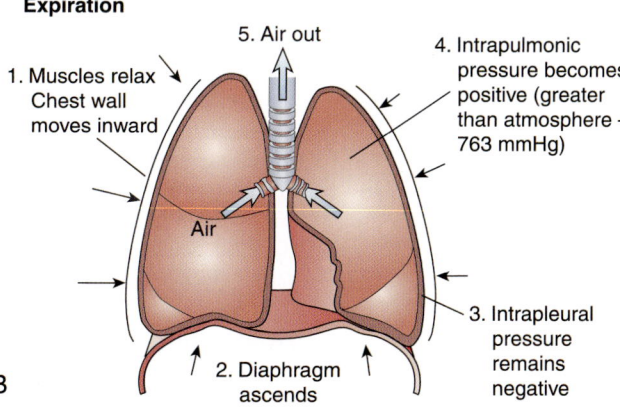

**Expiration**

5. Air out

1. Muscles relax Chest wall moves inward

4. Intrapulmonic pressure becomes positive (greater than atmosphere – 763 mmHg)

Air

2. Diaphragm ascends

3. Intrapleural pressure remains negative

B

**Fig. 4.1** Figure demonstrating (A) normal inspiration and (B) normal expiration.

The function of ventilation is to maintain blood gases at their optimum level, by delivering air to the alveoli where gas exchange can take place. Other physical properties of the lungs such as the recoil of the elastic tissues and airway resistance also influence the effectiveness of ventilation. It is important to understand the principles of ventilation, as many lung diseases affect the physical properties of the lung and therefore will result in impaired gas exchange.

## LUNG VOLUMES

The gas held by the lungs is subdivided into specific lung volumes which can be established when an individual performs pulmonary function tests. These lung volumes are summarized in Table 4.1. Fig. 4.2 displays how these lung volumes are measured from an instrument called a spirometer. Further detailed methods of measuring lung volumes, such as spirometry, nitrogen washout, helium dilution and plethysmography, can be found in Chapter 10.

**Table 4.1** Descriptions of lung volumes and capacities

| Air in lungs is divided into four volumes | |
| --- | --- |
| TV | Volume of air breathed in and out in a single breath: 0.5 L |
| Inspiratory reserve volume (IRV) | Volume of air breathed in by a maximum inspiration at the end of a normal inspiration: 3.3 L |
| Expiratory reserve volume (ERV) | Volume of air that can be expelled by a maximum effort at the end of a normal expiration: 1.0 L |
| RV | Volume of air remaining in lungs at end of a maximum expiration: 1.2 L |
| **Pulmonary capacities are combinations of two or more volumes** | |
| Inspiratory capacity (IC) = TV + IRV | Volume of air breathed in by a maximum inspiration at the end of a normal expiration: 3.8 L |
| Functional residual capacity (FRC) = ERV + RV | Volume of air remaining in lungs at the end of a normal expiration. Acts as buffer against extreme changes in alveolar gas levels with each breath: 2.2 L |
| VC = IRV + TV + ERV | Volume of air that can be breathed in by a maximum inspiration following a maximum expiration: 4.8 L |
| TLC = VC + RV | Only a fraction of TLC is used in normal breathing: 6.0 L |

*ERV, Expiratory reserve volume; IRV, inspiratory reserve volume; RV, residual volume; TLC, total lung capacity; TV, tidal volume; VC, vital capacity.*

## Residual volume and functional residual capacity

After breathing out, the lungs are not completely emptied of air. This is useful physiologically, as a completely deflated lung requires significantly more energy to inflate it than one in which the alveoli have not completely collapsed.

Even following a maximum respiratory effort (forced expiration), some air remains within the lungs as all the structures within the lungs (including the airways) are compressed by the positive intrapleural pressure. Consequently, the smaller airways collapse before the alveoli empty completely, meaning some air remains within the lungs. This is known as the residual volume (RV).

During normal breathing (quiet breathing), the lung volume oscillates between inhalation and exhalation. In quiet breathing, after the tidal volume has been expired:

- Pressure outside the chest is equal to alveolar pressure (i.e., atmospheric pressure).
- Elastic forces tending to collapse the lung are balanced by the elastic recoil trying to expand the chest.
- This creates a subatmospheric (negative) pressure in the intrapleural space.

The lung volume at this point is known as functional residual capacity (FRC). Both RV and FRC can be measured using nitrogen washout, helium dilution and plethysmography (see Chapter 10).

## Effects of respiratory disease on lung volumes

Disease affects lung volumes in specific patterns, depending on the pathological processes. Diseases can be classified as obstructive, restrictive or mixed, with each resulting in characteristic changes displayed by their corresponding lung volumes (Fig. 4.3).

### Obstructive disorders

This group of disorders is characterized by the obstruction of normal air flow caused by airway narrowing. If this process is not reversed, air is trapped behind closed airways, a process referred to as hyperinflation. The RV is therefore increased as trapped gas cannot leave the lung, and the RV:total lung capacity (TLC) ratio increases. In patients with severe obstruction, air trapping can be so extensive that vital capacity is decreased. An example of an obstructive lung disease where a patient develops gas trapping and hyperinflation is chronic obstructive pulmonary disease (COPD). See Fig. 4.4 for how this change in lung volume typically appears when measured using a spirometer.

### Restrictive disorders

Restrictive disorders result in stiffer lungs that cannot expand to normal volumes. All the subdivisions of volume are decreased and the RV:TLC ratio will be normal or increased (where vital

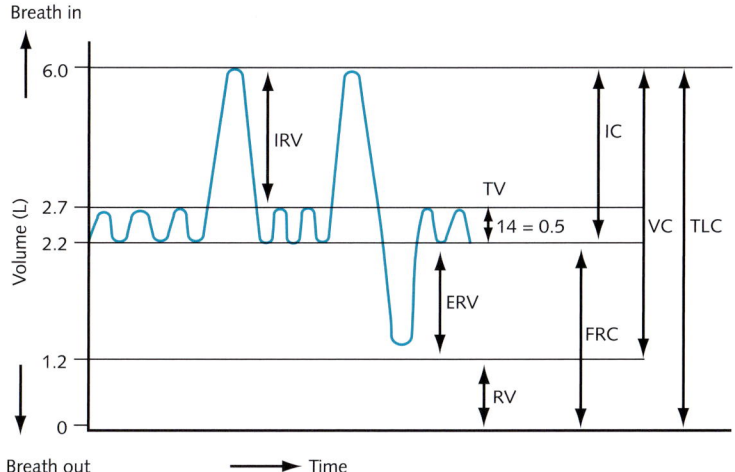

**Fig. 4.2** Lung volumes measured by a spirometer. *ERV*, Expiratory reserve volume; *FRC*, functional residual capacity; *IRV*, inspiratory reserve volume; *RV*, residual volume; *TLC*, total lung capacity; *TV*, tidal volume; *VC*, vital capacity.

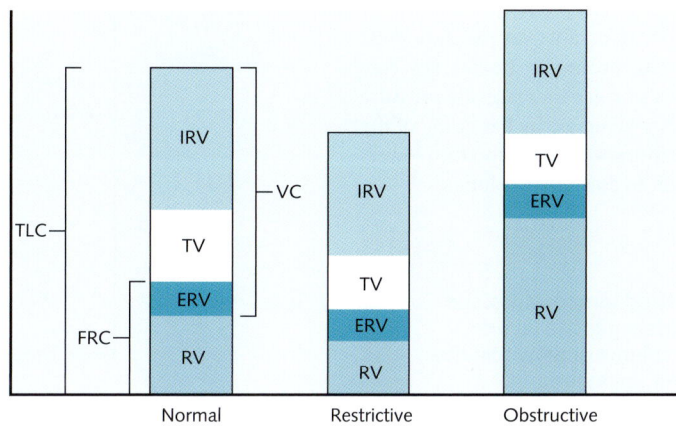

**Fig. 4.3** Effect of disease on lung volumes. *ERV*, Expiratory reserve volume; *FRC*, functional residual capacity; *IRV*, inspiratory reserve volume; *RV*, residual volume; *TLC*, total lung capacity; *TV*, tidal volume; *VC*, vital capacity.

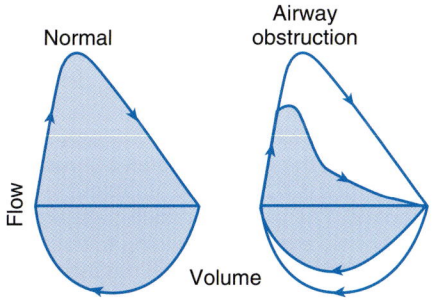

**Fig. 4.4** Flow–volume loop demonstrating the shape change that results from an obstructive lung disorder.

capacity has decreased more quickly than RV). An example of a restrictive lung disorder is interstitial lung disease such as idiopathic pulmonary fibrosis. See Fig. 4.5 for how this change in lung volume typically appears when measured using a spirometer.

## MECHANICS OF BREATHING

Pulmonary ventilation involves three different pressures:

Atmospheric pressure ($P_{atm}$): The pressure of air outside the body.
Intraalveolar pressure ($P_A$): The pressure inside the alveoli of the lungs.
Intrapleural pressure: The pressure within the pleural cavity.

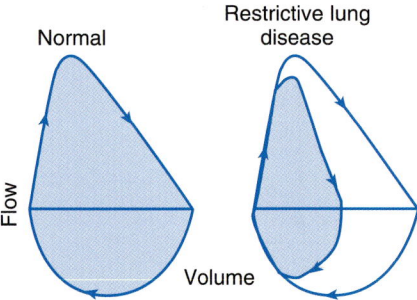

**Fig. 4.5** Flow–volume loop demonstrating the shape change that results from a restrictive lung disorder.

## Flow of air into the lungs

To achieve air flow into the lungs, we require a driving pressure (remember that air flows from a high to low pressure) (see Fig. 4.6).

- If $P_A = P_{atm}$, no air flow occurs (e.g., at FRC).
- If $P_A < P_{atm}$, air flows into the lungs.
- If $P_A > P_{atm}$, air flows out of the lungs.

As atmospheric pressure is constant, alveolar pressure must be altered to achieve air flow. According to Boyle's law (see Box 4.1), decreasing the volume of a gas increases its pressure and vice versa. In the lungs, this is achieved by flattening of the diaphragm, which increases the thoracic volume and thus lowers intrapleural pressure, allowing air to flow into the lungs.

---

### HINTS AND TIPS

Boyle's law states that at a fixed temperature, the pressure and volume of an ideal gas are inversely proportional, that is, as the volume of air within the lungs increases, the pressure decreases.

---

In expiration, relaxation of the chest wall muscles allows the elastic recoil of the lungs to cause contraction of the lungs, reducing thoracic volume and increasing intrapleural pressure and thus expulsion of gas.

## Intrapleural pressure

Intrapleural pressure drives air flow in and out of the lung during breathing. At FRC the elastic recoil of the lungs is balanced by the elastic recoil of the chest wall (which acts to expand the chest). These two opposing forces create a subatmospheric (negative) pressure within the intrapleural space. Because the alveoli communicate with the atmosphere, the pressure inside the lungs is higher than that of the intrapleural space, creating a pressure gradient, known as transmural pressure. This transmural pressure ensures that the lungs are held partially expanded in the thorax (like suspended balloons) with the chest wall. Intrapleural

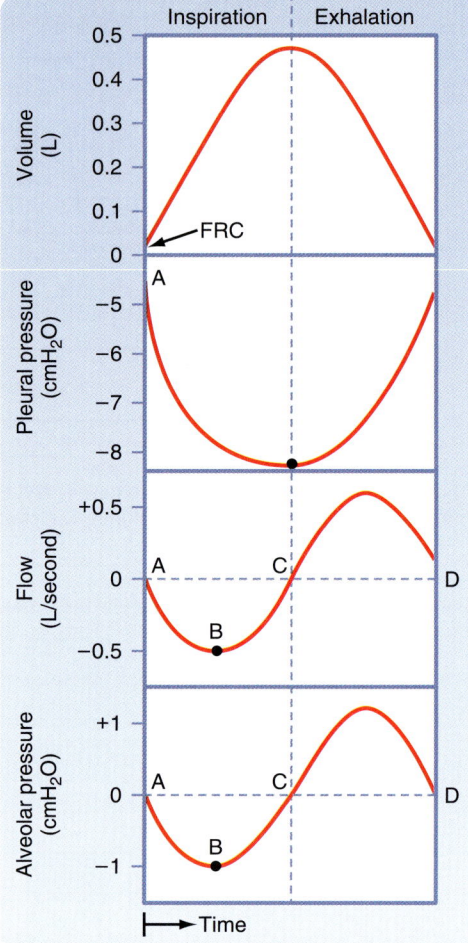

**Fig. 4.6** Changes in alveolar and pleural pressure during quiet breathing (tidal volume).

pressure fluctuates during breathing but is approximately 0.5 kPa at the end of quiet expiration.

During quiet breathing, intrapleural pressure is always negative. However, in forced expiration the intrapleural pressure becomes positive, forcing a reduction in lung volume and expulsion of air.

---

### CLINICAL NOTES

Puncture wounds through the thorax can mean that the intrapleural space is open to the atmosphere (a pneumothorax). The pressures equilibrate and the lungs are no longer held expanded, leading to collapse of the lung. This requires prompt medical management – see Chapter 20 for further information.

---

## BOX 4.1 LAW OF LAPLACE

Laplace's law states that 'The pressure within a bubble is equal to twice the surface tension divided by the radius'.

$$P = \frac{2T}{r}$$

where
P = pressure within bubble
T = surface tension
r = radius

- The smaller a bubble (i.e., the more curved the surface), the larger the radial component.
- The larger the radial component, the greater the tendency to collapse.
- Smaller bubbles must have a greater internal pressure to keep them inflated.

## Muscles of respiration

This section describes how the muscles of respiration bring about changes in lung volumes.

### Thoracic wall

The thoracic wall is made up of (from superficial to deep):

- Skin and subcutaneous tissue.
- Ribs, thoracic vertebrae, sternum and manubrium.
- Intercostal muscles: external, internal and thoracis transversus.
- Parietal pleura.

Situated at the thoracic outlet is the diaphragm, which attaches to the costal margin, xiphoid process and lumbar vertebrae.

### Intercostal muscles

The intercostal muscles pull the ribs closer together:

1. External intercostal muscles pull the ribs upwards.
2. Internal intercostal muscles pull the ribs downwards.

#### External intercostal muscles

External intercostal muscles (Fig. 4.7) span the space between adjacent ribs, originating from the inferior border of the upper rib, and attaching to the superior border of the rib below. The muscle attaches along the length of the rib, from the tubercle to the costal–chondral junction, and its fibres run forward and downwards.

#### Internal intercostal muscles

Internal intercostal muscles (Fig. 4.7) span the space between adjacent ribs, originating from the subcostal groove of the rib above, and attaching to the superior border of the rib below. The muscle attaches along the length of the rib from the angle of the rib to the sternum, and its fibres run downwards and backwards.

## Diaphragm

The diaphragm is the main muscle of respiration (Fig. 4.8). The central region of the diaphragm is tendinous; the outer margin is muscular, originating from the borders of the thoracic outlet.

The diaphragm has right and left domes. The right dome is higher than the left, to accommodate the liver below. There is a central tendon that sits below the two domes, attaching to the xiphisternum anteriorly and the lumbar vertebrae posteriorly.

Several important structures pass through the diaphragm:

- The inferior vena cava passes through the right dome at the level of the eighth thoracic vertebra (T8).
- The oesophagus passes through a sling of muscular fibres from the right crus of the diaphragm at the level of T10.
- The aorta pierces the diaphragm anterior to T12.

The diaphragm attaches to the costal margin anteriorly and laterally. Posteriorly, it attaches to the lumbar vertebrae by the crura (left crus at L1 and L2, right crus at L1, L2 and L3). In addition, the position of the diaphragm changes relative to posture: it is lower when standing than sitting.

The phrenic nerve innervates the diaphragm and its blood supply arises from pericardiophrenic and musculophrenic branches of the internal thoracic artery.

### HINTS AND TIPS

The phrenic nerve supplies the diaphragm (60% motor, 40% sensory). Remember, 'nerve roots 3, 4 and 5 keep the diaphragm alive'.

## Function of the muscles of respiration

Breathing can be classified by direction of air movement into inspiration and expiration and by activity level as quiet or forced.

### Inspiration
#### Quiet inspiration

In quiet inspiration, contraction of the diaphragm flattens its domes. This action increases the volume of the thorax, thus lowering intrapleural pressure and drawing air into the lungs. At the same time, the abdominal wall relaxes, allowing the abdominal contents to be displaced downwards as the diaphragm flattens. During quiet inspiration, the change in intrathoracic volume is mainly caused by the movement of the diaphragm downwards. Contraction of the diaphragm therefore comprises 75% of the energy expenditure during quiet breathing. However, the intercostal muscles are involved. With the first rib fixed, the intercostal muscles can expand the ribcage by two movements:

1. Forward movement of the lower end of the sternum.
2. Upward and outward movement of the ribs.

**Muscles of expiration**

**Quiet breathing**

Expiration results from passive recoil of lungs and rib cage

**Active breathing**

Internal intercostal mm., except interchondral part (aid forced expiration)

Abdominal mm. (depress lower ribs, compress abdominal contents, thus pushing up diaphragm, aiding forced expiration)

Rectus abdominis m.

External abdominal oblique m.

Internal abdominal oblique m.

Transversus abdominis m.

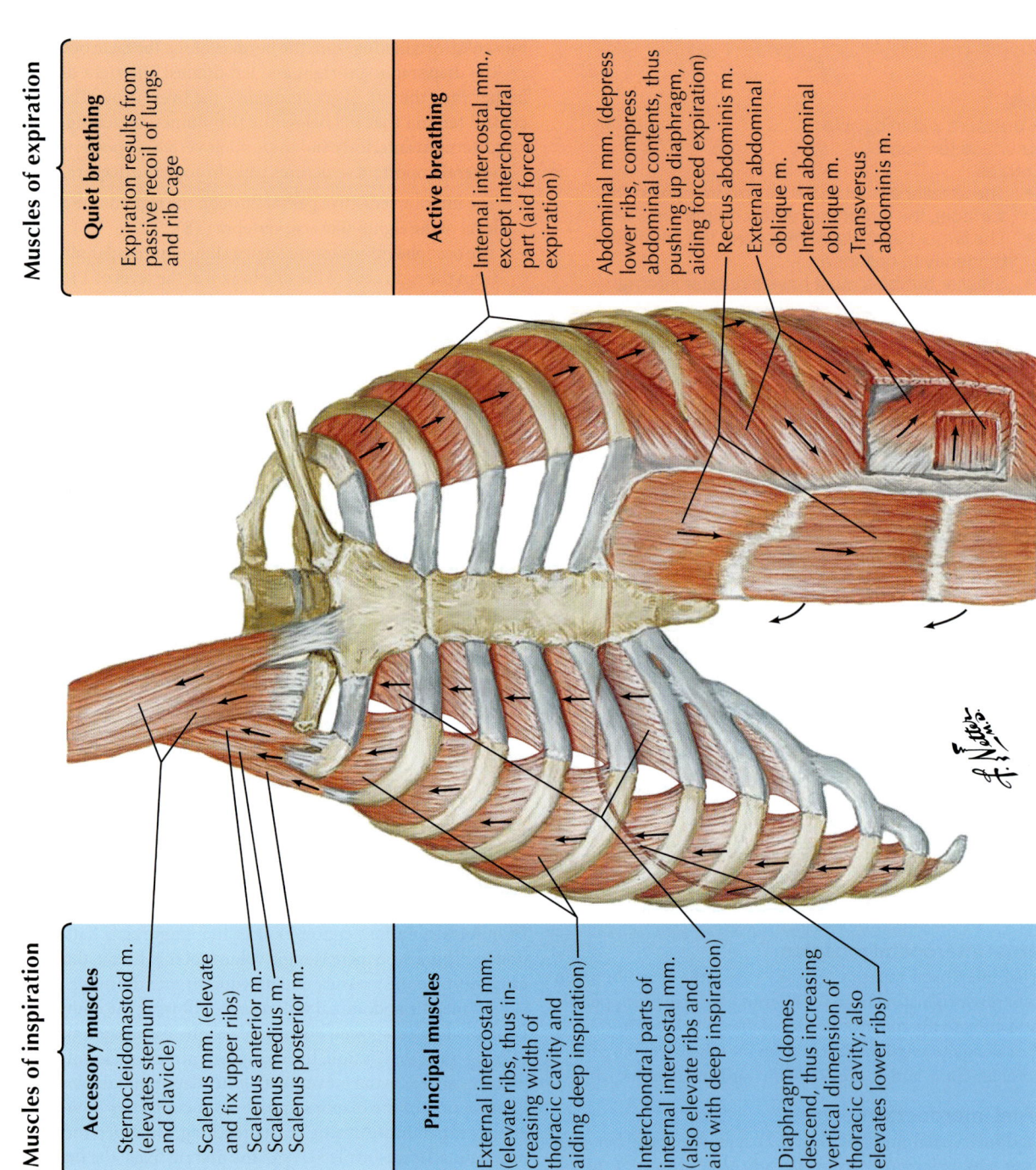

**Muscles of inspiration**

**Accessory muscles**

Sternocleidomastoid m. (elevates sternum and clavicle)

Scalenus mm. (elevate and fix upper ribs)

Scalenus anterior m.
Scalenus medius m.
Scalenus posterior m.

**Principal muscles**

External intercostal mm. (elevate ribs, thus increasing width of thoracic cavity and aiding deep inspiration)

Interchondral parts of internal intercostal mm. (also elevate ribs and aid with deep inspiration)

Diaphragm (domes descend, thus increasing vertical dimension of thoracic cavity; also elevates lower ribs)

**Fig. 4.7** Muscles of respiration.

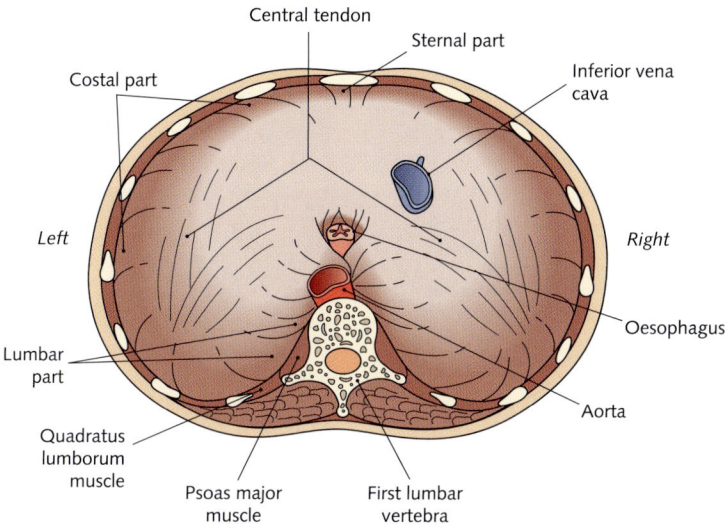

**Fig. 4.8** Anatomy of the diaphragm.

These actions are small and the intercostal muscles mainly prevent deformation of the tissue between the ribs, which would otherwise lower the volume of the thoracic cage (Fig. 4.9).

### Forced inspiration

In addition to the action of the diaphragm:

Scalene muscles and sternocleidomastoids raise the ribs anteroposteriorly, producing movement at the manubriosternal joint.

Intercostal muscles are more active and raise the ribs to a far greater extent than in quiet inspiration.

The 12th rib, which is attached to quadratus lumborum, allows forcible downward movement of the diaphragm.

Arching the back using erector spinae also increases thoracic volume.

During respiratory distress, the scapulae are fixed by trapezius muscles. The rhomboid muscles and levator scapulae, pectoralis minor and serratus anterior raise the ribs. The arms can be fixed (e.g., by holding the back of a chair), allowing the use of pectoralis major.

## Expiration

### Quiet expiration

Quiet expiration is passive and there is no direct muscle action. During inspiration, the lungs are expanded against their elastic recoil. This recoil is sufficient to drive air out of the lungs in expiration. Thus, quiet expiration involves the controlled relaxation of the intercostal muscles and the diaphragm.

### Forced expiration

Elastic recoil of the lungs is reinforced by contraction of the muscles of the abdominal wall. This forces the abdominal contents against the diaphragm, displacing the diaphragm upwards (Fig. 4.10).

**CLINICAL BOX**

The features of forced inspiration/expiration are important clinically. It is vitally important to detect patients needing to use their accessory muscles to breathe. These patients are in respiratory distress and, as active respiration is energy intensive, they will eventually tire. If you detect features of forced inspiration/expiration in a patient on the wards or in the emergency department, urgent action is required and you should alert the medical team.

In addition, quadratus lumborum pulls the ribs down, adding to the force at which the abdominal contents are pushed against the diaphragm. Intercostal muscles prevent outward deformation of the tissue between the ribs.

## VENTILATION AND DEAD SPACE

### Minute ventilation

Minute ventilation ($V_E$) is a measurement of the amount of air that is moved in and out of the lungs in 1 minute. To calculate ($V_E$) you need to know:

- The number of breaths per minute.
- The volume of air moved in and out with each breath (the tidal volume: $V_T$).

The normal frequency of breathing varies between 12 and 18 breaths per minute. Normal tidal volume is approximately 500 mL in quiet breathing. If a subject with a tidal volume of 500 mL took 12 breaths a minute, the minute ventilation would be $500 \times 12 = 6000$ mL/min.

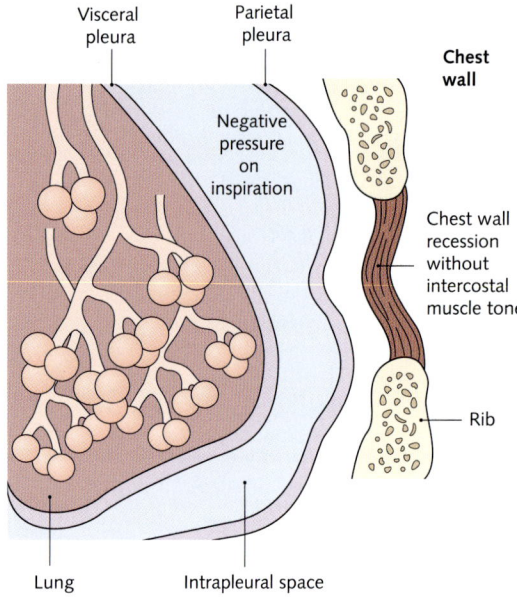

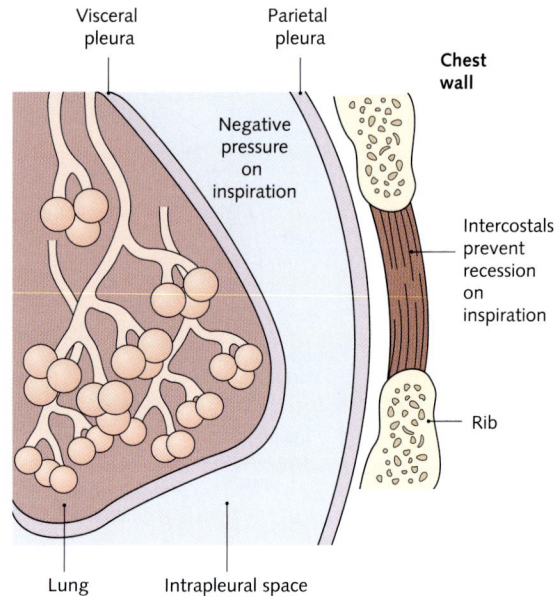

**Fig. 4.9** Action of the intercostal muscles during inspiration.

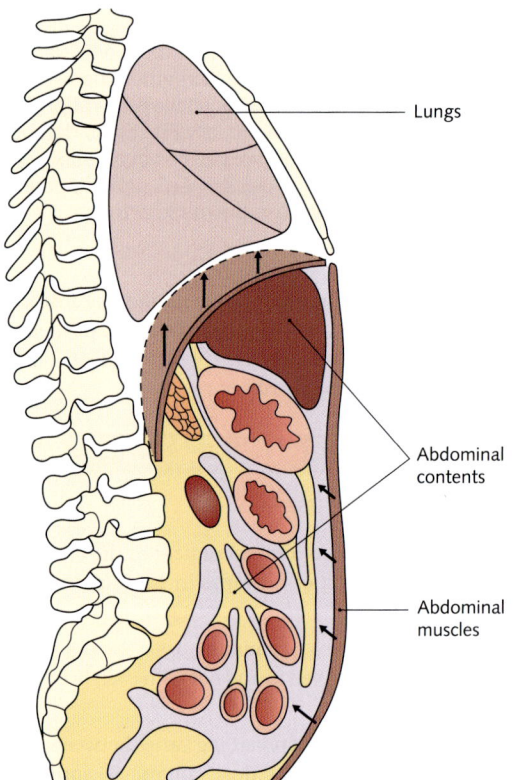

Abdominal contents pushing diaphragm upwards

**Fig. 4.10** Forced expiration.

Or, more generally:

$$V_E = V_T f$$

where $V_E$ = minute ventilation, $V_T$ = tidal volume and $f$ = the respiratory rate (breaths/minute).

## Alveolar ventilation

Not all inspired air reaches the alveoli; some stays within the trachea and other conducting airways (also known as dead space).

Therefore, two values of minute ventilation need to be considered:

1. Minute ventilation ($V_E$), as described above.
2. Minute alveolar ventilation ($V_E$), which is the amount of air that reaches the alveoli in 1 minute.

We can say that for one breath:

$$V_A = V_T - V_D$$

where $V_A$ = the volume reaching the alveolus in one breath, and $V_D$ = the volume of dead space. Hence, in 1 minute:

$$V_A = (V_T - V_D) f$$

## Anatomical dead space

Not all air entering the respiratory system actually reaches the alveoli and takes part in gas exchange. Anatomical dead space describes those areas of the airway not involved in gaseous exchange (i.e., the conducting zone). Included in this space are:

- Nose and mouth
- Pharynx and larynx

- Trachea, bronchi and bronchioles (including the terminal bronchioles).

The volume of the anatomical dead space ($V_D$) is approximately 150 mL (or 2 mL/kg of body weight). Anatomical dead space varies with the size of the subject and also increases with deep inspiration because greater expansion of the lungs lengthens and widens the conducting airways.

Anatomical dead space can be measured using Fowler's method, which is based on the single-breath nitrogen test (Fig. 4.11). The patient makes a single inhalation of 100% $O_2$ and exhales through a gas analyzer that measures $N_2$ concentration. On expiration, the nitrogen concentration is initially low as the patient breathes out the dead-space oxygen just inspired (100% $O_2$). The concentration of $N_2$ rises where the dead-space gas has mixed with alveolar gas (a mixture of nitrogen and oxygen). As pure alveolar gas is expired, nitrogen concentration reaches a plateau (the alveolar plateau).

If there were no mixing of alveolar and dead-space gas during expiration, there would be a stepwise increase in nitrogen concentration when alveolar gas is exhaled (Fig. 4.11A). In reality, mixing does occur, which means that the nitrogen concentration increases slowly, then rises sharply. The dead-space volume is defined as the midpoint of this curve (where the two shaded areas are equal in Fig. 4.11B).

## Physiological dead space

The physiological dead space includes the anatomical dead space and also gas in the alveoli that does not participate in gas exchange (i.e., alveolar dead space).

*Physiological dead space = anatomical dead space + alveolar dead space*

Alveolar dead space comes about because gas exchange is suboptimal in some parts of the lung. If each acinus (or end respiratory unit) were perfect, the amount of air received by each alveolus would be matched by the flow of blood through the pulmonary capillaries. In reality:

- Some areas receive less ventilation than others.
- Some areas receive less blood flow than others.

In a normal, healthy person, anatomical and physiological dead space are almost equal, with alveolar dead space being very small (<5 mL). However, when lung disease alters ventilation:perfusion relationships, the volume of alveolar dead space increases.

Physiological dead space can be measured using the Bohr equation. The method requires a sample of arterial blood and involves the analysis of carbon dioxide in expired air. Knowing that carbon dioxide is not exchanged in respiratory units that are

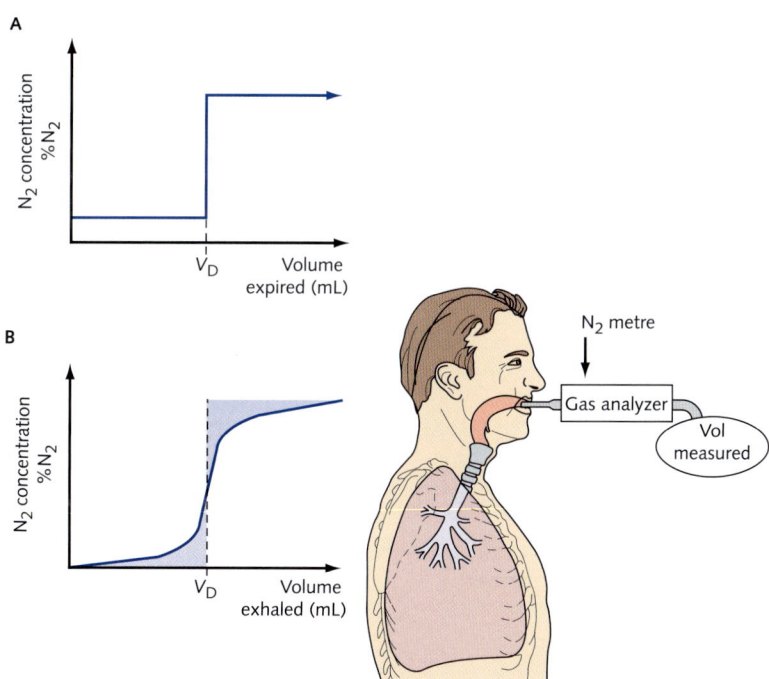

**Fig. 4.11** Measurement of anatomical dead space.

not perfused, and that carbon dioxide in air is almost zero, it is possible to calculate the volume of physiological dead space.

## Lung compliance and the role of surfactant

For ventilation to occur, the respiratory muscles must overcome the mechanical properties of the lungs and thorax, specifically the lung's tendency to elastic recoil.

The elastic properties of the lung are caused by:

- Elastic fibres and collagen in lung tissue.
- Surface tension forces in the lung created by the alveolar–liquid interface.

Compliance describes the distensibility or ease of stretch of lung tissue when an external force is applied to it. Elasticity (*E*) is the resistance to that stretch. Therefore:

$$C = 1/E$$

In respiratory physiology, we deal with:

- Compliance of the lung ($C_L$).
- Compliance of the chest wall ($C_W$).
- Total compliance ($C_{TOT}$) of the chest wall and lung together.

Lung compliance is the ease with which the lungs expand under pressure. The pressure to inflate arises from the transmural pressure (i.e., the difference between the intrapleural pressure and the intrapulmonary pressure); this is plotted against the change in volume on a pressure–volume curve (Fig. 4.12). Compliance represents the slope of the curve ($\Delta V{:}\Delta P$). You can see from the pressure–volume curve that expanding the lung is like blowing up a balloon. At first, high pressure is required for a small increase in volume. Then the slope becomes steeper before flattening out again.

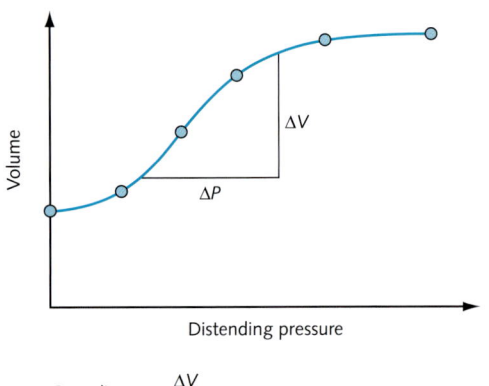

Compliance $= \dfrac{\Delta V}{\Delta P}$

**Fig. 4.12** The pressure–volume curve.

Lung compliance varies with lung volume; compliance is greatest at lower lung volumes and smallest at higher lung volumes. For these reasons, lung compliance is sometimes quoted as specific lung compliance ($sp.C_L$).

$$sp.C_L = C_L / V_L$$

This change in lung compliance helps explain the difference in ventilation between the apex and base of the lung. The lung volume at the base is less (because it is compressed) relative to the apex. Thus, the base of the lung has greater initial compliance than that of the apex. Because both the base and apex are subject to intrapleural pressure changes of the same magnitude during inspiration, the base of the lung will expand to a greater extent than the apex.

## Chest wall compliance

The chest wall has elastic properties; at FRC these are equal and opposite to those in the lung (i.e., act to expand the chest). During inspiration, elastic forces (acting to expand the chest wall) aid inflation; however, at approximately two-thirds of TLC, the chest wall reaches its resting position. Any expansion beyond this point requires a positive pressure to stretch the chest wall.

## Effect of disease on compliance

Emphysema and pulmonary fibrosis (Fig. 4.13) represent two extremes of lung compliance in disease. In emphysema the

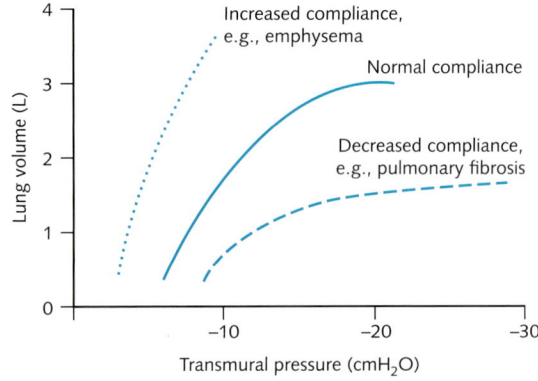

**Fig. 4.13** Pressure–volume curves in disease.

compliance of the lung is increased, that is, the lung becomes more easily distended. This is because the normal lung architecture is damaged, including the elastic fibres and collagen. Impaired elastic recoil means that the lungs do not deflate adequately, which contributes to air trapping. In diseases that cause fibrosis, scar tissue replaces normal interstitial tissue. As a result, the lungs become stiffer and compliance decreases. Structural changes in the thorax (e.g., kyphoscoliosis) can similarly alter chest wall compliance and reduce the ability of the chest wall to expand, thus producing a restrictive ventilatory defect.

## Surface tension and surfactant

The elasticity, and therefore lung compliance, is dependent on two factors:

1. Elastic fibres in lung tissue.
2. The surface tension of the alveolar lining (this lining is a thin film of liquid, the main component of which is surfactant).

Surface tension is a physical property of liquids that arises because fluid molecules have a stronger attraction to each other than to air molecules. Molecules on the surface of a liquid in contact with air are pulled close together and act like a skin. When molecules of a liquid lie on a curved surface (e.g., in a bubble), surface tension acts to pull that surface inwards. If the bubble is to be prevented from collapsing, there must be an equal and opposite force tending to expand it. This is provided by positive pressure within the bubble.

The alveoli are lined with liquid and are in contact with air. They can therefore be considered similar to tiny bubbles. Laplace's law (see Box 4.1) tells us that the smaller a bubble, the greater the internal pressure needed to keep it inflated. If a bubble of about the same size as an alveolus was lined with interstitial fluid and filled with air, it would require an internal pressure in the order of 3 kPa to prevent it from collapsing. The lungs would have a very low compliance and the forces involved in breathing would be extremely large. However, this is not the case because the alveoli are not lined with interstitial fluid, they are lined with surfactant.

## Surfactant

Surfactant is manufactured by type II pneumocytes. It is first stored intracellularly as lamellar bodies and then released as tubular myelin (the storage form of active surfactant). Once in the alveolar air space, the tubular myelin unravels to form a thin layer of surfactant over type I and type II pneumocytes.

Surfactant is 90% lipid (mostly a phospholipid called dipalmitoyl phosphatidylcholine) and 10% protein. The three mechanical functions of surfactant are:

1. Prevention of alveolar collapse (gives alveolar stability).
2. Increase in lung compliance by reducing surface tension of alveolar lining fluid.
3. Prevention of transudation of fluid into alveoli.

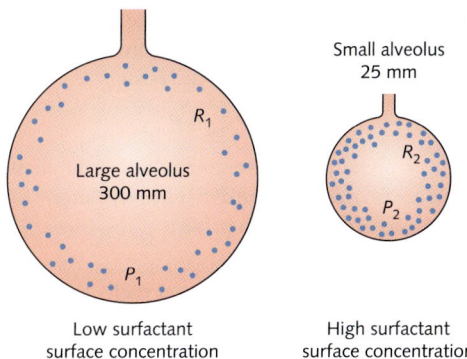

**Fig. 4.14** Surface tension in the alveoli. *R*, Radius; *P*, pressure.

Surfactant also has immunological functions, which are discussed in Chapter 2.

## Prevention of alveolar collapse

There are two properties of surfactant that ensure alveolar stability:

1. The surface tension of the alveolar lining fluid varies with surface area. This is because surfactant reduces surface tension in proportion to its surface concentration. Surfactant is insoluble in water and floats on the surface of the alveolar lining fluid. In larger alveoli the surfactant is more dilute and thus the surface tension is higher (Fig. 4.14).
2. There is interaction between adjacent groups of alveoli. Therefore, collapsing alveoli pull on adjacent alveoli, preventing further collapse. This is termed alveolar interdependence.

## Respiratory distress syndrome

Respiratory distress syndrome occurs in premature babies of less than 32 weeks' gestation. This results from deficiency of surfactant produced by type II pneumocytes. Difficulty in breathing occurs as alveoli collapse leading to low lung compliance. There is diffuse damage to alveoli with hyaline membrane formation. The neonate's breathing is rapid and laboured from the moment of delivery, often with an expiratory grunt. Treatment is with high-concentration oxygen therapy, and ventilator support if required. A course of corticosteroids can be given to a mother at risk of preterm delivery to decrease the risk of respiratory distress syndrome.

## Airway resistance

The previous section examined the elastic properties of the lungs (i.e., those caused by surface tension and tissue elasticity). However, in addition to overcoming the elastic properties of the lung during breathing, dynamic resistance to lung inflation must be overcome in order to provide effective ventilation.

The total pressure difference ($P_{TOT}$) required to inflate the lungs is the sum of the pressure to overcome lung compliance and the pressure to overcome dynamic resistance:

$$P_{TOT} = P_{COM} + P_{DYN}$$

where $P_{COM}$ = pressure to overcome lung compliance and $P_{DYN}$ = pressure to overcome the dynamic resistance.

Dynamic resistance itself comprises:

- Airway resistance.
- Resistance to tissues as they slide over each other – viscous tissue resistance.

$$P_{DYN} = P_{AR} + P_{VTR}$$

where $P_{AR}$ = pressure to overcome airways resistance and $P_{VTR}$ = pressure to overcome viscous tissue resistance.

Viscous tissue resistance comprises approximately 20% of the total dynamic resistance, that is, the vast majority of the total resistance is provided by the airways.

Airway resistance is an important concept because it is increased in common diseases such as asthma and COPD. It is defined as the resistance to flow of gas within the airways of the lung.

Before we discuss airway resistance further, it is important to outline pattern of flow.

## Pattern of flow

The pattern of air flowing through a tube (e.g., an airway) varies with the velocity and physical properties of the airway (Fig. 4.15).

### Laminar flow

Laminar flow is described by Poiseuille's law (see Box 4.2). In basic terms, Poiseuille's law means that the wider the tube, the lower the resistance to air flow. Importantly, the change in width is not directly proportional to the change in resistance: for a given reduction in the radius, there is a 16-fold increase in resistance. Narrower or longer pipes have a higher resistance to flow and so flow rate is reduced.

### Turbulent flow

Turbulent flow is much more likely to occur with:

- High velocities (e.g., within the airways during exercise).
- Larger-diameter airways.
- Low-viscosity, high-density fluids.

Branching or irregular surfaces can also initiate turbulence.

## Sites of airway resistance

When breathing through the nose, approximately one-half of the resistance to air flow occurs in the upper respiratory tract. This is significantly reduced when mouth breathing. Thus, approximately one-half of the resistance lies within the lower respiratory tract. Assuming laminar air flow, Poiseuille's law predicts that major resistance to air flow would occur in airways with a smaller radius. This is not the case because, although the individual diameter of each airway is small, the total cross-sectional area for flow increases (i.e., there are a large number of small airways further down the tracheobronchial tree).

**HINTS AND TIPS**

Remembering Poiseuille's law isn't drastically important, but understanding it is! So, remember that, in laminar flow, a small change in radius significantly affects either flow rate or pressure drop required to achieve the same flow. An example of this is bronchoconstriction in asthma.

- Flow varies directly with pressure drop.
- Flow varies inversely with viscosity.

**A**

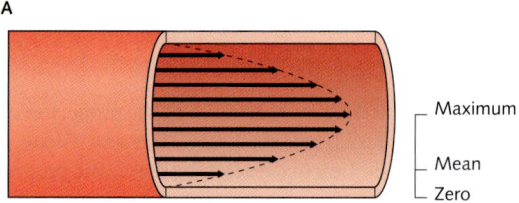

Maximum

Mean

Zero

**B**

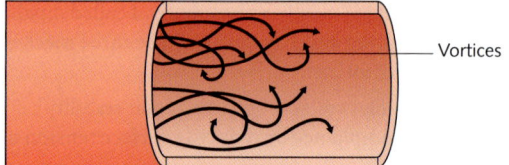

Vortices

**Fig. 4.15** (A) Laminar and (B) turbulent air flow.

In exercise, the airway resistance may increase significantly, owing to high air flows inducing turbulence. It is normal under these conditions to switch to mouth breathing to reduce airway resistance.

It is important to note that resistance of the smaller airways is difficult to measure. Thus, these small airways may be damaged by disease and it may be some time before this damage is detectable, thus representing a 'silent' zone.

## Factors determining airway resistance
Factors affecting airway resistance are:

- Lung volume
- Bronchial smooth-muscle tone
- Altered airway calibre
- Change in density and viscosity of inspired gas.

### Lung volume
Airways are supported by radial traction of lung parenchyma and thus their diameter and resistance to flow are affected by lung volume:

- Low lung volumes tend to collapse and compress the airways, reducing their diameter and thus increasing resistance to flow.
- High lung volumes tend to increase radial traction, increasing the length and diameter of airways.

### Bronchial smooth-muscle tone
Motor innervation of the smooth muscle of the airways is via the vagus nerve. The muscle has resting tone determined by the autonomic nervous system. This tone can be affected by a number of factors (Fig. 4.16). Factors acting to decrease the airway diameter include:

- Irritant and cough receptors, C-fibre reflex.
- Pulmonary stretch receptors.
- Mediator release – inflammatory mediators (histamine, leukotrienes, etc.) cause bronchoconstriction.

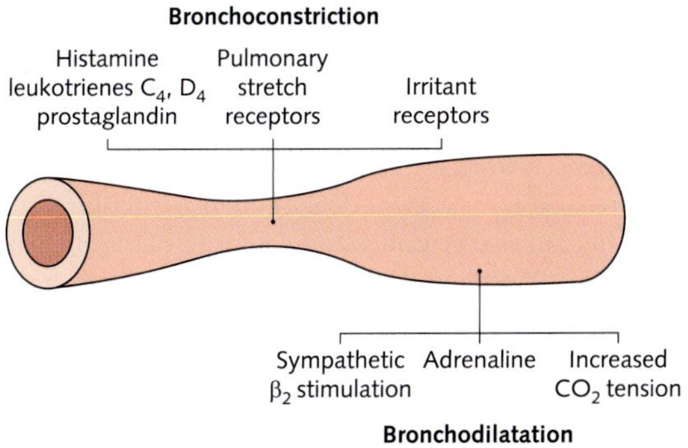

Factors acting to increase the airway diameter include:

- Carbon dioxide
- Catecholamine release
- Other nerves – nonadrenergic, noncholinergic nerves cause bronchodilatation.

Increased smooth-muscle tone is very important in asthma. Inflammatory mediators act to narrow the airways and increase airway resistance.

### HINTS AND TIPS

Things to remember:
- The major site of airway resistance is medium-sized bronchi.
- Eighty percent of the resistance of the upper respiratory tract is presented by the trachea and bronchi.
- Less than 20% of airway resistance is caused by airways less than 2 mm in diameter.

## Effect of transmural pressure on airway resistance
The pressure difference between the gas in the airway and the pressure outside the airway is known as the transmural pressure difference. The pressure outside the airway reflects the intrapleural pressure.

### During inspiration
The pressure within the pleural cavity is always negative and the alveolar pressure is greater than intrapleural pressure. The transmural pressure difference is always positive; thus the airway is distended (radial traction) (Fig. 4.17A).

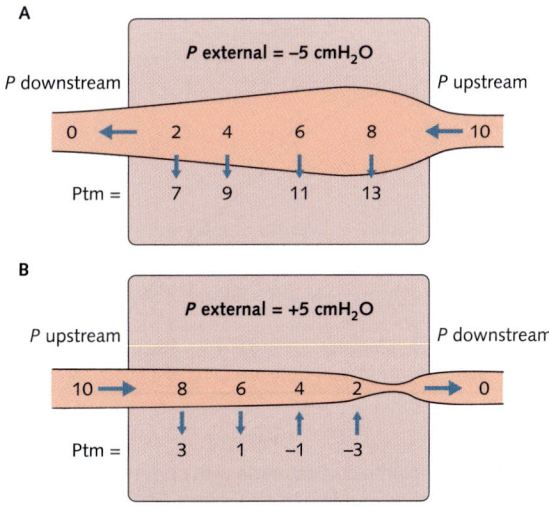

**Fig. 4.17** Transmural pressure *(Ptm)* in (A) inspiration and (B) forced expiration.

**Bronchoconstriction**

Histamine leukotrienes $C_4$, $D_4$ prostaglandin | Pulmonary stretch receptors | Irritant receptors

Sympathetic $\beta_2$ stimulation | Adrenaline | Increased $CO_2$ tension

**Bronchodilatation**

**Fig. 4.16** Factors affecting bronchial smooth-muscle tone.

## During expiration

The pressure within the alveolus is positive with respect to the intrapleural pressure; hence, the alveolus stays open. The transmural pressure difference, however, is dependent upon expiratory flow rate and intrapleural pressure.

During forced expiration, the positive intrapleural pressure is transmitted through the lungs to the external wall of the airways. In addition, there is a dynamic pressure drop from the alveolus to the airway caused by airway resistance. This is greater at high expiratory flow rates. Thus, the pressure in the lumen of the airway may be lower than the external wall pressure (negative transmural pressure), leading to airway collapse.

Thus, the harder the subject tries to exhale forcibly, the more the airways are compressed, so the rate of expiration does not rise as the increased pressure gradient (from alveoli to atmospheric pressure) is offset by the reduced airway calibre. This phenomenon is known as dynamic compression of airways (Fig. 4.17B).

Dynamic compression of airways is greater at lower lung volumes because the effect of radial traction holding the airways open is less. Thus it can be seen that, for a specific lung volume, there is a maximum expiratory flow rate caused by dynamic compression of the airways (Fig. 4.18). Any rate of expiration below this flow rate is dependent on how much effort is made to expel the air from the lungs and the flow is said to be effort dependent. At maximum expiratory flow rate, any additional effort does not alter the expiratory flow rate (because of dynamic compression of airways) and the flow is said to be effort independent.

### Dynamic compression in disease

In patients with COPD, dynamic compression limits expiratory flow, even in tidal breathing. The main reasons for this are:

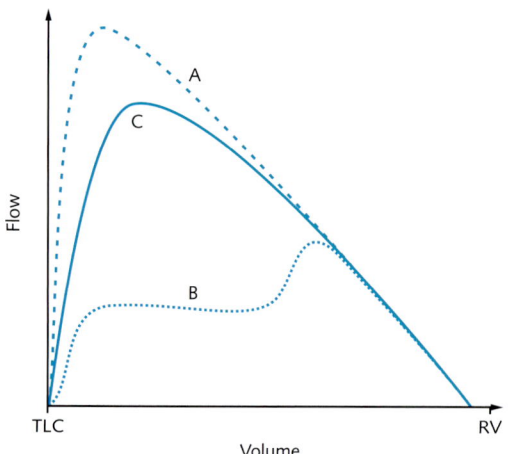

**Fig. 4.18** Flow–volume curves made with spirometer. (A) Maximum inspiration and forced expiration. (B) Slow expiration initially, then forced. (C) Expiratory flow almost to maximum effort. *RV*, Residual volume; *TLC*, total lung capacity.

- Loss of radial traction (owing to destruction of lung architecture). This means the airways are more readily compressed.
- Increased lung compliance, leading to lower alveolar pressure and less force driving air out of the lungs.

The clinical consequences are airway collapse on expiration and air trapping in the alveoli. Patients sometimes demonstrate pursed-lip breathing as they attempt to increase pressure on expiration and reduce the amount of air trapped.

## Measuring airway resistance

Airway resistance can be measured by plethysmography. In practice, estimates of airway resistance are made every day using simpler methods which rely on the relationship between resistance and air flow. Peak expiratory flow rate measures the maximum air flow achieved in a rapid, forced expiration. Spirometry measures the volume exhaled in a specified time (e.g., the forced expired volume in 1 second or $FEV_1$).

# The work of breathing

The work of breathing describes the work done by the respiratory muscles to overcome the forces described above, that is, resistance to air flow and the elastic recoil of the lungs.

The work done ($W$) to change a volume ($\Delta V$) of gas at constant pressure ($P$) is shown by the relationship below:

$$W = P\Delta V$$

Work done is measured in joules: a volume change of 10 L at a pressure of 1 cm $H_2O$ = 1 J of energy.

Respiration normally represents just a small fraction of the total cost of metabolism (approximately 2%). However, the work required to inflate the lungs, along with this percentage, will rise if:

- Lungs are inflated to a larger volume (e.g., COPD and chronic severe asthma).
- Lung compliance decreases (e.g., fibrotic lungs).
- Airway resistance increases (e.g., COPD and asthma).
- Turbulence is induced in the airways (e.g., in high flow rates experienced during strenuous exercise).

In contrast, the work of breathing is reduced by bronchodilators, which act to decrease airway resistance.

The increased work requirement can be dramatic in patients with severe COPD, as a great deal of energy is required to just breathe. This can also be understood in terms of the efficiency of ventilation (i.e., the amount of work done divided by the required energy expenditure). Efficiency of normal quiet breathing is low (about 10%), even in health. In COPD, ventilation efficiency decreases, so that all the oxygen supplied from increasing ventilation is consumed by the respiratory muscles. The work of breathing can be illustrated by volume–pressure curves (Fig. 4.19).

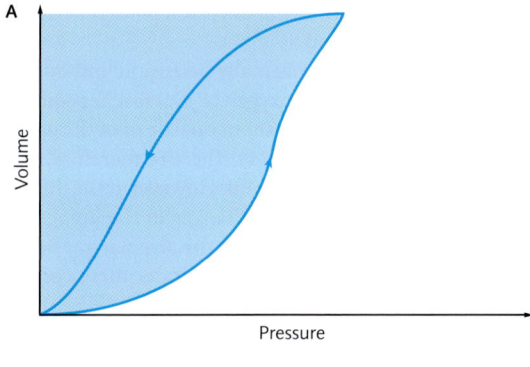

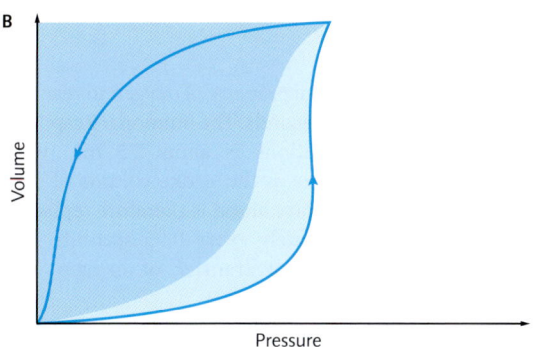

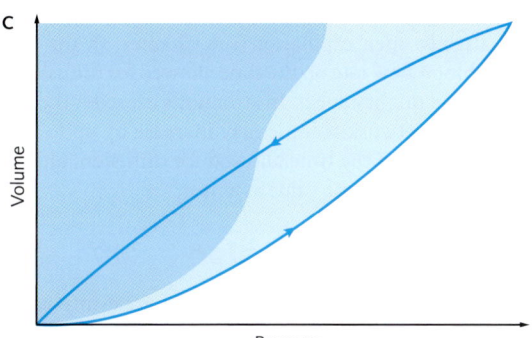

**Fig. 4.19** The work of breathing. (A) Graph of normal lung volume against trans-lung pressure; (B) increased airway resistance (e.g., in asthma); (C) decreased compliance (e.g., in fibrotic lung disease).

**HINTS AND TIPS**

Try to relate these concepts to respiratory failure. A patient with lung disease may be able to respond to impaired gas exchange by raising the ventilatory rate, leading to rapid, shallow breaths. This increases the work of breathing. If lung disease is severe, the work of breathing may become unsustainable. Respiratory muscles tire, ventilatory failure ensues and the patient must be mechanically ventilated to reduce the work of breathing.

## GASEOUS EXCHANGE IN THE LUNGS

This section discusses how gas is transferred from the alveoli to the bloodstream and from the bloodstream to the alveoli.

### Diffusion

Gas exchange between alveolar air and blood in the pulmonary capillaries takes place by diffusion.

- Diffusion occurs from an area of high concentration to an area of low concentration. Thus, the driving force for diffusion is the concentration difference ($\Delta C$).
- Diffusion will occur until the concentration in the two areas is equalized (i.e., net movement has ceased). Random movement of particles continues to occur and this is known as a dynamic equilibrium.

Diffusion in the lungs occurs across a membrane and is therefore governed by Fick's law. Fick's law tells us that the rate of diffusion of a gas increases:

- As the surface area of the membrane increases.
- The thinner the membrane.
- The greater the partial pressure gradient across the membrane.
- The more soluble the gas.

It is clear that the blood–gas interface, with its large surface area of 50–100 m$^2$ and average thickness of 0.4 μm, permits the high rate of diffusion required by the body.

The rate of diffusion across the alveoli is directly dependent upon the difference in partial pressures.

**HINTS AND TIPS**

The following will decrease the rate of oxygen diffusion into the blood:

- Reduction in the overall alveolar surface area (e.g., emphysema).
- Increased distance for diffusion (e.g., emphysema).
- Increased thickness of the alveolar wall (e.g., fibrosing alveolitis).
- Reduction in the alveolar partial pressure of oxygen (e.g., high altitude).
- Partial pressures are also expressed in kPa: 1 kPa is 7.5 mmHg.

### Perfusion and diffusion limitation

At the gas exchange surface, gas transfer occurs through a membrane into a flowing liquid. There are two processes occurring (Fig. 4.20):

- Diffusion across the alveolar–capillary membrane.
- Perfusion of blood through pulmonary capillaries.

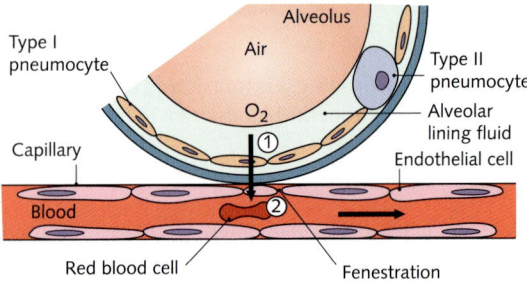

**Fig. 4.20** Gas transfer across the alveolar–capillary membrane. (1) Diffusion across membrane; (2) perfusion of blood through pulmonary capillaries.

Uptake of a gas into the blood is dependent on its solubility and the chemical combination (e.g., with haemoglobin). If the chemical combination is strong, the gas is taken up by the blood with little rise in arterial partial pressure.

The solubility of nitrous oxide ($N_2O$) in the blood is low, and it does not undergo chemical combination with any component of the blood. Thus, rate of transfer of gas into the liquid phase is slow and partial pressure of the gas in the blood rises rapidly (Fig. 4.21). This reduces the partial pressure difference between alveolar gas and the blood and hence is the driving force for diffusion. Nitrous oxide is, therefore, an example of a gas that is said to be perfusion limited. Thus, the amount of nitrous oxide taken up by the blood is dependent almost solely upon the rate of blood flow through the pulmonary capillaries.

In the case of carbon monoxide (CO), the gas is taken up rapidly and bound tightly by haemoglobin; hence the arterial partial pressure rises slowly (Fig. 4.21). Thus, there is always a driving force (partial pressure difference) for diffusion (even at low perfusion rates) and the overall rate of transfer will be dependent on the rate of diffusion. This type of transfer is said to be diffusion limited. Thus, the amount of carbon monoxide taken up by the

blood is dependent on the rate of diffusion of carbon monoxide from the alveoli to the blood.

The transfer of oxygen is normally perfusion limited because the arterial partial pressure of oxygen ($P_aO_2$) reaches equilibrium with the alveolar gas ($P_AO_2$) by about one-third of the way along the pulmonary capillary (Fig. 4.21). There is, therefore, no driving force for diffusion after this point. However, if the diffusion is slow because of emphysematous changes in the lung, then the $P_aO_2$ may not reach equilibrium with the alveolar gas before the blood reaches the end of the capillary. Under these conditions, the transfer of oxygen is diffusion limited.

## Oxygen uptake in the capillary network

The time taken for the partial pressure of oxygen to reach its plateau is approximately 0.25 seconds. The pulmonary capillary volume under resting conditions is about 75 mL, which is approximately the same size as the stroke volume of the right ventricle. Pulmonary capillary blood is therefore replaced with every heartbeat, approximately every 0.75 seconds. This far exceeds the time needed for transfer of oxygen into the bloodstream.

During exercise, however, the cardiac output increases and the flow rate through the pulmonary capillaries also increases. Because the lungs have the ability to recruit new capillaries and distend already open capillaries (see Chapter 3), the effect of increased blood flow rate on the time allowed for diffusion is not as great as one might expect. In strenuous exercise, the pulmonary capillary network volume may increase by up to 200 mL. This helps maintain the time allowed for diffusion, although it cannot keep it to the same value as at rest.

## Carbon dioxide transfer

Diffusion rates of gas in blood are also of great importance in respiratory medicine. Diffusion in liquids is directly dependent upon the solubility of the gas, but inversely proportional to the square root of its molecular weight. Carbon monoxide diffuses 20 times more rapidly than oxygen, but has a similar molecular weight. Thus, the difference in rates of diffusion is caused by the much higher solubility of carbon dioxide.

Under normal conditions, the transfer of carbon dioxide is not diffusion limited.

## Measuring diffusion

Carbon monoxide is the gas most commonly used to study diffusing capacity. Because carbon monoxide is taken up into the liquid phase very quickly, the rate of perfusion of pulmonary capillaries does not significantly affect the partial pressure difference between alveolar gas and the bloodstream. In addition, carbon

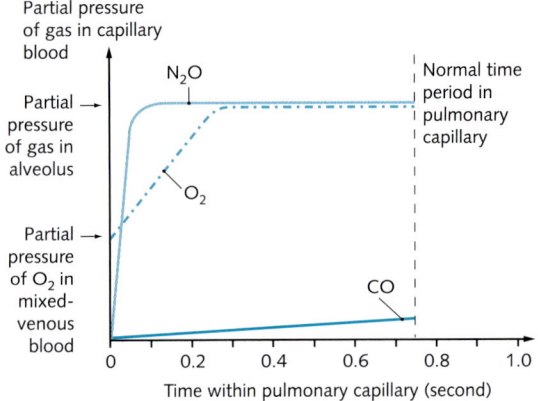

**Fig. 4.21** Partial pressures of respiratory gases.

monoxide binds irreversibly to haemoglobin and is not taken up by the tissues.

In contrast, oxygen is not a good candidate for calculating diffusing capacity because it binds reversibly to haemoglobin; thus, mixed-venous partial pressure may not be the same as that of blood entering the pulmonary capillary bed. In addition, because oxygen is taken up less quickly than carbon monoxide, perfusion has more of an effect.

We therefore use the diffusing capacity of carbon monoxide ($D_L CO$) as a general measure of the diffusion properties of the lung.

One of the methods used to measure diffusion across the blood–gas interface is the single-breath method. A single breath of a mixture of carbon monoxide and air is taken. The breath is then held for approximately 10 seconds. The difference between inspiratory and expiratory concentrations of carbon monoxide are measured and therefore the amount of carbon monoxide taken up by the blood in 10 seconds is known. If the lung volume is also measured by the helium dilution method, it is possible to

determine the transfer coefficient ($KCO$) or diffusion rate per unit of lung volume. This is a more useful measure of diffusion where lung volume has been lost: for example, after surgery or in pleural effusion. Because there can be many causes of a reduction in diffusing capacity, it is not a specific test for lung disease. It is, however, a sensitive test: it is able to demonstrate minor impediments to gas diffusion.

Factors that decrease the rate of diffusion include:

- Thickening of the alveolar–capillary membrane (e.g., in fibrosing alveolitis).
- Oedema of the alveolar capillary walls.
- Increased lining fluid within the alveoli.
- Increased distance for gaseous diffusion (e.g., in emphysema).
- Reduced area of alveolar–capillary membrane (e.g., in emphysema).
- Reduced flow of fresh air to the alveoli from terminal bronchioles.

## Chapter Summary

- The function of ventilation is to maintain blood gases at their optimum level by delivering air to the alveoli where gas exchange can take place.
- The gas held by the lungs is subdivided into specific lung volumes. Lung volumes are important in clinical practice and are measured through pulmonary function testing. See Fig. 4.1 and Table 4.1.
- The muscles involved in respiration include the diaphragm, internal and external intercostal muscles and the abdominal wall muscles.
- Minute ventilation ($V_E$) is the volume of gas moved in and out of the lungs in 1 minute. Minute alveolar ventilation ($V_E$), which is the amount of air that reaches the alveoli in 1 minute.
- Anatomical dead space describes those areas of the airway not involved in gaseous exchange (i.e., the conducting zone). The volume of the anatomical dead space ($V_D$) is approximately 150 mL.
- Lung compliance is the ease with which the lungs expand under pressure. The pressure to inflate arises from the transmural pressure (the difference between the intrapleural pressure and the intrapulmonary pressure).
- Alveoli are lined with surfactant. Surfactant prevents alveolar collapse, and increases lung compliance.
- Gas exchange between alveolar air and blood in the pulmonary capillaries takes place by diffusion from an area of high concentration to low concentration. The driving force for diffusion is concentration difference.

**MLA Conditions**
Chronic obstructive pulmonary disease
Interstitital lung disease
Pneumothorax

**MLA Presentations**
Nil

# Perfusion and gas transport

## OVERVIEW

The pulmonary circulation is a highly specialized system adapted to accommodate the entire cardiac output, both at rest and during exercise, facilitated by its low pressure, low resistance and ability to recruit more vessels with only a slight increase in arterial pulmonary pressure.

However, good perfusion is not enough to ensure that the blood is adequately oxygenated. The most important determinant in arterial blood gas composition is the way in which ventilation (V) and perfusion (Q) are matched to each alveolus. V:Q mismatching is the main problem in many common lung diseases.

The ability of the lungs to change minute ventilation, and therefore alter the rate of excretion of carbon dioxide, gives the respiratory system a key role in maintaining the body's acid–base status. This chapter therefore also reviews the fundamentals of acid–base balance and discusses the common acid–base disturbances.

## THE VENTILATION–PERFUSION RELATIONSHIP

### Basic concepts

To achieve efficient gaseous exchange, it is essential that the flow of gas (V) and the flow of blood (Q) are closely matched. The ideal situation would be where:

- All alveoli are ventilated equally with gas of identical composition and pressure.
- All pulmonary capillaries in the alveolar wall are perfused with equal amounts of mixed-venous blood.

Unfortunately, this is not the case, as neither ventilation nor perfusion is uniform throughout the lung. This carries certain clinical implications, as outlined further in the chapter.

The partial pressure of oxygen in the alveoli determines the amount of oxygen transferred to blood. Two factors affect the partial pressure of oxygen in the alveoli:

1. The amount of ventilation (i.e., the addition of oxygen to the alveolar compartment).
2. The perfusion of blood through pulmonary capillaries (i.e., the removal of oxygen from the alveolar compartment).

It is the ratio of ventilation to perfusion that determines the concentration of oxygen in the alveolar compartment.

## Ventilation:perfusion ratio

By looking at the V:Q ratio, we can see how well ventilation and perfusion are matched. By definition:

$$\text{Ventilation : perfusion ratio} = V_A/Q$$

where $V_A$ = alveolar minute ventilation (usually about 4.2 L/min) and $Q$ = pulmonary blood flow (usually about 5.0 L/min). Thus, normal $V_A/Q = 0.84$ (i.e., approximately 1).

This is an average value across the lung. Different V:Q ratios are present throughout the lung from apex to base.

## Extremes of ventilation:perfusion ratio

Looking at the V:Q ratio, there are two extremes to this relationship. These extremes were introduced in Chapter 1. Either there is:

1. No ventilation (a shunt): $V_A/Q = 0$.
2. No perfusion (dead space): $V_A/Q = \infty$.

### Right-to-left shunt

A right-to-left shunt is when the pulmonary circulation bypasses the ventilation process, meaning deoxygenated blood from the right side of the heart travels to the left side of the heart without gas exchange or oxygenation. This process (Fig. 5.1) occurs by either:

1. Bypassing the lungs completely (e.g., transposition of great vessels).
2. Perfusion of a nonventilated lung area.

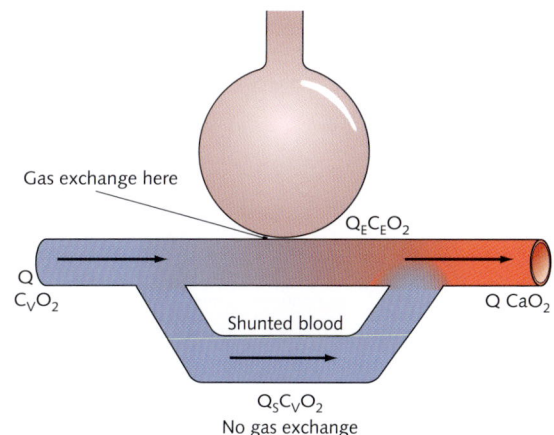

**Fig. 5.1** Shunted blood. The shunted blood has a low oxygen concentration (i.e., of venous blood) and is known as the venous admixture. *a*, arterial; *C*, capillary; *E*, exchange; *Q*, perfusion/blood flow; *S*, shunted; *v*, venous.

The shunted blood will not have been oxygenated or able to give up its carbon dioxide; thus its levels of $PO_2$ and $PCO_2$ are those of venous blood. When added to the systemic circulation, this blood will proportionately decrease arterial $PO_2$; it is called the venous admixture.

In normal physiology, there is only a very small amount of shunting (about 1%). However, right-to-left shunting makes a significant contribution to abnormal gas exchange in some disease states, notably:

- Cyanotic congenital heart disease: group of conditions with changes in the anatomy of the heart/vasculature that increase the venous admixture.
- Eisenmenger syndrome: ASD/VSD that also increases venous admixture.
- Pulmonary oedema: reduces ventilation of lung areas.
- Severe pneumonia: reduces ventilation of lung areas.

## Regional variation of ventilation and perfusion

Both ventilation and perfusion increase towards the lung base because of the effects of gravity.

Because the blood has a greater density than air, the gravitational effects on perfusion are much greater than on ventilation. This leads to a regional variation (Fig. 5.2) in the $V:Q$ ratio from lung apex (high $V/Q$) to lung base (low $V/Q$).

These regional variations are caused by the lung being upright; thus, changes in posture will alter the $V:Q$ ratio throughout the lung. For example, when lying down, the posterior area of the lung has a low $V:Q$ ratio and the anterior area has a high $V:Q$ ratio.

The effect of high and low $V:Q$ ratios on carbon dioxide and oxygen in the alveolus and blood is highlighted in Fig. 5.3, described below and summarized in Table 5.1.

## At low ventilation:perfusion ratios (e.g., at the lung base)

### Effect on carbon dioxide concentrations

Carbon dioxide diffuses from the blood to alveoli; however, because ventilation is low, carbon dioxide is not rapidly taken away. Thus, carbon dioxide tends to accumulate in the alveolus until a new, higher steady-state $P_ACO_2$ is reached.

Assuming that the overall lung function is normal, this regional variation in $P_ACO_2$ will not affect overall $P_vCO_2$. Thus, reducing the $V:Q$ ratio will not increase $P_aCO_2$ above the mixed-venous value.

### Effect on oxygen concentrations

Oxygen diffuses from the alveolus into the blood; however, because ventilation is low, oxygen taken up by the blood and metabolized is not replenished fully by new air entering the lungs. Oxygen in the alveolus is depleted until a new, lower steady-state $P_AO_2$ is reached. Because diffusion continues until equilibrium is achieved, the $P_aO_2$ of this unit will also be low (Fig. 5.4A).

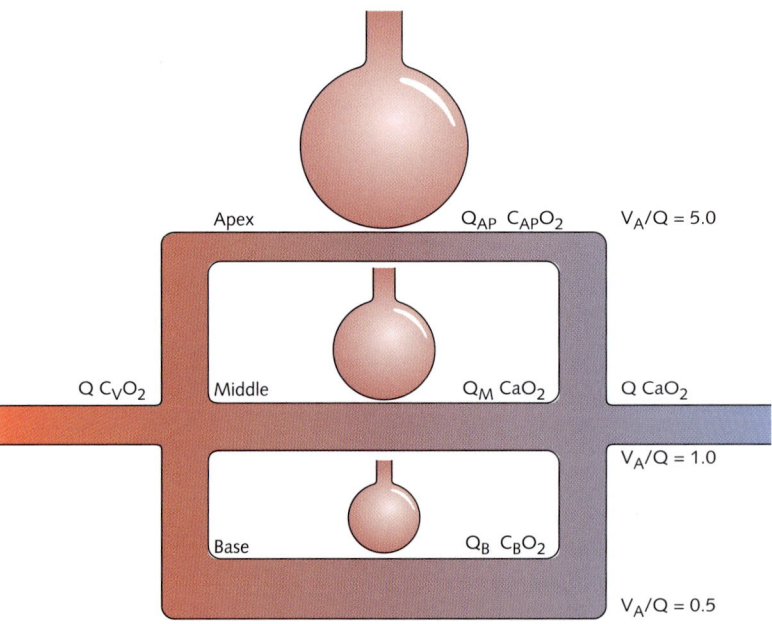

**Fig. 5.2** Ventilation ($V$) and perfusion ($Q$) at the lung apex, middle and base. $C$, capillary; $Q$, blood flow.

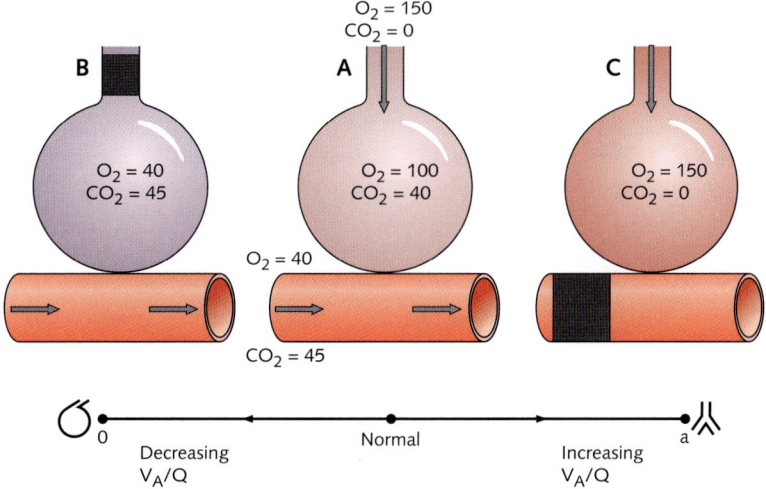

**Fig. 5.3** The effect of altering the ventilation:perfusion ($V{:}Q$) ratio on the $P_AO_2$ and $P_ACO_2$ in a lung unit: (A) normal lung; (B) lung unit is not ventilated – $O_2$ falls and $CO_2$ rises within lung unit; (C) lung unit is not perfused – $O_2$ is not taken up and $CO_2$ does not diffuse into the alveolus.

## At high ventilation:perfusion ratios (e.g., at the lung apex)

### Effect on carbon dioxide concentrations

The carbon dioxide diffusing from the blood is nearly all removed; carbon dioxide in the alveolus is depleted until a new, lower steady-state $P_ACO_2$ is reached. Diffusion continues until equilibrium is achieved: $P_aCO_2$ will also be low.

### Effect on oxygen concentrations

Oxygen diffusing from the alveolar gas is not taken away by the blood in such large amounts because the relative blood flow is reduced; in addition, oxygen is replenished with each breath.

Thus, oxygen tends to accumulate in the alveolus until a new steady-state concentration is reached (Fig. 5.4B). Diffusion occurs until a new higher equilibrium is achieved; thus, $P_aO_2$ is also higher.

## Measurement of ventilation and perfusion

### Ventilation:perfusion scans

In clinical practice, $V{:}Q$ ratios are assessed primarily by means of radioisotope scans. Ventilation is detected by inhalation of a gas or aerosol labelled with a radioisotope, of which the most widely used is technetium-99m DTPA. The

**Table 5.1**  Summary of the effects of low and high ventilation:perfusion ratios on carbon dioxide and oxygen concentrations

| | Effect on carbon dioxide concentrations | Effect on oxygen concentrations |
|---|---|---|
| Low ventilation:perfusion ratios (e.g., lung base) | $CO_2$ diffuses from blood → alveoli but due to low ventilation, $CO_2$ is not rapidly removed | $O_2$ diffuses from alveolus → blood but due to low ventilation, $O_2$ is not replenished fully |
| | $CO_2$ accumulates in alveolus until a higher steady-state alveolar $CO_2$ pressure is reached | $O_2$ is depleted in alveolus until a lower steady-state alveolar $O_2$ pressure is reached → diffusion is ongoing until equilibrium reached hence the arterial $O_2$ pressure is also lower |
| High ventilation:perfusion ratios (e.g., lung apex) | $CO_2$ diffusing from the blood is rapidly removed | $O_2$ diffusing from alveolus is not taken away by blood in large amounts |
| | $CO_2$ is depleted in alveolus until a lower steady-state alveolar $CO_2$ pressure is reached → diffusion is ongoing until equilibrium reached hence the arterial $CO_2$ pressure is also low | $O_2$ accumulates in alveolus until a higher steady-state alveolar $O_2$ pressure is reached → diffusion is ongoing until equilibrium reached hence the arterial $O_2$ pressure is also higher |

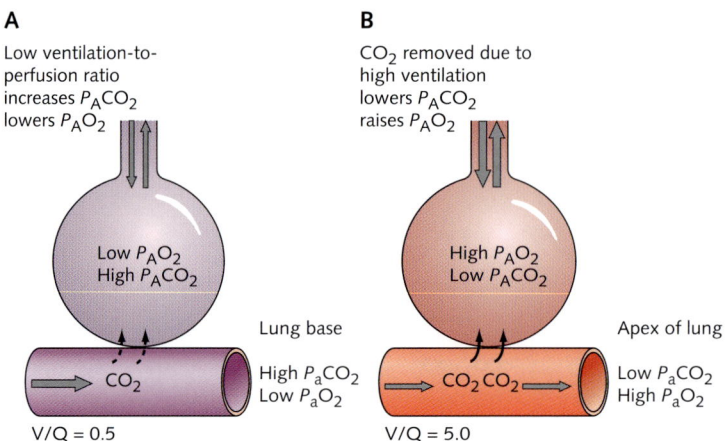

**A**

Low ventilation-to-perfusion ratio increases $P_ACO_2$ lowers $P_AO_2$

Low $P_AO_2$
High $P_ACO_2$

Lung base

High $P_aCO_2$
Low $P_aO_2$

$CO_2$

$V/Q = 0.5$

**B**

$CO_2$ removed due to high ventilation lowers $P_ACO_2$ raises $P_AO_2$

High $P_AO_2$
Low $P_ACO_2$

Apex of lung

Low $P_aCO_2$
High $P_aO_2$

$CO_2$ $CO_2$

$V/Q = 5.0$

**Fig. 5.4** Ventilation (V) and perfusion (Q) at lung base (A) and apex (B). At the lung base, perfusion is high and the V/Q ratio is low. This reduces alveolar $O_2$ and raises $CO_2$. At the apex, the V/Q ratio is higher, leading to a high alveolar $O_2$ and more $CO_2$ blown off.

distribution of pulmonary blood flow is tested with an intravenous injection of $^{99m}$Tc-labelled macroaggregated albumin (MAA). These radioactive particles are larger than the diameter of the pulmonary capillaries and they remain lodged for several hours. A gamma camera is then used to detect the position of the MAA.

The two scans are then assessed together for 'filling defects' or areas where ventilation and perfusion are not matched. The technique has previously been used to detect pulmonary emboli. However, spiral computed tomography scans have largely superseded this technique in most clinical areas, although they can be used in pregnant patients or as an alternative in those with an allergy to contrast or severe renal impairment. Fig. 5.5 shows a lung scan following pulmonary embolism.

## GAS TRANSPORT IN THE BLOOD

### Oxygen transport

Oxygen is carried in the blood in two forms:

1. Dissolved in plasma.
2. Bound to haemoglobin.

### Dissolved oxygen

To meet the body's metabolic demands, large amounts of oxygen must be carried in the blood. We have seen that the amount of gas dissolved in solution is proportional to the partial pressure of

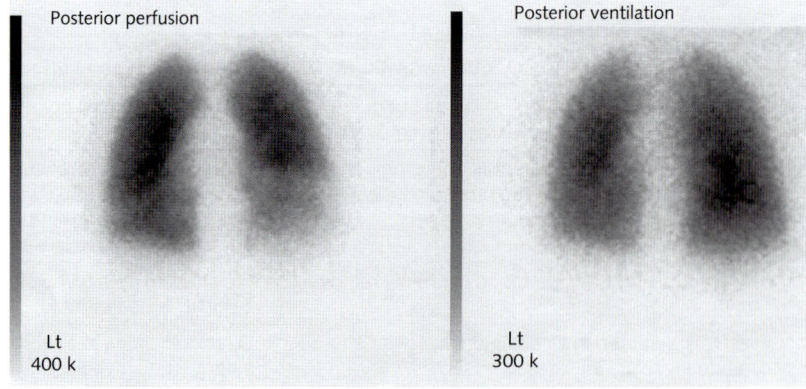

Posterior perfusion

Lt
400 k

Posterior ventilation

Lt
300 k

**Fig. 5.5** Ventilation:perfusion scan following pulmonary embolus. (Courtesy Jones I and the Nuclear Medicine staff, Derriford Hospital, Plymouth.)

the gas (Henry's law). Thus, with a normal arterial $P_aO_2$ (100 mmHg; 13.3 kPa), for each 100 mL of blood, there is only 0.003 mL of dissolved oxygen. Based on a 5 L cardiac output, this is 15 mL of oxygen per minute ($100 \times 0.003 \times 5000/100$). At rest, the body requires approximately 250 mL of oxygen per minute. Thus, if all the oxygen in the blood were carried in the dissolved form, cardiac output would meet only 6% of the demand.

Therefore, most of the oxygen must be carried in chemical combination, not in simple solution. Oxygen is thus combined with haemoglobin.

## Haemoglobin

Haemoglobin is found in red blood cells and is a conjugated protein molecule, containing iron within its structure. The molecule consists of four polypeptide subunits, two α and two β. Associated with each polypeptide chain is a haem group that acts as a binding site for oxygen. Haemoglobin is thus capable of binding up to four molecules of oxygen.

The haem group consists of a porphyrin ring containing iron and is responsible for binding of oxygen:

- Haemoglobin contains iron in a ferrous ($Fe^{2+}$) or ferric ($Fe^{3+}$) state.
- Only haemoglobin in the ferrous form can bind oxygen.
- Methaemoglobin (containing iron in a ferric state) cannot bind oxygen.

The quaternary structure of haemoglobin determines its ability to bind oxygen. In its deoxygenated state, haemoglobin (known as reduced haemoglobin) has a low affinity for oxygen. The binding of one oxygen molecule to haemoglobin causes a conformational change in its protein structure; this positive cooperativity allows easier access to the other oxygen-binding sites, thus increasing haemoglobin's affinity for further binding of oxygen.

It should be noted that, during this reaction, the iron atom of the haem group remains in the ferrous ($Fe^{2+}$) form. It is not oxidized to the ferric ($Fe^{3+}$) form. The interaction of oxygen with haemoglobin is oxygenation, not oxidation.

The main function of haemoglobin is to take up oxygen at the alveolar–capillary membrane and to transport the oxygen within the blood and release it into the tissues. However, haemoglobin also has other functions:

- Buffering of $H^+$ ions.
- Transport of carbon dioxide as carbamino compounds.

## Haemoglobin binding

Haemoglobin has four binding sites; the amount of oxygen carried by haemoglobin in the blood depends on how many of these binding sites are occupied. Therefore, the haemoglobin molecule can be said to be saturated or partially saturated:

- Saturated – all four binding sites are occupied by oxygen.
- Partially saturated – some oxygen has bound to haemoglobin, but not all four sites are occupied.

If completely saturated, the maximum binding of oxygen to haemoglobin we could expect is:

$$150 \times 1.34 = 201\text{mL of oxygen per litre of blood}$$

This is calculated from approximating 150 g of haemoglobin in 1 L of blood and knowing that 1 gram of haemoglobin can bind 1.34 mL of oxygen.

In addition, there is approximately 10 mL of oxygen in solution. The total (210 mL) is called the oxygen capacity; the haemoglobin is said to be 100% saturated ($SO_2 = 100\%$). The actual amount of oxygen bonded to haemoglobin and dissolved in the blood at any one time is called the oxygen content.

The oxygen saturation ($SO_2$) of the blood is defined as the amount of oxygen carried in the blood, expressed as a percentage of oxygen capacity:

$$SO_2 = O_2 \text{ content} / O_2 \text{ capacity} \times 100$$

## Cyanosis

Haemoglobin absorbs light of different wavelengths depending on whether it is in the reduced or oxygenated form. Oxyhaemoglobin appears bright red, whereas reduced haemoglobin appears purplish, giving a bluish pallor to skin. This is called cyanosis, which can be described as either central or peripheral. Cyanosis depends on the absolute amount of deoxygenated haemoglobin in the vessels, not the proportion of deoxygenated:oxygenated haemoglobin. In central cyanosis, there is more than 5 g/dL deoxygenated haemoglobin in the blood and this can be seen in the peripheral tissues and other body parts (e.g., lips, tongue). Peripheral cyanosis has a local cause (e.g., vascular obstruction of a limb).

## Oxygen dissociation curve

How much oxygen binds to haemoglobin is dependent upon the partial pressure of oxygen in the blood. This relationship is represented by the oxygen dissociation curve (Fig. 5.6A); this is an equilibrium curve at specific conditions:

- 150 g of haemoglobin per litre of blood
- pH 7.4
- Temperature 37°C.

### Factors affecting the oxygen dissociation curve

The shape of the curve, and therefore oxygen delivery to the tissues, is affected by a number of factors, including:

- pH
- Carbon dioxide

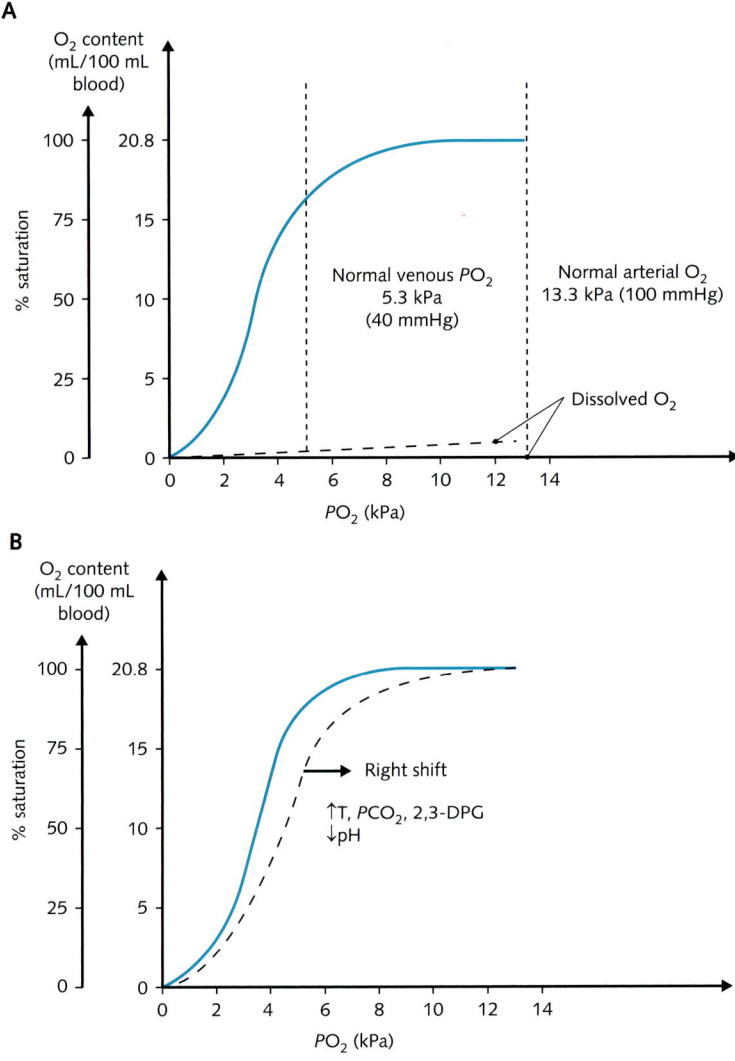

**Fig. 5.6** (A) Oxyhaemoglobin dissociation curve. (B) The effect of temperature ($T$), $PCO_2$, pH and 2,3-diphosphoglycerate (*2,3-DPG*) on the oxyhaemoglobin dissociation curve.

- Temperature
- Other forms of haemoglobin.

These factors shift the oxygen dissociation curve to the right or to the left:

- A shift to the right allows easier dissociation of oxygen (i.e., lower oxygen saturation at any particular $PO_2$) and increases the oxygen release from oxyhaemoglobin.
- A shift to the left makes oxygen binding easier (i.e., higher oxygen saturation at any particular $PO_2$) and increases the oxygen uptake by haemoglobin.

The following factors shift the curve to the right (Fig. 5.6B):

- Increased $PCO_2$ and decreased pH (increased hydrogen ion concentration), known as the Bohr shift.
- Increased temperature.
- Increase in 2,3-diphosphoglycerate (2,3-DPG), which binds to the β chains.

2,3-DPG is a product of anaerobic metabolism. Red blood cells possess no mitochondria and therefore carry out anaerobic metabolism to produce energy. 2,3-DPG binds more strongly to reduced haemoglobin than to oxyhaemoglobin. Concentrations

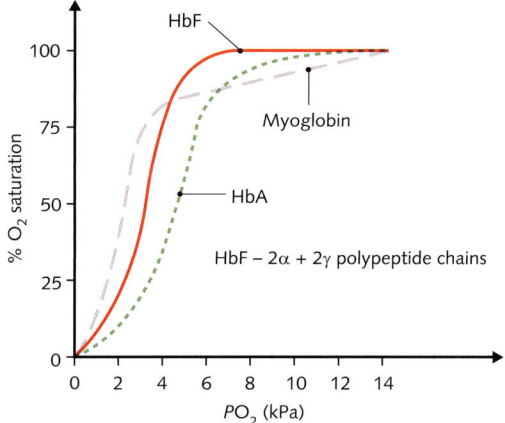

**Fig. 5.7** Comparison of oxygen dissociation curves for myoglobin, foetal haemoglobin (*HbF*) and adult haemoglobin (*HbA*).

of 2,3-DPG increase in chronic hypoxia, e.g., in patients with chronic lung disease or at high altitude.

## Other forms of haemoglobin

### Foetal haemoglobin

Foetal haemoglobin differs from adult haemoglobin by having two γ chains instead of two β chains (Fig. 5.7).

Foetal haemoglobin has a higher affinity for oxygen because its γ chains bind 2,3-DPG less avidly than the β chains of adult haemoglobin and are therefore able to bind oxygen at lower partial pressures (maternal venous $P_vO_2$ is low: <40 mmHg).

Release of carbon dioxide from foetal haemoglobin causes a shift to the left of the foetal oxyhaemoglobin dissociation curve, thus increasing its affinity for oxygen. This released carbon dioxide binds to maternal haemoglobin, causing a shift to the right of maternal haemoglobin, thus reducing the affinity of the latter for oxygen. Oxygen is therefore released by maternal haemoglobin and bound by foetal haemoglobin. This is known as the double Bohr shift.

### Haemoglobin S

Haemoglobin S is a form of haemoglobin found in sickle cell anaemia. Sickle cell anaemia is an autosomal recessive disorder in which there is a defect in the β-globulin chain of the haemoglobin molecule.

There is a substitution of the amino acid valine for glutamine at position 6 of the β chain, forming haemoglobin S. The heterozygote has sickle cell trait and the homozygote has sickle cell anaemia. The abnormal haemoglobin S molecules polymerize when deoxygenated and cause the red blood cells

containing the abnormal haemoglobin to sickle. The fragile sickle cells haemolyze and may block vessels, leading to ischaemia and infarction. The heterozygous patient usually has asymptomatic anaemia, and the homozygote has painful crises with bone and abdominal pain; there may also be intrapulmonary shunting.

### Thalassaemia

The thalassaemias are autosomal recessive disorders with decreased production of either the α or the β chain of haemoglobin. There are two genes for the β chain and, depending on the number of normal genes, the thalassaemia is quoted as major or minor. There are four genes which code for the α chain, leading to various clinical disorders depending on the genetic defect. $HbA_2$ is present in a small amount in the normal population and consists of two α and two δ chains. It is markedly raised in β-thalassaemia minor.

### Carboxyhaemoglobin (carbon monoxide poisoning)

Carbon monoxide (CO) displaces oxygen from oxyhaemoglobin because the affinity of haemoglobin for carbon monoxide is more than 200 times that for oxygen. This changes the shape of the oxyhaemoglobin dissociation curve. Fig. 5.8 shows the effects of carbon monoxide poisoning:

- In this instance, oxygen capacity is 50% of normal (i.e., 50% $HbO_2$ and 50% HbCO). The actual value will depend

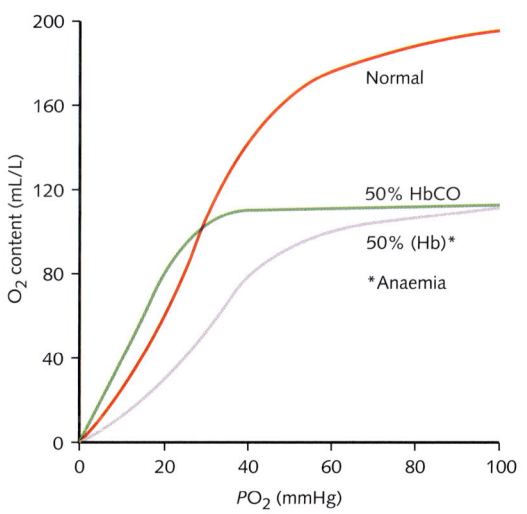

**Fig. 5.8** Oxyhaemoglobin curve showing effects of anaemia and carbon monoxide poisoning (50% HbCO and anaemia* compared with normal haemoglobin [*Hb*]).

on the partial pressure of carbon monoxide (e.g., with a PCO of 16 mmHg, 75% of haemoglobin will be in the form of HbCO).

- Saturation is achieved at a $PO_2$ of < 40 mmHg (below venous $PO_2$).
- HbCO causes a shift to the left for the oxygen dissociation curve (i.e., HbCO has a higher affinity for oxygen than normal $HbO_2$).
- Carbon monoxide binds to two of the four available haem groups.

Carbon monoxide takes a long time to be cleared, but this can be sped up by ventilation with 100% oxygen. Additionally, the patient is not cyanosed because HbCO is cherry-red, and oxygen saturation levels recorded by a pulse oximeter are unable to differentiate HbCO and $HbO_2$, meaning the patient's saturations can read as normal while they are grossly under-oxygenated.

## Carbon dioxide transport

There are three ways in which carbon dioxide can be transported in the blood:

1. Dissolved in plasma
2. As bicarbonate ions
3. As carbamino compounds.

### Dissolved carbon dioxide

The solubility of carbon dioxide in the blood is much greater than that of oxygen (20 times greater); so, unlike oxygen, a significant amount (approximately 10%) of carbon dioxide is carried in solution.

## Bicarbonate ions

Approximately 60% of carbon dioxide is transported as bicarbonate ions. Dissolved carbon dioxide interacts with water to form carbonic acid as follows:

$$CO_2 + H_2O \rightleftharpoons H_2CO_3 \tag{1}$$

Carbonic acid rapidly dissociates into ions:

$$H_2CO_3 \rightleftharpoons H^+ + HCO_3^- \tag{2}$$

The total reaction being:

$$CO_2 + H_2O \rightleftharpoons H_2CO_3 \rightleftharpoons H^+ + HCO_3^-$$

The first reaction is very slow in plasma, but within the red blood cell, it is dramatically sped up by the enzyme carbonic anhydrase. Reaction 2 is very fast, but, if allowed to proceed alone, a large amount of $H^+$ would be formed, slowing down or halting the reaction. Haemoglobin has the property that it can bind $H^+$ ions and act as a buffer, thus allowing the reaction to go on rapidly.

$$H^+ + HbO_2^- \rightleftharpoons HHb + O_2$$
$$H^+ + Hb^- \rightleftharpoons HHb$$

The bicarbonate produced in the red blood cells diffuses down its concentration gradient into the plasma in exchange for chloride ions $(Cl^-)$. This process is known as the chloride shift (Fig. 5.9).

### Carbamino compounds

Carbon dioxide is capable of combining with proteins, interacting with their terminal amine groups to form carbamino compounds (Fig. 5.9). The most important protein involved is haemoglobin,

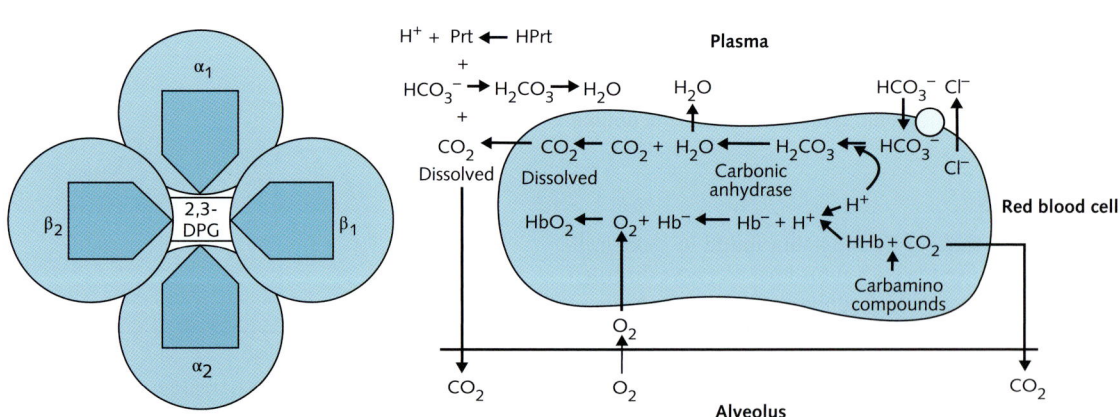

**Fig. 5.9** The exchange of $CO_2$ and $O_2$ that occurs between the blood and the alveolar air. Bicarbonate ions ($HCO_3^-$) enter the red blood cell in exchange for chloride ions (which are transported out). Carbonic acid is formed once the $O_2$ is bound to haemoglobin (*Hb*). Carbonic acid is converted to $CO_2$ and $H_2O$. The $CO_2$ is then excreted from the cell. $CO_2$ stored in carbamino compound form can be excreted from the cell passively without the involvement of an enzyme. *2,3-DPG,* 2,3-Diphosphoglycerate.

as it is the most abundant in the blood. Approximately 30% of carbon dioxide is carried as carbamino compounds.

## Haldane effect

Carriage of carbon dioxide is increased in deoxygenated blood because of two factors:

1. Reduced haemoglobin has a greater affinity for carbon dioxide than does oxyhaemoglobin.
2. Reduced haemoglobin is less acidic (i.e., a better proton acceptor: $H^+$ buffer) than oxyhaemoglobin.

The Haldane effect minimizes changes in the pH of blood when gaseous exchange occurs. The decrease in pH caused by the oxygenation of haemoglobin is offset by the increase that results from the loss of carbon dioxide to the alveolar air. The reverse occurs in the tissues. This is an important effect because:

- In peripheral capillaries, the unloading of oxygen from haemoglobin aids the binding of carbon dioxide to haemoglobin.
- In pulmonary capillaries, the loading of oxygen on haemoglobin reduces the binding of carbon dioxide to haemoglobin.

This allows efficient gaseous exchange of carbon dioxide in the tissues and the lungs.

### Carbon dioxide dissociation curve

The carriage of carbon dioxide is dependent upon the partial pressure of carbon dioxide in the blood. This relationship is described by the carbon dioxide dissociation curve. Compared with the oxygen dissociation curve:

- The carbon dioxide curve is more linear.
- The carbon dioxide curve is much steeper than the oxygen curve (between venous and arterial partial pressure of respiratory gases).
- The carbon dioxide curve varies according to oxygen saturation of haemoglobin.

## GAS TRANSPORT AND RESPIRATORY FAILURE

### Hypoventilation and hyperventilation

If $P_aCO_2$ is a measure of ventilation, it is appropriate in a review of carbon dioxide transport to consider two key concepts in respiratory medicine: hypoventilation and hyperventilation. For the body to function normally, ventilation must meet the metabolic demand of the tissues (Table 5.2). Thus, metabolic tissue consumption of oxygen must be equal to the oxygen taken up in the blood from alveolar gas. Or, metabolic tissue production of carbon dioxide must be equal to the amount of carbon dioxide blown off at the alveoli.

### Hypoventilation

The term 'hypoventilation' refers to a situation when ventilation is insufficient to meet metabolic demand.

### Hyperventilation

The term 'hyperventilation' refers to a situation where ventilation is excessive to metabolic demand, thus blowing off carbon dioxide from the lungs.

## Hypocapnia and hypercapnia

### Hypocapnia

A low partial pressure of carbon dioxide in the blood ($P_aCO_2$ < 40 mmHg) is termed 'hypocapnia'.

### Hypercapnia

A high partial pressure (concentration) of carbon dioxide in the blood ($P_aCO_2$ > 45 mmHg) is termed 'hypercapnia', or $P_aCO_2$ ≥ 6 kPa as per BTS guidelines.

**Table 5.2** Comparison of hypoventilation and hyperventilation

| Respiratory physiological state | Causes | Consequences |
| --- | --- | --- |
| Hypoventilation | Obstruction:<br>• Chronic obstructive airways disease<br>• Foreign body (e.g., peanut)<br>Brainstem lesion<br>Respiratory muscle weakness<br>Trauma (e.g., fractured rib)<br>Drugs, notably opioids | Ventilation is too low for metabolic demand<br>Not enough $CO_2$ is blown off at the lungs<br>$P_aCO_2$ > 45 mmHg |
| Hyperventilation | Anxiety<br>Brainstem lesion<br>Drugs, e.g., salicylate overdose<br>Compensation for metabolic acidosis | Ventilation too great for metabolic demand<br>Too much $CO_2$ blown off from lungs<br>$P_aCO_2$ < 40 mmHg |

**Table 5.3** Summary of type I and type II respiratory failure

| Type I respiratory failure | Type II respiratory failure |
|---|---|
| $P_aCO_2 < 6$ kPa (may be normal or low)<br>$P_aO_2 < 8$ kPa | $P_aCO_2 > 6$ kPa (high)<br>$P_aO_2 < 8$ kPa |
| Represents $V:Q$ mismatch | Indicates poor ventilation of lungs |

# Respiratory failure

Hypocapnia and hypercapnia are important concepts in the assessment of respiratory failure. Respiratory failure is defined as a $P_aO_2 < 8$ kPa (60 mmHg) and is divided into type I and type II, depending on the $P_aCO_2$ (Table 5.3).

In type I respiratory failure, $P_aCO_2 < 6$ kPa (45 mmHg). $P_aO_2$ is low (hypoxaemic), but $P_aCO_2$ may be normal or low; this represents a $V:Q$ mismatch.

In type II respiratory failure, $P_aCO_2 > 6$ kPa. Both $P_aO_2$ and $P_aCO_2$ indicate that the lungs are not well ventilated.

The significance of this classification is that in type II respiratory failure, the patient may have developed tolerance to increased levels of $P_aCO_2$; in other words, the drive for respiration no longer relies on hypercapnic drive (high $P_aCO_2$) but on hypoxic drive (low $P_aO_2$). Thus, if the patient is given high-concentration oxygen therapy, the hypoxic drive for ventilation may decrease and the patient may stop breathing.

# Hypoxia

This is a condition in which the metabolic demand for oxygen cannot be met by the circulating blood.

## Causes of hypoxia

Many cells can respire anaerobically; however, the neurons in the brain cannot and therefore need a constant supply of oxygen to maintain normal function. A severe shortage of oxygen to the brain can lead to unconsciousness and even death. Therefore, treatment of hypoxic patients is critically important. There are four principal types of hypoxia:

1. Hypoxic hypoxia
2. Anaemic hypoxia
3. Stagnant hypoxia (or static hypoxia)
4. Cytotoxic hypoxia (or histotoxic hypoxia).

### Hypoxic hypoxia

This occurs when the arterial $P_aO_2$ is significantly reduced, so that haemoglobin in the blood exiting the lungs is not fully saturated with oxygen.

**CAUSES OF HYPOXIC HYPOXIA**

**Physiological**
- At high altitude where there is a low oxygen tension in inspired air, the $P_AO_2$ and, accordingly, the $P_aO_2$ will fall.

**Pathological**
- Hypoventilation:
  - Respiratory muscle weakness, e.g., chronic obstructive pulmonary disease, myasthenia gravis and poliomyelitis patients.
  - Iatrogenic causes, e.g., general anaesthetics and analgesics (opiates), which act upon the respiratory centres in the medulla to decrease respiratory muscle activity.
- Abnormal $V/Q$ matching, e.g., airway obstruction, pulmonary embolism.
- Impaired diffusing capacity, e.g., pulmonary oedema, as seen in left ventricular failure.
- Right-to-left shunting, e.g., cyanotic congenital heart diseases, severe pneumonia.

The haemoglobin saturation is reduced in patients with hypoxic hypoxia. Most forms of hypoxic hypoxia can be corrected if patients are given hyperbaric oxygen to breathe. The high concentration of oxygen will increase the $P_AO_2$, and thus the $P_aO_2$, improving the oxygen saturation status of haemoglobin. In patients with right-to-left shunt, hyperbaric oxygen may not have any benefit, because the $P_AO_2$ will be normal, but since the blood is being shunted away from the alveoli the $P_aO_2$ will remain low.

## Anaemic hypoxia

This occurs when there is a significant reduction in the concentration of haemoglobin, so the oxygen content of the arterial blood will be abnormally reduced. There are numerous causes of anaemia. It can be due to:

- Blood loss (e.g., large haemorrhage).
- Reduced synthesis of haemoglobin (e.g., vitamin $B_{12}$ deficiency, bone marrow failure).
- Abnormal haemoglobin synthesis owing to a genetic defect (e.g., sickle cell anaemia).

The $P_AO_2$ in anaemic patients is usually normal and the haemoglobin saturation is also normal. Patients become hypoxic because there is a reduction in the oxygen content in the blood as there is less haemoglobin than normal. Treating anaemic patients with hyperbaric oxygen will be of limited benefit because the blood leaving the lung will already be fully saturated. Anaemic patients will not appear cyanosed because the amount of deoxygenated blood leaving the respiring tissue will not be higher than normal.

## Stagnant hypoxia

This is the result of low blood flow, and hence a reduction in oxygen supply to the tissues. This may occur with a reduced blood flow along an artery to a specific organ, with only that organ being affected; alternatively, reduced blood flow to all organs can occur if the cardiac output is significantly reduced (e.g., because of heart failure). There is usually nothing wrong with the lungs in terms of ventilation and perfusion in stagnant hypoxia, so the $P_AO_2$ and the $P_aO_2$ will be normal. Since the blood flow to the respiring tissues is slow, the tissues will try to extract as much available oxygen as possible from the arterial supply, so the venous $PO_2$ will be lowered and hence give rise to peripheral cyanosis.

Treatment with hyperbaric oxygen will not be beneficial to these patients as the blood leaving the lung will already be fully saturated. Only a slight rise in the level of oxygen dissolved within the blood plasma will occur.

## Cytotoxic hypoxia

This occurs when the respiring cells within the tissues are unable to use oxygen, mainly due to poisoning of the oxidative enzymes of the cells. For example, in cyanide poisoning, cyanide combines with the cytochrome chain and prevents oxygen from being used in oxidative phosphorylation.

In cytotoxic hypoxia, both the $P_AO_2$ and the $P_aO_2$ are normal and so, again, treating these patients with oxygen will be of limited value. Since the oxygen is unable to be utilized by the tissues, the venous $PO_2$ will be abnormally high and cyanosis will not occur in these patients.

## ACID–BASE BALANCE

## Normal pH

The pH of the intracellular and extracellular compartments must be tightly controlled for the body to function efficiently, or at all. The normal arterial pH lies within a relatively narrow range: 7.35–7.45 ($H^+$ range, 45–35 mmol/L). An acid–base disturbance arises when arterial pH lies outside this range. If the blood pH is less than 7.35, an acidosis is present; if pH is greater than 7.45, the term alkalosis is used. Although a larger variation in pH can be tolerated (pH 6.8–7.8) for a short time, recovery is often impossible if blood remains at pH 6.8 for long.

Such a tight control of blood pH is achieved by a combination of blood buffers and the respiratory and renal systems, which make adjustments to return pH towards its normal levels.

## Key concepts in acid–base balance

### Metabolic production of acids

Products of metabolism (carbon dioxide, lactic acid, phosphate, sulphate, etc.) form acidic solutions, thus increasing the hydrogen ion concentration and reducing pH. We also have an intake of acids in our diet (approximately 50–100 mmol $H^+$ per day). We rely on three methods to control our internal hydrogen ion concentration:

1. Dilution of body fluids.
2. The physiological buffer system.
3. Excretion of volatile and nonvolatile acids.

### Buffers

A buffer is a substance that can either bind or release hydrogen ions, therefore keeping the pH relatively constant even when considerable quantities of acid or base are added. There are four buffers of the blood:

1. Haemoglobin
2. Plasma proteins
3. Phosphate
4. Bicarbonate.

It is the bicarbonate system that acts as the principal buffer and which is of most interest in respiratory medicine.

We have already seen that carbon dioxide dissolves in water and reacts to form carbonic acid, and that this dissociates to form bicarbonate and protons:

$$CO_2 + H_2O \rightleftharpoons H_2CO_3 \rightleftharpoons H^+ + HCO_3^-$$

This equilibrium tells us that changes in either $CO_2$ or $HCO_3^-$ will have an effect on pH. For example, increasing $CO_2$ will drive the reaction to the right, increasing $H^+$ ion concentration.

As changes in carbon dioxide and bicarbonate can alter pH, controlling these elements allows the system to control acid–base

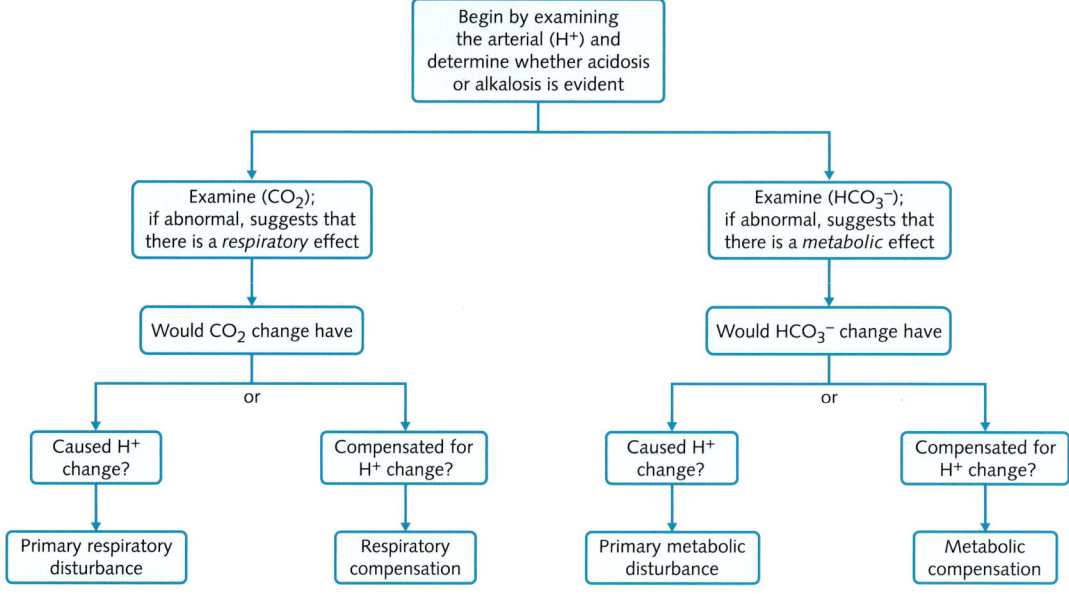

**Fig. 5.10** Differentiating between acid–base disorders.

equilibrium. This is why the bicarbonate buffer system is so useful; the body has control over both elements:

- Carbon dioxide is regulated through changes in ventilation.
- Bicarbonate concentrations are determined by the kidneys.

## Acid–base disturbances

As noted above, blood pH can either be lower than normal (acidosis) or higher (alkalosis). Acidosis can be caused by either:

- A rise in $PCO_2$
- A fall in $HCO_3^-$.
  Similarly, alkalosis can occur through:
- A fall in $PCO_2$
- A rise in $HCO_3^-$.

Where the primary change is in carbon dioxide, we term the disturbance 'respiratory', whereas a disturbance in bicarbonate is termed 'metabolic'. This allows us to classify four types of disturbance, outlined in Fig. 5.10:

1. Respiratory acidosis
2. Respiratory alkalosis
3. Metabolic acidosis
4. Metabolic alkalosis.

The disturbance was described as *primary* because the kidneys and lungs may try to return the acid–base disturbance towards normal values. This is called compensation and means that even in respiratory disturbances, it may not be just carbon dioxide that is abnormal; bicarbonate may have altered too. Similarly, carbon dioxide may be abnormal in a metabolic disturbance. The ways in which the two systems compensate are:

- The respiratory system alters ventilation; this happens quickly.
- The kidney alters the excretion of bicarbonate; this takes 2–3 days.

It is now clear that lung disease that affects gas exchange, and therefore $PCO_2$, will have major effects on the body's acid–base status. It is also clear that, while the respiratory system can act quickly to compensate for metabolic disturbances, it will take time for compensation to take place in respiratory disease; the renal system cannot act as quickly. We see this in clinical practice: a change in bicarbonate is characteristic of chronic lung disease, rather than acute lung disease.

Full details of assessment of acid–base status and interpretation of arterial blood gases can be found in Chapter 10.

## Assessing acid–base disturbances

Assessing acid–base disorders is relatively simple if you approach the problem in stages.

1. Start with the pH: is it outside the normal range?
2. If there is an acidosis or alkalosis, can it be explained by a change in carbon dioxide?
3. If so, then it is a primary disturbance with a respiratory cause.
4. Now look at bicarbonate – has this changed to return the ratio to normal?
5. If so, it is a respiratory disorder with metabolic compensation.

# Respiratory acidosis

Respiratory acidosis results from an increase in $PCO_2$ caused by:

- Hypoventilation (less carbon dioxide is blown off).
- $V:Q$ mismatch.

From the Henderson–Hasselbach equation, we see that an increase in $PCO_2$ causes an increase in hydrogen ion concentration (i.e., a reduction in pH). Thus, plasma bicarbonate concentration increases to compensate for the increased hydrogen ion concentration.

## Renal compensation

The increase in hydrogen ion concentration in the blood results in increased filtration of hydrogen ions at the glomeruli, thus:

- Increasing $HCO_3^-$ reabsorption
- Increasing $HCO_3^-$ production.

Thus, plasma $HCO_3^-$ rises, compensating for the increased $H^+$, i.e., renal compensation raises pH towards normal.

## Causes of respiratory acidosis

Mechanisms reducing ventilation or causing $V/Q$ mismatch include:

- Chronic obstructive pulmonary disease.
- Asthma (severe exacerbation).
- Obesity hypoventilation syndrome.
- Neuromuscular disorders, e.g., Amyotrophic lateral sclerosis (ALS), motor neurone disease, Guillain–Barré syndrome, myasthenia gravis.
- Drugs that reduce respiratory drive (ventilation), including morphine, barbiturates and general anaesthetics.
- Central nervous system depression – neurological disease, e.g., trauma, brainstem lesion, infection (encephalitis), drug induced (above).

# Respiratory alkalosis

Respiratory alkalosis results from a decrease in $PCO_2$ generally caused by alveolar hyperventilation (more carbon dioxide is blown off). This causes a decrease in hydrogen ion concentration and thus an increase in pH.

## Renal compensation

The reduction in hydrogen ion concentration in the blood results in decreased hydrogen ion filtration at the glomeruli, thus:

- Reducing $HCO_3^-$ reabsorption
- Reducing $HCO_3^-$ production.

Thus, plasma $HCO_3^-$ falls, compensating for the reduced $H^+$; i.e., renal compensation reduces pH towards normal.

## Causes of respiratory alkalosis

The causes of respiratory alkalosis include:

- Increased ventilation – caused by hypoxic drive in pneumonia, diffuse interstitial lung diseases, high altitude, mechanical ventilation, etc.
- Hyperventilation – brainstem damage, infection causing fever, drugs (e.g., aspirin), pain, anxiety.

# Metabolic acidosis

Metabolic acidosis results from an excess of hydrogen ions in the body, which reduces bicarbonate concentration (shifting the equation below to the left). Respiration is unaffected; therefore, $PCO_2$ is initially normal.

## Respiratory compensation

$$CO_2 + H_2O \rightleftharpoons H_2CO_3 \rightleftharpoons H^+ + HCO_3^-$$

The reduction in pH is detected by the peripheral chemoreceptors. This causes an increase in ventilation, which lowers $PCO_2$. Also:

- The above equation is driven further to the left, reducing hydrogen ion concentration and bicarbonate.
- The decrease in hydrogen ion concentration raises pH towards normal.

Respiratory compensation cannot fully correct the values of $PCO_2$, $HCO_3^-$ and $H^+$, as there is a limit to how far $PCO_2$ can fall with hyperventilation. Correction can be carried out only by removing the excess hydrogen ions from the body or restoring the lost bicarbonate (i.e., correcting the metabolic fault).

## Causes of metabolic acidosis

Causes of metabolic acidosis are:

- Exogenous acid loading (e.g., aspirin overdose).
- Endogenous acid production (e.g., ketogenesis in diabetes).
- Loss of $HCO_3^-$ from the kidneys or gut (e.g., diarrhoea).
- Metabolic production of hydrogen ions. The kidneys may not be able to excrete the excess hydrogen ions immediately, or at all (as in renal failure).

## Metabolic alkalosis

Metabolic alkalosis results from an increase in bicarbonate concentration or a fall in hydrogen ion concentration. Removing hydrogen ions from the right of the equation below drives the reaction to the right, increasing bicarbonate concentration. Decrease in hydrogen ion concentration raises pH; initially, $PCO_2$ is normal.

### Respiratory compensation

$$CO_2 + H_2O \rightleftharpoons H_2CO_3 \rightleftharpoons H^+ + HCO_3^-$$

The increase in pH is detected by the peripheral chemoreceptors. This causes a decrease in ventilation which raises $PCO_2$. Also:

- The above equation is driven further to the right, increasing hydrogen ion and bicarbonate concentrations.
- The decrease in hydrogen ion concentration raises pH towards normal.

Respiratory compensation is through alveolar hypoventilation but ventilation cannot reduce enough to correct the disturbance. This can only be carried out by removing the problem either of reduced hydrogen ion concentration or increased bicarbonate concentration. This is done by reducing renal hydrogen ion secretion.

More bicarbonate is excreted because more is filtered at the glomerulus and less is reabsorbed in combination with hydrogen ions.

### Causes of metabolic alkalosis

The causes of metabolic alkalosis include:

- Vomiting (hydrochloric acid loss from the stomach).
- Ingestion of alkaline substances.
- Potassium depletion, e.g., diuretic, excess aldosterone (low potassium results in the body's cells taking in $H^+$ ions in exchange for $K^+$ – this has the effect of increasing $K^+$ concentration as well as blood pH).

### ● Chapter summary

- The ventilation:perfusion ratio is defined as the ratio between alveolar ventilation $V_A$ and perfusion to the alveoli by pulmonary capillaries (Q). The $V/Q$ ratio averages 1 in healthy individuals, with better ventilation at the lung apices and better perfusion at the lung bases.
- Oxygen binds to haemoglobin to be transported in the blood. The amount of oxygen bound to haemoglobin is dependent upon the partial pressure of oxygen in the blood, demonstrated by the oxygen dissociation curve.
- Hypoxia is a condition in which the metabolic demand for oxygen cannot be met by the circulating blood.
- Type I respiratory failure is defined as hypoxaemia with a low/normal $P_aCO_2$, representing a ventilation:perfusion mismatch.
- Type II respiratory failure is defined as hypoxaemia with a raised $P_aCO_2$, indicating inadequate ventilation.
- Normal arterial pH is 7.35–7.45 and is controlled by respiratory and metabolic variation. Understanding the physiological changes to pH allows you to calculate whether there is a primary metabolic, respiratory or combined pathology in disease states.

# Control of respiratory function

6

## CONTROL OF VENTILATION

## Control within the respiratory system

When considering control of breathing, the main control variable is $P_aCO_2$. We try to control this value near to 40 mmHg or approximately 5.3 kPa, which can be carried out by adjusting the respiratory rate, the tidal volume, or both.

By controlling $P_aCO_2$, we are effectively controlling alveolar ventilation and thus $P_ACO_2$.

Although $P_aCO_2$ is the main control variable, $P_aO_2$ is also controlled, but normally to a much lesser extent than $P_aCO_2$. However, the $P_aO_2$ control system can take over and become the main controlling system when the $P_aO_2$ drops below 50 mmHg (~6.7 kPa).

Control can be brought about by:

- Metabolic demands of the body (metabolic control) – tissue oxygen demand and acid–base balance. This acts in a feedback system whereby the brainstem looks at the measured level of $P_aCO_2$ and relates this to the desired level, adjusting it as necessary through methods such as increasing respiratory rate.
- Behavioural demands of the body (behavioural control) – singing, coughing, laughing (i.e., control is voluntary). This system will not be dealt with in this book.

## Metabolic control of breathing

Metabolic control of breathing is a function of the brainstem (pons and medulla). The controller can be considered as specific groups of neurones (previously called respiratory centres).

### Pontine neurones

The pontine respiratory group consists of expiratory and inspiratory neurones. Their role is to regulate (i.e., affect the activity of) the dorsal respiratory group and possibly the ventral respiratory group (neurone groups in the medulla).

### Medullary neurones

It is believed that the medulla is responsible for respiratory rhythm.

Three groups of neurones associated with respiratory control have been identified in the medulla:

1. The dorsal respiratory group, situated in the nucleus tractus solitarius.
2. The ventral respiratory group, situated in the nucleus ambiguus and the nucleus retroambigualis.
3. The Bötzinger complex, situated rostral to the nucleus ambiguus.

These groups receive sensory information, which is compared with the desired value of control; adjustments are made to respiratory muscles to rectify any deviation from ideal.

- The dorsal respiratory group contains neurone bodies of inspiratory upper motor neurones. These inhibit the activity of expiratory neurones in the ventral respiratory group and have an excitatory effect on lower motor neurones to the respiratory muscles, increasing ventilation.
- Ventral respiratory group neurones contain inspiratory upper motor neurones that go on to supply, through their lower motor neurones, external intercostal muscles and accessory muscles.
- The Bötzinger complex contains only expiratory neurones. It works by inhibiting inspiratory neurones of the dorsal and ventral respiratory groups and through excitation of expiratory neurones in the ventral respiratory group.

## Effectors (muscles of respiration)

The major muscle groups involved are the diaphragm, internal and external intercostals and abdominal muscles.

The strength of contraction and coordination of these muscles is set by the central controller. If the muscles are not coordinated, abnormal breathing patterns will result.

## Sensors (receptors)

Sensors report to the central controller current values, or discrepancies from ideal values, for the various variables being controlled (e.g., $P_aCO_2$, $P_aO_2$ and pH). There are many types of sensors and receptors involved with respiratory control:

- Chemoreceptors – central and peripheral.
- Lung receptors – slowly adapting stretch receptors, rapidly adapting stretch receptors and C-fibres.
- Receptors in the chest wall – muscle spindles and Golgi tendon organs.
- Other receptors – nasal, tracheal and laryngeal receptors, arterial baroreceptors, pain receptors.

# Chemoreceptors

Chemoreceptors monitor blood gas tensions, $P_aCO_2$, $P_aO_2$ and pH, and help keep minute volume appropriate to the metabolic demands of the body. Therefore, chemoreceptors respond to:

- Hypercapnia
- Hypoxia
- Acidosis.

## Central chemoreceptors

Central chemoreceptors are tonically active and vital for maintenance of respiration; 80% of the drive for ventilation is a result of stimulation of the central chemoreceptors. When they are inactivated, respiration ceases. These receptors are readily depressed by drugs (e.g., opiates and barbiturates).

The receptors are located in the brainstem on the ventrolateral surface of the medulla, close to the exit of cranial nerves IX and X. They are anatomically separate from the medullary respiratory control centre.

Central chemoreceptors respond to hydrogen ion concentration within the surrounding brain tissue and cerebrospinal fluid (CSF).

- Raised hydrogen ion concentration increases ventilation, increasing the removal of $CO_2$ and thus reducing the acidity of blood.
- Lowered hydrogen ion concentration decreases ventilation.

Diffusion of ions across the blood–brain barrier is poor. Blood levels of hydrogen ions and bicarbonate have little short-term effect on the concentrations of hydrogen ions and bicarbonate in the CSF and thus have little effect on the central chemoreceptors.

Carbon dioxide, however, can pass freely by diffusion across the blood–brain barrier. On entering the CSF, the increase in carbon dioxide increases the free hydrogen ion concentration. This increase in hydrogen ion concentration stimulates the central chemoreceptors. Thus:

- Central chemoreceptors are sensitive to $P_aCO_2$, not arterial hydrogen ion concentration.
- Central chemoreceptors are not sensitive to $P_aO_2$.
- Because there is less protein in the CSF (<0.4 g/L) than in the plasma (60–80 g/L), a rise in $P_aCO_2$ has a larger effect on pH in the CSF than in the blood (CSF has lower buffering capacity).

Long-standing raised $P_aCO_2$ causes the pH of the CSF to return towards normal. This is because prolonged hypercapnia alters the production of bicarbonate by the glial cells and allows bicarbonate to cross the blood–brain barrier. It can therefore diffuse freely into the CSF and alter the CSF pH. This is seen in patients with chronic respiratory failure, e.g., those with severe chronic obstructive pulmonary disease (COPD).

## Peripheral chemoreceptors

Chemoreceptors are located around the carotid sinus and aortic arch. These are the carotid bodies and aortic bodies, respectively. Stimulation of peripheral chemoreceptors has both cardiovascular and respiratory effects. Of the two receptor groups, the carotid bodies have the greatest effect on respiration.

### Carotid bodies

The carotid bodies contain two different types of cells. Type I cells are stimulated by hypoxia; they connect with afferent nerves to the brainstem. Type II cells are supportive (structural and metabolic), similar to glial cells of the central nervous system.

There is a rich blood supply to the carotid bodies (blood flow per mass of tissue far exceeds that to the brain); venous blood flow, therefore, remains saturated with oxygen.

The exact mechanism of action of the carotid bodies is not known. It is believed that type I (glomus) cells are activated by hypoxia and release transmitter substances that stimulate afferents to the brainstem.

Peripheral chemoreceptors are sensitive to:

- $P_aO_2$
- $P_aCO_2$
- pH
- Blood flow
- Temperature.

The carotid bodies are supplied by the autonomic nervous system, which appears to alter their sensitivity to hypoxia by regulating blood flow to the chemoreceptor:

- Sympathetic action vasoconstricts, increasing sensitivity to hypoxia.
- Parasympathetic action vasodilates, reducing sensitivity to hypoxia.

The relationship between $P_aO_2$ and the response from the carotid bodies is not a linear one. At a low $P_aO_2$ (<50 mmHg or 6.7 kPa), a further decrease in arterial oxygen tension

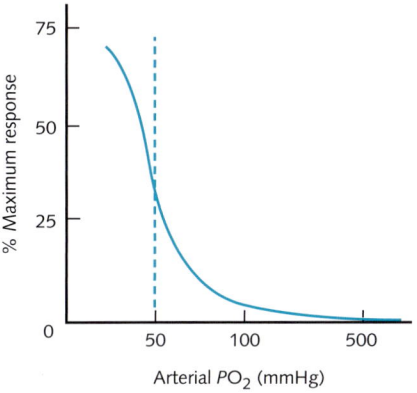

**Fig. 6.1** Response of ventilation to $P_aO_2$. The response to a lowered $P_aO_2$ is small until the $P_aO_2$ falls below a value of 50 mmHg, after which point the response increases dramatically.

significantly increases ventilation (Fig. 6.1). However, at levels of oxygen tension close to 100 mmHg, changes have little effect on ventilation. If $P_aO_2$ increases above 100 mmHg/13.3 kPa (achieved when breathing high-concentration oxygen), ventilation is only slightly reduced.

Unlike central chemoreceptors, peripheral chemoreceptors are directly stimulated by blood pH. Although peripheral chemoreceptors are stimulated by $P_aCO_2$, their response is much less (<10% of the effect) than that of central chemoreceptors.

## Receptors in the lung

Afferent impulses arising from receptors in the lung travel via the vagal nerve to the respiratory centres of the brain, where they influence the control of breathing. There are three main types of afferent receptors:

1. Rapidly adapting receptors.
2. Slowly adapting receptors.
3. C-fibre receptors – formerly juxtapulmonary or J receptors.

Their characteristics are described in Table 6.1 and their function is discussed below.

### Rapidly adapting receptors

Rapidly adapting receptors are involved in lung defence and form part of the cough reflex. This is reflected in their location in the upper airways. They produce only transitory responses and may

**Table 6.1** Characteristics of the three principal types of afferent receptors in the lung

| Receptor type | Stretch receptors | | C-fibre receptors |
| --- | --- | --- | --- |
| | Rapidly adapting stretch receptor (RAR) | Slowly adapting stretch receptor (SAR) | |
| Location in airway | Primarily upper airways – nasopharynx, larynx, trachea, carina | Trachea and main bronchus | Throughout airways |
| Location in airway wall | Just below epithelium | Airway smooth muscle | Alveolar wall and bronchial mucosa |
| Structure | Small myelinated fibres | Small myelinated fibres | Free nerve endings |
| Conduction speed | Fast | Fast | Slower |
| Stimuli | Mechanical deformation Chemical irritants and noxious gases Inflammatory stimuli | Inflation | Chemical mediators – histamine and capsaicin (an extract of chilli peppers and the 'C' that gives 'C-fibres' their name) Inflation and forced deflation Pulmonary vascular congestion Oedema – interstitial fluid in the alveolar wall |

be sensitized by inflammatory mediators, making them more sensitive to stimulation.

### Slowly adapting receptors

Slowly adapting receptors are important in the control of breathing, not the cough reflex, and produce sustained responses. They are stimulated by inflation (which stretches the lungs):

- Inflation leads to decreased respiration (inflation reflex or Hering–Breuer reflex).
- Deflation leads to increased respiration (deflation reflex).

These reflexes are active in the first year of life, but are weak in adults. Therefore, they are not thought to determine the rate and depth of breathing in adults. However, these reflexes are seen to be more active if the tidal volume increases above 1.0 L and therefore might have a role in exercise.

Afferent fibres travel to the respiratory centres through the vagus nerve. The functions of these receptors are:

- The termination of inspiration.
- Regulation of the work of breathing.
- Reinforcement of respiratory rhythm in the first year of life.

However, if the nerve is blocked by anaesthesia, there is no change seen in the rate and depth of breathing.

### C-fibres

Stimulation of C-fibres results in:

- Closure of the larynx
- Rapid, shallow breathing
- Bradycardia
- Hypotension.

C-fibres also contribute to the breathlessness of heart failure, and although they are afferent nerve endings, C-fibres are able to release inflammatory mediators (neurokinins and substance P).

### Receptors in the chest wall

Receptors in the chest wall consist of:

- Joint receptors – measure the velocity of rib movement.
- Golgi tendon organs – found within the muscles of respiration (e.g., diaphragm and intercostals) and detect the strength of muscle contraction.
- Muscle spindles – monitor the length of muscle fibres both statically and dynamically (i.e., detect muscle length and velocity).

These receptors help to minimize changes to ventilation imposed by an external load (e.g., lateral flexion of the trunk). They achieve this by modifying motor neurone output to the respiratory muscles. The aim is to achieve the most efficient respiration in terms of tidal volume and frequency. It is thought that stimulation of mechanoreceptors in the chest wall, along with hypercapnia and hypoxaemia, leads to increased respiratory effort in a patient with sleep apnoea. It is this sudden respiratory effort that then wakes the patient up.

Thus, reflexes from muscles and joints stabilize ventilation in the face of changing mechanical conditions.

### Arterial baroreceptors

Hypertension stimulates arterial baroreceptors, which inhibit ventilation. Hypotension has the opposite effect.

### Pain receptors

Stimulation of pain receptors causes a brief apnoea, followed by a period of hyperventilation.

## COORDINATED RESPONSES OF THE RESPIRATORY SYSTEM

### Response to carbon dioxide

Carbon dioxide is the most important factor in the control of ventilation. Under normal conditions, $P_aCO_2$ is held within very tight limits and ventilatory response is very sensitive to small changes in $P_aCO_2$.

The response of ventilation to carbon dioxide has been measured by inhalation of mixtures of carbon dioxide, raising the $P_aCO_2$ and observing the increase in ventilation (Fig. 6.2).

Note that a small increase in $P_ACO_2$ causes a significant increase in ventilation. The response to $P_ACO_2$ is also dependent upon the arterial oxygen tension. At lower values of $P_aO_2$, the ventilatory response is more sensitive to changes in $P_aCO_2$ (steeper slope) and ventilation is greater for a given $P_aCO_2$. If the $P_aCO_2$ is reduced, this causes a significant reduction in ventilation.

Factors that affect ventilatory response to $P_aCO_2$ are:

- $P_aO_2$
- Blood pH
- Genetics
- Age
- Fitness
- Anixety/agitation

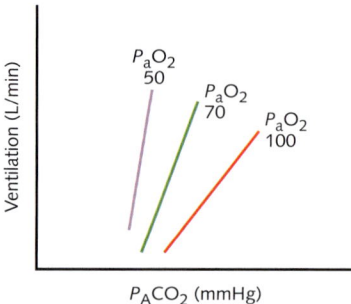

**Fig. 6.2** The response of ventilation to $CO_2$. Note that at higher levels of $P_aO_2$, an increase in $P_ACO_2$ has less effect on ventilation (the curve is less steep).

- Drugs (e.g., opiates, such as morphine and diamorphine, which reduce respiratory and cardiovascular drive).

## Response to oxygen

As mentioned previously, the response to reduced $P_aO_2$ is by stimulation of the peripheral chemoreceptors. This response, however, is not significant until the $P_aO_2$ drops to around 50 mmHg (6.7 kPa). The relationship between $P_aO_2$ and ventilation has been studied by measuring changes in ventilation while a subject breathes hypoxic mixtures (Fig. 6.3). It is assumed that end-expiratory $P_AO_2$ and $P_ACO_2$ are equivalent to arterial gas tensions.

The response to $P_AO_2$ is also seen to change with different levels of $P_ACO_2$.

- The greater the carbon dioxide tension, the earlier the response to low oxygen tension.
- Therefore, at high $P_ACO_2$, a decrease in oxygen tension below 100 mmHg (13.3 kPa) causes an increase in ventilation.

Under normal conditions, $P_aO_2$ does not fall to values of around 50 mmHg (6.7 kPa) and, therefore, daily control of ventilation does not rely on hypoxic drive. However, under conditions of severe lung disease, or at high altitude, hypoxic drive becomes increasingly important. A patient with COPD may rely almost entirely on hypoxic drive alone, having lost ventilatory response to carbon dioxide (described previously). Central chemoreceptors have become unresponsive to carbon dioxide; in addition, ventilatory drive from the effects of reduced pH on peripheral chemoreceptors is lessened by renal compensation for the acid–base abnormality. Administration of high-concentration oxygen therapy (e.g., 100% $O_2$) may abolish any hypoxic drive that the patient was previously relying upon, depressing ventilation and worsening the patient's condition.

## Response to pH

Remember that hydrogen ions do not cross the blood–brain barrier and therefore affect only peripheral chemoreceptors. It is difficult to separate the response from increased $P_aCO_2$ and decreased pH. Any change in pH may be compensated for in the long term by the kidneys and therefore has less effect on ventilation than might be expected.

An example of how pH may drive ventilation is seen in the case of metabolic acidosis. The patient will try to achieve a reduction in hydrogen ion concentration by blowing off more carbon dioxide from the lungs. This is achieved by increasing ventilation and is seen in diabetic ketoacidosis as Kussmaul breathing.

## Response to exercise

As human beings, we are capable of a huge increase in ventilation in response to exercise: approximately 15 times the resting level. In moderate exercise, the carbon dioxide output and oxygen uptake are well matched. Increases in respiratory rate and tidal volume do not cause hyperventilation, and the subject is said to be hyperpnoeic (i.e., have increased depth of breathing):

- $P_aCO_2$ does not increase, but may fall slightly.
- $P_aO_2$ does not decrease.
- In moderate exercise, arterial pH varies very little.

So where does the drive for ventilation come from? Many causes have been suggested for the increase in ventilation seen during exercise, but none is completely satisfactory:

- Carbon dioxide load within venous blood returning to the lungs affects ventilation.
- There is a change in the pattern of oscillations of $P_aCO_2$ (Fig. 6.4).
- Central control of $P_aCO_2$ is reset to a lower value and held constant during exercise.
- Movement of limbs activates joint receptors, which contribute to increased ventilation.
- Increase in body temperature during exercise may also stimulate ventilation.
- The motor cortex stimulates respiratory centres.
- Adrenaline released in exercise also stimulates respiration.

### The possible role of oscillations of $P_aCO_2$

It is suggested that there are cyclical changes of $P_aCO_2$, with inspiration and expiration. Although mean $P_aCO_2$ does not change during moderate exercise, the amplitude of these oscillations may increase, providing the stimulus for ventilation.

In heavy exercise, there can be measurable changes in $P_aO_2$ and $P_aCO_2$, which stimulate respiration. In addition, the pH falls because anaerobic metabolism leads to production of lactic acid

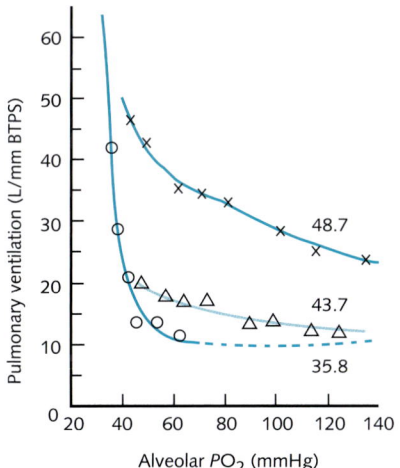

**Fig. 6.3** The response of ventilation to $P_AO_2$ at three values of $P_ACO_2$ (35.8, 43.7, 48.7 mmHg). Lowered $P_AO_2$ has a much greater effect on ventilation when increased values of $P_ACO_2$ are present. *BTPS,* Body temperature pressure saturated.

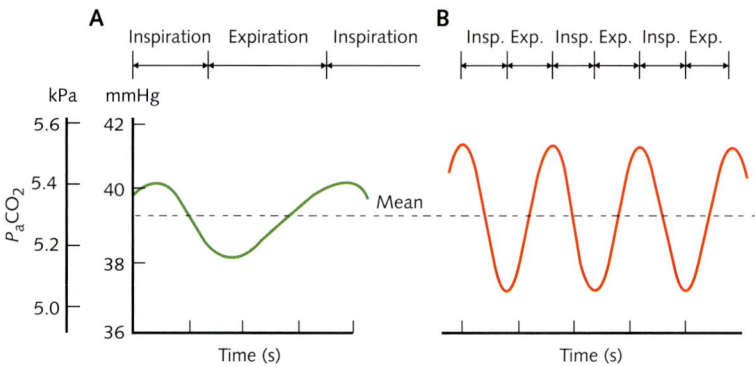

**Fig. 6.4** Cyclical changes of $P_aCO_2$ with inspiration and expiration: (A) at rest; (B) during exercise. Larger oscillations are thought to alter ventilation.

(blood lactate levels increase 10-fold). This lactic acid is not oxidized because the oxygen supply cannot keep up with the demands of the exercising muscles (i.e., an 'oxygen debt' is incurred). Rises in potassium ion concentration and temperature may also contribute to the increase in ventilation.

When exercise stops, respiration does not immediately return to basal levels. It remains elevated to provide an increased supply of oxygen to the tissues to oxidize the products of anaerobic metabolism ('repaying the oxygen debt').

## Abnormalities of ventilatory control

### Cheyne–Stokes respiration

In Cheyne–Stokes respiration, ventilation alternates between progressively deeper breaths and progressively shallower breaths in a cyclical manner. Ventilatory control is not achieved and the respiratory system appears to become unstable:

- Arterial carbon dioxide and oxygen tensions vary significantly.
- Tidal volumes wax and wane (Fig. 6.5).
- There are short periods of apnoea separated by periods of hyperventilation.

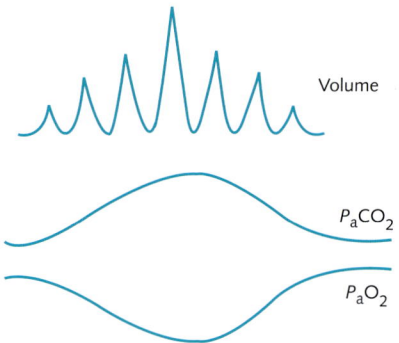

**Fig. 6.5** Cheyne–Stokes respiration.

Cheyne–Stokes breathing is observed at various times:

- At altitude – often when asleep.
- During sleep.
- During periods of hypoxia.
- After voluntary hyperventilation.
- During disease, particularly with combined right and left heart failure and uraemia.
- Secondary to brainstem lesions or compression.

## RESPIRATORY RESPONSE TO EXTREME ENVIRONMENTS

### Response to high altitude

At high altitude, the barometric pressure is much lower than at sea level. Hence, the partial pressure of oxygen is lower.

In addition, the partial pressure of water vapour is constant, because inspired air is saturated at body temperature. Therefore, the partial pressure of oxygen in the alveoli (and in the blood) is significantly lower than at sea level.

The carriage of oxygen in the blood is dependent on:

- Partial pressure of oxygen in the blood.
- Haemoglobin concentration.
- The oxyhaemoglobin dissociation curve.

At altitude the partial pressure of oxygen in the blood is lowered. This would tend to limit the amount of oxygen carriage. To combat this problem, the body can:

- Hyperventilate in an attempt to decrease the partial pressure of carbon dioxide in the alveoli and therefore increase the partial pressure of oxygen.
- Increase the amount of haemoglobin in the blood (polycythaemia), thereby increasing oxygen carriage (oxygen capacity).

- Shift the oxygen dissociation curve.
- Alter the circulation.
- Increase anaerobic metabolism in tissues, increase cytochrome oxidase activity and increase myoglobin in muscle tissue.

As a result of the physiological adjustments made at altitude, a number of unique medical problems can occur in high-altitude environments, including hyperventilation, altitude sickness, pulmonary and cerebral oedema.

## Scuba diving

Scuba diving is an increasingly popular recreational activity, as well as a scientific tool for underwater discovery. Scuba diving is performed with a compressed air system to deliver adequate oxygenation while swimming underwater at varying depths. The resulting barometric pressure effects created at increasing depths create unique challenges for human physiology. Hypoxia can occur with air delivery failures, while hypercapnia can occur with inadequate ventilation with the aim to conserve oxygen supply, compounded by inhaling higher than normal carbon dioxide concentrations in dead air space systems. The result is that hypoxic and hypercapnic states are dangerous realities requiring prompt recognition and treatment in an underwater environment.

The increasing pressure on descent causes compression of all gases in the body, with lung volume being reduced as per the pressure–volume relationship described by Boyle's law. This compression effect is counteracted by the process of equalization and pressurized air systems, but can cause significant morbidity, especially in free diving. By the same principle, ascent causes compressed gases to expand which, without controlled ascent to allow adjustment, leads to rapid expansion of all gases in tissues throughout the body. In the lungs, barotrauma through rapid re-expansion is common, exacerbating existing lung conditions and can be complicated by a pneumothorax, arterial air embolism, subcutaneous emphysema and many other life-threatening conditions. While the take-home message for any medical exam is that if you have ever had a pneumothorax, you are banned from diving for life (the risk of recurrence is high), diving medicine is a complex multisystem speciality requiring a strong understanding of the control of respiratory function.

---

### ● Chapter Summary

- Breathing is controlled centrally by the medulla and pons, with control regulated by central and peripheral chemoreceptors.
- Peripheral chemoreceptors are located in the carotid and aortic bodies. They are sensitive to $P_aO_2$, $P_aCO_2$, pH, blood flow and temperature changes.
- Carbon dioxide is the most important factor in the control of ventilation in the healthy individual, regulated largely by central chemoreceptors and kept within a tight range.
- In pathological states of chronic hypercapnia, such as in severe chronic obstructive pulmonary disease, the regulation of ventilation is instead largely determined by the oxygen concentration, known as the hypoxic drive.
- Huge levels of compensation in ventilation are possible, owing to changes made during exercise. Separate compensations are also made at high altitude and while scuba diving.

#### MLA Conditions

Acid–base abnormality
Chronic obstructive pulmonary disease
Obstructive sleep apnoea
Polycythaemia

#### MLA Presentations

Breathlessness

# Basic pharmacology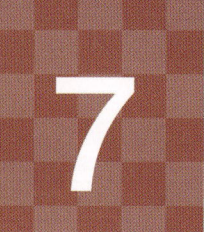

## OVERVIEW

The aim of this chapter is to introduce classes of drugs that are commonly prescribed in respiratory medicine, particularly inhaled drugs used in airways disease and medication used in smoking cessation. Drugs used to treat specific conditions are covered within the relevant clinical chapters.

## BRONCHODILATORS

Bronchodilators are medications that reduce the resistance to air flow in the respiratory tract, thus increasing air flow to the lungs. They are most commonly used in asthma and chronic obstructive pulmonary disease (COPD) and can be grouped as follows (with Table 7.1 providing a summary):

- Short-acting $\beta_2$-agonists
- Long-acting $\beta_2$-agonists
- Short-acting muscarinic antagonists
- Long-acting muscarinic antagonists
- Theophylline.

### Short-acting $\beta_2$-agonists

Bronchial smooth muscle contains numerous $\beta_2$-receptors, which act through an adenylate cyclase/cyclic adenosine monophosphate (cAMP) second-messenger system to cause smooth-muscle relaxation and hence bronchodilatation (Fig. 7.1). Examples of short-acting $\beta_2$-agonists are:

- Salbutamol
- Terbutaline sulphate.

These drugs are usually inhaled as an aerosol, a powder or a nebulized solution but can also be given intravenously in life-threatening asthma. They are used for acute symptoms and act within minutes, producing effects lasting 4–5 hours. When used in asthma, they are commonly referred to as 'reliever inhalers'.

The $\beta_2$-agonists are not completely specific and have some $\beta_1$-agonistic effects, especially in high doses:

- Tachycardia
- Fine tremor
- Nervous tension
- Headache.

At the doses given by aerosol, these side effects seldom occur. Tolerance may occur with high repeated doses.

### Long-acting $\beta_2$-agonists

Like the short-acting $\beta_2$-agonists, these drugs also relax bronchial smooth muscle. They differ from the short-acting drugs in that:

- Their effects last for much longer (up to 24 hours)
- The full effect is only achieved after regular administration of several doses and, generally, less desensitization occurs.

For these reasons, long-acting $\beta_2$-agonists are not used to treat acute attacks of asthma. The main long-acting $\beta_2$-agonists are:

- Salmeterol (partial agonist)
- Formoterol (full agonist)
- Indacaterol
- Olodaterol
- Vilanterol.

Long-acting $\beta_2$-agonists should not be used as monotherapy in asthma, but can be used alone in patients with COPD. They are available in a combined preparation with a corticosteroid which is used in asthma and COPD. Combination inhalers are more convenient and there may also be pharmacological advantages when administered together. Commonly used combination inhalers are:

- Salmeterol and fluticasone (Seretide)
- Formoterol and budesonide (Symbicort)
- Formoterol and beclometasone (Fostair).

Due to the differing $\beta$-agonist drug profiles, only combination inhalers containing a full, rather than a partial $\beta$-agonist can be used as maintenance and reliever therapy (MART) for asthma. More details can be found in Chapter 14.

### Muscarinic antagonists (antimuscarinics)

Muscarinic antagonists (or antimuscarinics) are competitive antagonists of muscarinic acetylcholine receptors and are a subtype of anticholinergics. They therefore block the vagal control of bronchial smooth-muscle tone in response to irritants and reduce reflex bronchoconstriction. Ipratropium bromide and tiotropium bromide are both antimuscarinics; they have two mechanisms of action:

- Reduction of reflex bronchoconstriction (e.g., from dust or pollen) by antagonizing muscarinic receptors on bronchial smooth muscle.
- Reduction of mucus secretions by antagonizing muscarinic receptors on goblet cells.

Antimuscarinics are available in short-acting forms, e.g., ipratropium, which reach their maximum effect within 60–90 minutes

**Table 7.1** Summary of bronchodilator therapies

| Bronchodilator therapy | Examples | Key points |
| --- | --- | --- |
| Short-acting β2-agonists (SABAs) | Salbutamol Terbutaline sulphate | • Used for acute symptoms – 'reliever' in asthma<br>• Acts within minutes, effects last for a few hours<br>• Side effects: fine tremor, tachycardia, headache |
| Long-acting β2-agonists (LABAs) | Salmeterol (partial agonist) Formoterol (full agonist) | • Effects last for 24 hours<br>• Can be used as monotherapy in COPD<br>• May be combined with ICS for MART (to use one inhaler rather than two) |
| Short-acting muscarinic antagonists (SAMAs) | Ipratropium bromide | • SAMA: works between 1 and 6 hours<br>• LAMA: effects last for 24 hours<br>• Side effects: dry mouth, urinary retention, constipation<br>• Can be used as add-on therapy in moderate–severe asthma |
| Long-acting muscarinic antagonists (LAMAs) | Tiotropium bromide | |
| Theophylline | Theophylline: oral Aminophylline: intravenous | • Theophylline has a small therapeutic window – regular blood tests are important<br>• Aminophylline may be given in severe asthma cases that have not responded to steroids or other bronchodilators (senior decision)<br>• Side effects of aminophylline: arrhythmias, hypotension, central nervous system stimulation leading to seizures – to avoid, must give it slowly |

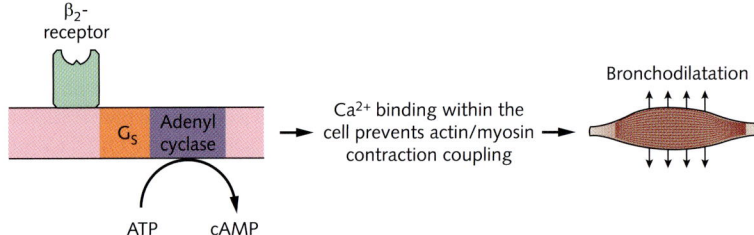

**Fig. 7.1** Mechanisms of action of β$_2$-agonists—relaxation of bronchial muscle (which leads to bronchodilatation) and inhibition of mast cell degranulation (β-receptors on mast cell). *ATP,* Adenosine triphosphate; *cAMP,* cyclic adenosine monophosphate; *G$_S$,* alpha subunit.

and act for 4–6 hours. Long-acting forms, e.g., tiotropium, aclidinium, glycopyrronium and umeclidinium, exert their effects for up to 24 hours. They are poorly absorbed orally and are therefore given by aerosol via an inhaler or nebulizer.

Antimuscarinics as monotherapy are not the first-choice bronchodilator in asthma treatment because they only reduce the vagally mediated element of bronchoconstriction, having no effect on other important causes of bronchoconstriction such as inflammatory mediators. However, they are licensed as add-on therapy in patients with moderate to severe asthma. There is some evidence that antimuscarinics are effective when given together with a β$_2$-agonist in severe acute asthma by nebulized therapy. Contrastingly, in COPD, cholinergic hyperactivity significantly contributes to bronchoconstriction and therefore monotherapy with antimuscarinics is more effective than bronchodilators.

Side effects are rare as systemic absorption is poor, but can include:

- Dry mouth
- Urinary retention
- Constipation.

Long-acting muscarinic antagonists are also available as combination therapy with long-acting β$_2$-agonists for use in patients with COPD, where complementary additive effects of both drugs may allow better bronchodilation than either drug alone. Commonly used combination inhalers are:

- Olodaterol and tiotropium (Spiolto)
- Vilanterol and umeclidinium (Anoro)
- Indacaterol and glycopyrronium (Ultibro)
- Formoterol and aclidinium (Duaklir).

## Theophylline

Theophylline appears to work by inhibiting phosphodiesterase, thereby preventing the breakdown of cAMP (Fig. 7.2). The amount of cAMP within the bronchial smooth-muscle cells is therefore increased, which causes bronchodilation in a similar way to β$_2$-agonists.

Theophylline is metabolized by cytochrome P450 enzymes in the liver and there is considerable variation in half-life between individuals. Theophylline therefore has a small therapeutic

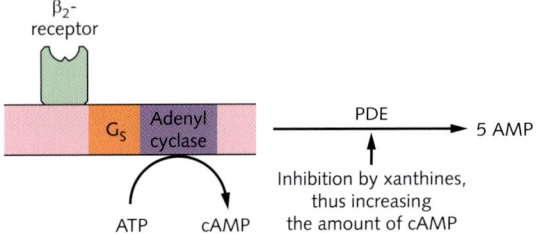

**Fig. 7.2** Xanthines. The inhibition of phosphodiesterase (*PDE*) leads to an increase in cellular cyclic adenosine monophosphate (*cAMP*). *AMP*, Adenosine monophosphate; *ATP*, adenosine triphosphate; $G_S$, alpha subunit.

**Table 7.2** Factors altering theophylline clearance

| Increased clearance (lower serum levels) | Decreased clearance (high serum levels) |
|---|---|
| Cytochrome P450 enzyme-inducing drugs, e.g., rifampicin | Cytochrome P450 enzyme-inhibiting drugs, e.g., clarithromycin |
| Smoking | Liver disease |
| Alcohol | Viral infections |
| Young age | Old age |

window, meaning the therapeutic dose is close to the toxic dose. Consequently, blood serum levels must be checked in patients admitted unwell on theophylline or after drug initiation. Some factors that alter theophylline clearance are shown in Table 7.2.

Oral theophylline has modest symptomatic benefit when given as a bronchodilator in stable COPD. It can be given intravenously in the form of aminophylline (theophylline with ethylenediamine), but must be administered slowly to prevent side effects. Side effects include arrhythmias, hypotension, central nervous system stimulation leading to seizures and gastrointestinal effects, including diarrhoea and nausea. Aminophylline may be given in cases of severe asthma that do not respond to initial treatment with bronchodilators and steroids following senior input.

## GLUCOCORTICOIDS

Corticosteroids reduce the formation, release and action of many different mediators involved in inflammation. Their mode of action is complex and involves gene modulation after binding to steroid receptors in the cytoplasm of cells and translocation of the active receptor into the nucleus. This has a number of effects, including:

- Downregulation of proinflammatory cytokines and mediators, e.g., phospholipase $A_2$.
- Production of antiinflammatory proteins.

Corticosteroids in respiratory treatment may be topical (inhaled) or systemic (oral or parenteral).

## Inhaled corticosteroids

These include:

- Beclometasone dipropionate
- Budesonide
- Ciclesonide
- Fluticasone propionate
- Fluticasone furoate.

Side effects of inhaled steroids in adults include a hoarse voice, oral candidiasis, skin bruising and possibly pneumonia in patients with COPD. Corticosteroid inhalers in asthma are commonly known as 'preventer inhalers'.

## Oral steroids

The primary oral steroid is prednisolone. Side effects of systemic steroids include:

- Adrenal suppression
- Myopathy
- Effects on bones (including growth retardation in children and osteoporosis in adults)
- Diabetes mellitus
- Increased susceptibility to infection
- Weight gain
- Effects on skin (e.g., bruising and atrophy)
- Mood changes.

Because of these side effects, regular oral steroids are avoided wherever possible.

## MUCOLYTICS

Mucolytics (e.g., carbocisteine) are designed to reduce the viscosity of sputum. They have limited research evidence to support their use, however, carbocisteine is used commonly in COPD and bronchiectasis, both during stable and acute disease, to aid sputum expectoration. The main side effect is gastric ulceration and it should be avoided in those with active ulceration.

## DRUG DELIVERY DEVICES

### Inhalers

These are devices used to deliver drugs to the bronchial tree. Despite inhalers being the most commonly prescribed drugs in the United Kingdom, up to 80% of asthmatics do not use their inhaler device correctly. The percentage of drug delivered with each dose ranges from 15% to 40%, assuming good technique. In the last few years, there has been an explosion of new types of inhaler devices onto the market, to try to improve drug delivery (Fig. 7.3). Factors including advancing age, use of multiple devices and lack of education all contribute to poor inhaler usage. Common errors with use include problems with the inhalation rate and duration, coordination of breath with actuation, preparation prior to dose, poor exhalation prior to inhalation and difficulties with breath holding. For example, an elderly patient with arthritis may struggle to coordinate pressing a device with their breathing. Prior to starting therapy, patients should have the chance to try a full range of inhalers to find the correct device for them. They should have an education session prior to starting treatment and regular inhaler technique checks once established. All devices have different methods for priming and for counting the number of doses left until empty, and patients need to be aware of how their specific inhaler works.

Broadly, inhalers exist in two types as detailed below, with different techniques for use.

## Pressurized metered-dose inhaler

The medication is stored in a pressurized canister with propellant. As these inhalers are pressurized, inhaler technique should include a 'slow and steady' inspiratory breath coordinated with actuation of the device. Classic pressurized metered-dose inhalers (pMDIs) require coordinated inspiration with depression of the medicated canister. Where possible, to improve drug delivery, classic MDIs should be used in conjunction with a valve-holding chamber or spacer device. Newer devices such as Autohaler and Easi-breathe devices can be primed and breath activated, removing the need for complex coordination. Of note, pMDIs contain propellants compared to soft mist inhalers and dry powder inhalers (below) which do not. Therefore, pMDIs have a larger carbon footprint and so are worse for the environment.

## Soft mist inhaler

Soft mist inhalers are aerosol delivery devices that release an aerosolized measured dose of a medication by pressing a button. Like a pressurized MDI, the inhalation technique should include a slow and steady inspiratory breath coordinated with pressing the dose release button. An example of this inhaler type is the Respimat soft mist inhaler.

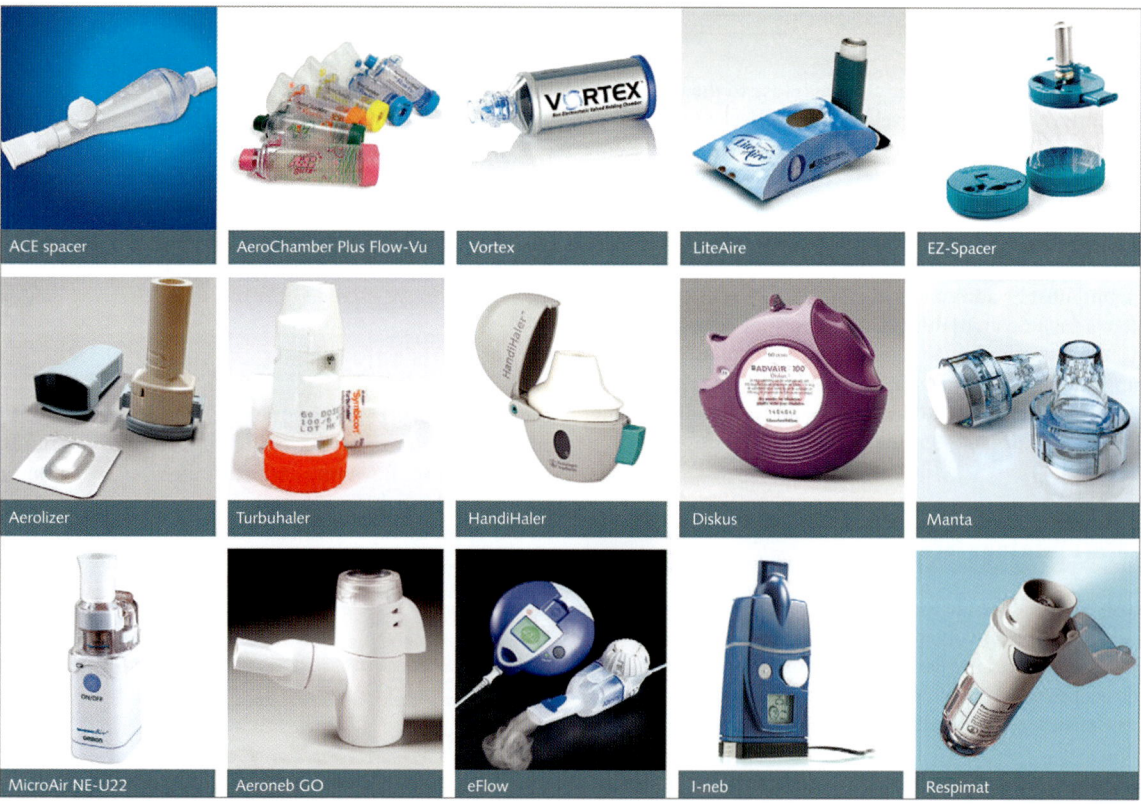

**Fig. 7.3** Inhaler device examples. (From Dolovich MB, Dhand R. Aerosol drug delivery: developments in device design and clinical use. *Lancet*. 2011;377(9770):1032–1045.)

## Dry powder inhaler

Examples of dry powder inhalers are Accuhaler, Turbohaler, Diskhaler, Nexthaler and Easyhaler.

These inhalers release dry powdered medication to the lungs and require a 'fast and deep' inhalation by the patient. The delivery of medication is dependent on the patient's inspiratory effort and therefore unsuitable for patients with poor inspiratory flow.

---

### HINTS AND TIPS

#### HOW TO USE A METERED-DOSE INHALER

Demonstrating inhaler technique to a patient is an important medical skill and commonly appears in 'OSCE' examinations at medical school. Helpful videos demonstrating different devices can be found on the Asthma + Lung UK website (asthmaandlung.org.uk). It is worth spending time with an asthma nurse who can demonstrate different devices.

---

## Nebulizers

Nebulizers are driven by air or oxygen and aerosolized liquid medication for inhalation. They are used in patients with:

1. Acute respiratory illnesses
2. Very severe disease
3. Patients who are unable to use inhalers.

Occasionally patients are prescribed nebulizers at home; however, guidelines advocate the use of an MDI with spacer in the majority of outpatient clinical scenarios and patients should therefore be seen by a respiratory physician prior to starting nebulized treatment at home.

---

### RED FLAG

#### SMOKING CESSATION

According to the Office for National Statistics, in 2022, 6.4 million adults (approximately 13%) in the United Kingdom smoke tobacco. It remains the leading cause of preventable death and illness worldwide. Four percent of hospital admissions are attributable to smoking. The National Smoking Cessation Audit 2019 found that only one in eight patients who smoke were referred to community- or hospital-based smoking cessation services. When assessing any patient, remember:

1. ASK – do you smoke? Have you ever smoked? When did you stop? And calculate pack years (number of years smoking × number of cigarettes smoked in one day/20).
2. ADVISE – provide advice on cognitive and pharmacological methods of smoking cessation.
3. ACT – refer to local smoking cessation providers.

---

## DRUGS USED IN SMOKING CESSATION

A combination of motivational interviewing and pharmacotherapy has been shown to be more successful than monotherapy alone for smoking cessation. The three main drugs used are:

1. Nicotine replacement therapy (NRT)
2. Varenicline
3. Bupropion.

NRT products (gums, patches, inhalators and nasal sprays) are classified as over-the-counter medicines and have been shown to be effective in treating tobacco withdrawal and dependence. Long-acting preparations such as patches should be used in combination with short-acting preparations such as lozenges to both prevent and treat cravings as they arise. Current guidance suggests that e-cigarettes can be used as NRT as an aid in smoking cessation. As the long-term effects of e-cigarettes are not yet known, potential harm from long-term use cannot be excluded and is therefore not advised.

Varenicline is a nicotine receptor partial agonist available as an oral preparation that helps relieve cravings and prevent withdrawal symptoms by decreasing the 'reward' from smoking. When used with NRT and motivational interviewing, it may double a person's chance of quitting. It should be started 2 weeks prior to stopping smoking and the dose increased over the first weeks of treatment. Side effects include nausea, and the dose should be decreased in renal failure.

Bupropion is an oral medication that helps decrease the urge to smoke. Similarly to varenicline, it should be started prior to stopping. It should be avoided in patients at risk of seizures as it can lower seizure threshold.

## E-cigarettes

Electronic cigarettes are battery-operated devices that deliver nicotine via vapour that can be inhaled in a similar manner to a cigarette. They do not contain tobacco; however, they contain nicotine, propylene glycol or glycerine, and flavourings. Use of e-cigarettes is increasing, especially in the form of vapes. In 2023, Action for Smoking and Health (ASH) estimated that the proportion of the UK population using e-cigarettes is 9.1% (approximately 4.7 million adults) which is the highest rate ever. What is more striking is the increasing use of vapes among children with a 50% increase in vape experimentation from 2022 to 2023.

E-cigarettes are generally considered to be less harmful than smoking tobacco as they contain fewer harmful components than traditional cigarettes, and are therefore generally accepted to have a role in smoking cessation. However, there is limited research evidence currently to support their role in smoking cessation. There are concerns that the long-term risks of e-cigarette smoking are as yet unknown and so never-smokers should be encouraged to not begin vaping.

## PALLIATIVE MEDICATIONS USED IN RESPIRATORY MEDICINE

Some respiratory diseases are progressive and incurable, and palliative care at the end stage of life of these patients can improve quality of life for both patients and families. The emphasis is on pre-empting and treating symptoms and preventing suffering. This is achieved by a combination of pharmacological measures and psychosocial support. Specialist palliative care services should be involved early.

The main pharmacological treatments used are:

- Opiates – used for analgesia and, in much smaller doses, to relieve dyspnoea.

- Benzodiazepines – used to treat anxiety associated with dyspnoea, in conjunction with complementary therapies and relaxation techniques.
- Steroids – used in low doses to encourage appetite in those with anorexia, in conjunction with nutritional support. Also used in higher doses to reduce cerebral oedema from intracranial metastases from malignant disease.

These medications have side effects, particularly respiratory depression for opiates and benzodiazepines, therefore caution must be taken when prescribing.

### Chapter Summary

- Bronchodilator medications reduce resistance to airflow in the respiratory tract and increase airflow into the lungs. Commonly prescribed inhaled bronchodilators include $\beta_2$-agonists and antimuscarinics.
- Drug delivery devices for inhaled medications include inhalers (pressurized metered-dose inhalers [pMDIs], soft mist inhalers, dry powder inhalers) and nebulizers.
- It is crucial to check a patient's inhaler technique during each inpatient hospital stay, at outpatient reviews and regularly in the community, via their specialist nurse.
- A combination of motivational interviewing and pharmacotherapy with medications (including nicotine replacement therapy and varenicline) has been shown to be most successful for smoking cessation.
- E-cigarettes are less harmful than smoking tobacco and may have a role in smoking cessation; however, the long-term effects of their use are as yet unknown.

| MLA Conditions | MLA Presentations |
|---|---|
| Asthma | Breathlessness |
| COPD | Disease prevention |
| | End of life care/symptoms of terminal illness |

# Section 2

# CLINICAL ASSESSMENT

# Taking a respiratory history

## INTRODUCTION

Taking a good history is the most important part of any clinical assessment. The key to identifying and successfully treating the respiratory patient is to understand the interplay between the underlying pathophysiology and the principal symptoms of respiratory disease. The symptoms of breathlessness, cough, haemoptysis, wheeze and chest pain are common to many different conditions but a good history focusing on the time course and progression of the illness can enable you to narrow down the differential diagnoses.

## GENERAL STEPS

A good history takes into account the patient's ideas and concerns, and addressing these will lay a foundation of trust, which is vital in treating the patient as a whole.

The respiratory history follows the same format as for the other systems, and at every stage, the goal is to ask questions to either rule in or rule out diagnoses. Remember that common things are common, and asking questions on red flag symptoms helps to rule out acute pathology. Ensure you are as prepared as possible for the patient encounter and have set distractions aside. Preferably find a quiet venue for taking the history; if things are busy on the ward, consider taking the patient to the day room.

Select an appropriate time if possible – avoiding drug rounds and meal times. Sometimes patients are confused or too unwell to provide a clear history, in which case a collateral history from a relative, friend or carer can give you the valuable information you need.

In the clinical setting (as opposed to an exam), it is often useful to find out as much about the patient as you can before you see them: read the referral letter, review old notes and look up any electronic records of medication lists, discharge summaries or previous clinic letters. This may give you valuable details of previous encounters and keep you up to speed with current pending or completed investigations and treatments received.

Introduce yourself to the patient and confirm the patient's name and date of birth. Explain what you wish to do and gain consent.

## HISTORY OF PRESENTING COMPLAINT

Start by finding out why the patient has come to seek medical advice. Ask open questions and allow the patient time to talk to describe their problems before moving on to closed questions. A good clinician is a good listener, and clues to the diagnosis will often be in how the patient describes their unique symptoms. Below is information on the most commonly presenting respiratory complaints.

## BREATHLESSNESS

Breathlessness, or dyspnoea, is difficulty or distress in breathing and is a symptom of many different diseases. Breathlessness is a very common reason for referral to a respiratory clinic.

The patient may describe the symptom in a variety of ways. Common terms used are 'puffed', 'can't get enough air' and 'feeling suffocated'. A number of physiological factors underlie this sensation and sometimes several mechanisms coexist to cause breathlessness. See Table 8.1 for common presentations of breathlessness, and associated symptoms and signs that point towards common illnesses.

Key points to ask:

- the time course and speed of the onset of breathlessness i.e., is it sudden, come on over days, weeks, months or longer
- the severity and progression of the breathlessness
- the variability in breathlessness (e.g., at rest or during activity, or at different times in the day or is it worse when lying flat at night)
- any exacerbating and relieving factors or response to prior treatments
- respiratory risk factors (preexisting respiratory disease, family history, occupational exposure)

The above history-taking can help to establish the severity of the underlying disease process: e.g., shortness of breath at rest suggests worse disease than in patients who experience exertional breathlessness.

Breathlessness may be episodic, and the diurnal variation (severity altering at different times of day) is characteristic of asthma.

Orthopnoea (breathlessness on lying flat) is a common feature of pulmonary oedema but is seen in any severe respiratory disease.

Paroxysmal nocturnal dyspnoea (waking up breathless in the night) is classic of pulmonary oedema but also of asthma, with differentiation made by extra features and clinical context.

Nonrespiratory causes of breathlessness include anaemia, heart failure, cardiac arrhythmias, anxiety or even a sign of respiratory compensation in diabetic ketoacidosis.

**Table 8.1** Common breathlessness patterns and associated diagnoses

| Description of symptoms | Diagnosis |
|---|---|
| Breathlessness variable in intensity and timing, associated with history of atopy<br>May have audible wheeze and raised eosinophils<br>Chest X-ray and spirometry may be normal | Asthma |
| Progressive breathlessness associated with exertion and smoking history (>10 pack years)<br>Chest X-ray may show hyperinflation and spirometry demonstrates an obstructive pattern | Chronic obstructive pulmonary disease |
| Progressive breathlessness at rest or on exertion associated +/− chronic productive cough and productive sputum<br>Chest X-ray may be normal or show dilated bronchi or thickened walls<br>Spirometry may demonstrate an obstructive pattern | Bronchiectasis |
| Progressive exertional breathlessness<br>Body mass Index > 30 kgm$^2$<br>Epworth score > 10 and excessive daytime sleepiness<br>Examination may be normal | Obesity/sleep apnoea |
| Exertional breathlessness may be associated with palpitations, presyncope, syncope, fatigue<br>ECG may be abnormal<br>Thyroid function tests may be abnormal | Arrhythmias |
| Breathlessness on exertion, nocturnal dyspnoea, orthopnoea, ankle oedema<br>Jugular venous pressure may be raised, audible fine crepitations<br>Chest X-ray may show cardiomegaly, upper lobe diversion and ECG may be abnormal | Heart failure |
| Progressive exertional breathlessness and fatigue<br>Pale, may be jaundiced<br>Haemoglobin low, MCV low, check haematinics | Anaemia |

Quantifying exertional breathlessness can provide valuable prognostic information and often guide treatment options, with several scoring systems in place to grade its symptom severity (see Table 8.2 for the Medical Research Council Dyspnoea Scale). It is vital to ask patients about the impact of breathlessness on their quality of life, as severe symptoms can lead to depression and poorer outcomes.

## COUGH

Everybody produces airway secretions. In a healthy nonsmoker, approximately 100–150 mL of mucus is produced every day. Normally, this mucus is transported up the airway's ciliary mucus escalator and swallowed. This process is not normally perceived. Coughing is a physiological mechanism of removing

**Table 8.2** Medical Research Council Dyspnoea Scale[a]

| Grade | Degree of breathlessness related to activity |
|---|---|
| 1 | Not troubled by breathlessness except on strenuous exercise |
| 2 | Short of breath when hurrying on a level or when walking up a slight hill |
| 3 | Walks slower than most people on the level, stops after a mile or so, or stops after 15 minutes walking at own pace |
| 4 | Stops for breath after walking 100 yards, or after a few minutes on level ground |
| 5 | Too breathless to leave the house, or breathless when dressing/undressing |

[a]A widely used tool for grading the impact of breathlessness on patients' lives.

excess sputum or foreign material by creating large positive pressure within the thorax to create a sharp forceful expiration. This results from irritation of the respiratory tract by infection, inflammation, excess sputum production, acid reflux or inhaled irritants such as smoking or other foreign bodies (see airway clearance in Chapter 2 for more details).

Sputum may be classified as:

- Mucoid: clear, grey or white.
- Serous: watery or frothy.
- Mucopurulent: a yellowish tinge.
- Purulent: dark green/yellow.

Always try to inspect the sputum and ask about the volume (teaspoon/tablespoon/eggcup/sputum pot full), colour, how easy it is to clear and its odour. These details can provide clues as to the underlying pathology. An increase in sputum production or a change in colour usually indicates infection and is caused by myeloperoxidase produced by eosinophils or neutrophils. Sputum in asthmatics may contain high numbers of eosinophils and can be abnormally coloured without underlying infection. Chronic bronchitis (an important component of chronic obstructive pulmonary disease [COPD]) has traditionally been defined as a cough productive of sputum for most days during at least three consecutive months, for more than two successive years. A summary of the differences between cough in asthma and that in chronic bronchitis is shown in Table 8.3.

**Table 8.3** Patterns of cough in asthma and chronic bronchitis

| | Asthma | Chronic bronchitis |
|---|---|---|
| Timing | Worse at night | Worse in the morning |
| Nature | Dry (may be green sputum) | Productive |
| Chronicity | Intermittent | Persistent |
| Response to treatment | Associated wheeze is reversible | Associated wheeze is irreversible |

Bronchogenic carcinomas commonly cause irritation of the respiratory tract and hence stimulate the cough reflex. The exception is the rare alveolar cell carcinoma, which does directly lead to copious amounts of mucoid sputum.

Coughing is reliant on the adequate closure of the vocal cords while intrathoracic pressure is raised. Invasion of the recurrent laryngeal nerve by a bronchial tumour can cause incomplete vocal cord closure and a characteristic 'bovine cough'. Persistent cough is the most common presenting symptom in lung cancers and hence any unexplained cough warrants an urgent referral for a chest X-ray.

Key points to ask:

- Do you cough up sputum from your chest on most mornings?
- Would you say you cough up sputum on most days for as much as 3 months a year?
- Do you often need antibiotics from your GP in winter?
- Do you currently smoke or have you ever smoked? (Chronic bronchitis is significantly more common in smokers.)

Nonrespiratory causes of cough include gastroesophageal reflux (laryngeal irritation and sometimes aspiration), postnasal drip secondary to sinusitis or drug induced (classically, angiotensin-converting enzyme inhibitors can cause a chronic dry cough).

## HAEMOPTYSIS

Haemoptysis is the coughing up of blood, but needs to be differentiated from other sources of bleeding within the oral cavity and haematemesis (vomiting blood). This distinction is usually obvious from the history. Haemoptysis is not usually a solitary event but can be a serious and often alarming symptom that requires immediate investigation. A chest radiograph is mandatory in a patient with haemoptysis. Despite appropriate investigations, often no obvious cause can be found and the episode is attributed to a simple bronchial infection. Important respiratory causes of haemoptysis are:

- Bronchial carcinoma
- Pulmonary embolism
- Tuberculosis (TB)
- Pneumonia (particularly pneumococcal)
- Bronchiectasis
- Acute/chronic bronchitis
- Pulmonary vasculitis (e.g., Goodpasture syndrome, granulomatosis with polyangiitis).

Key points to ask:

- ask about any preceding events such as respiratory infection
- ask about a history of deep vein thrombosis
- establish the frequency and volume, whether it is fresh or altered blood and if clots are present
- establish risk factors for a particular differential diagnosis; therefore ask about smoking history (bronchial carcinoma),

foreign travel and infective contacts (TB), recent immobilization owing to a long-haul flight or surgery (pulmonary embolism), rashes, joint pains and upper respiratory tract symptoms (vasculitis) and a history of recurrent chest infections requiring treatment (bronchiectasis)

## WHEEZE

Wheezing is a common complaint, complicating many different disease processes. Establish exactly what a patient means by 'wheeze'; when used correctly, the term describes musical notes heard mainly on expiration, caused by narrowed airways. It is important to differentiate wheeze as a symptom and wheeze as a clinical sign.

Wheeze as a physical sign can be classified as either polyphonic (of many different notes) or monophonic (just one note) and occurs during expiration. These are indistinguishable by history alone and require physical examination (Chapter 9). Polyphonic wheeze is common in widespread airflow obstruction and it is the characteristic wheeze heard in asthmatics. A localized monophonic wheeze suggests that a single airway is partially obstructed which can also occur in asthma (e.g., by a mucus plug) but may be caused by a tumour.

Key points

- ask about triggers for wheeze (weather, exercise, allergens)
- ask if it comes on at night
- ask if it occurs on inspiration or expiration

The symptom of wheezing is not diagnostic of asthma, but asthma and COPD are usually the commonest causes. In asthma, the wheeze is often worse first thing in the morning, or results from exposure to cold air or on physical exertion. Wheezing may be worse during the week and better on weekends, if that person is suffering with occupational asthma. Wheezing can also occur in pulmonary oedema, from airway oedema due to excessive fluid leakage. Stridor is an audible inspiratory noise and requires urgent investigation. It indicates partial obstruction of the upper, larger airways, such as the larynx, trachea and main bronchi. Causes of obstruction include tumour, epiglottitis and inhalation of a foreign body.

## CHEST PAIN

Pain can originate from most of the structures in the chest and can be classified as central or lateral. Make sure you ask specifically about the pain's relationship to deep breathing, coughing or movement; if it is made worse by these factors, it is likely to be pleural in origin. Pleural pain is sharp and stabbing in character and may be referred to the shoulder tip if the diaphragmatic pleura is involved. It can be very severe and often leads to shallow

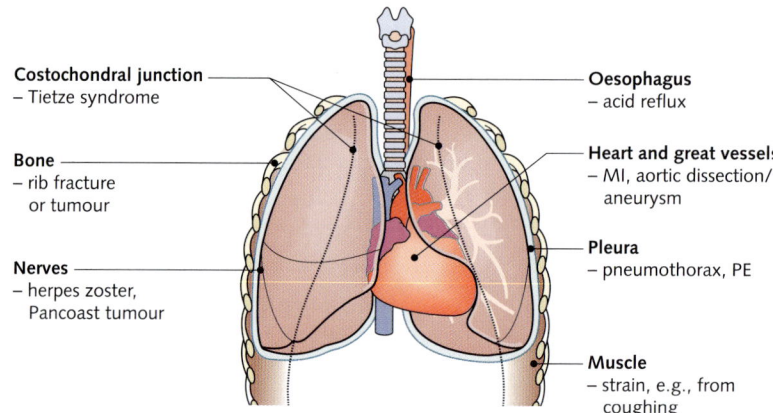

**Fig. 8.1** Summary of causes of chest pain. *MI,* Myocardial infarction; *PE,* pulmonary embolism.

breathing, avoidance of movement and cough suppression. The commonest causes of pleural pain are pulmonary embolus or pleural infection. Fig. 8.1 summarizes the main causes of chest pain, including nonrespiratory causes.

Key points to ask:

- As with pain anywhere in the body, enquire about **S**ite, **O**nset, **C**haracter, **R**adiation, **A**ssociated factors, **T**ime, **E**xacerbating/**R**elieving factors and **S**everity (SOCRATES).

Respiratory causes of central, or retrosternal, chest pain include bronchitis and acute tracheitis. This pain is often made worse by coughing and may be relieved when the patient coughs up sputum.

## OTHER ASSOCIATED SYMPTOMS

In addition to the principal presentations, there are several other symptoms that you should note.

### Hoarseness

Inquire whether the patient has noticed any changes in their voice recently. If there have been changes, ask if there were any events leading up to this, such as excessive voice use or a previous thyroidectomy. It's possible that the cause of hoarseness is simple and benign, such as:

- Cigarette smoking
- Acute laryngitis as part of an acute upper respiratory tract infection
- Use of inhaled steroids.

However, there may be a more sinister cause: like the bovine cough that can result from a lung tumour compressing the recurrent laryngeal nerve. Therefore in a smoker, any change in voice lasting longer than a few days should be investigated urgently to rule out malignancy.

### Weight loss

Unintentional weight loss is always an important sign, raising suspicion of carcinoma. Establish how much weight the patient has lost, over what period, and whether there is any loss of appetite. Note, however, that it is common for patients with severe emphysema or with severe infection (such as TB) to also lose weight. Additional features to suggest TB include chronic cough, night sweats and recent travel to/emigration from a country or region with a high prevalence of the disease.

### Ankle swelling

Patients with COPD may comment that their ankles swell during or independently of acute exacerbations. Ask about this and check for peripheral oedema as part of your overall examination. It is an important sign of cor pulmonale, which is the development of right-sided heart failure secondary to chronic lung disease.

### Fevers and sweats

Fevers and rigors are classically associated with infection, and a patient can experience sudden changes in temperature – shivering followed by fevers, as their temperature increases. Night sweats can occur without rigors and describe when the patient becomes drenched with sweat, often soaking through clothes or bedsheets. Night sweats suggest an underlying malignancy or a more chronic infective process such as TB.

## SYSTEMS REVIEW

Go through a systems review to ensure no other key information is missed.

## PAST MEDICAL HISTORY

Ask about any illnesses and/or operations the patient has had in the past (medical and surgical history). Does the patient see the general practitioner (GP) for anything regularly?

If a patient tells you he or she has a diagnosis of a respiratory disease, then explore this. The patient's current presentation may or may not be related to this, however. Patients may know considerably more than you about their condition; try not to let this disturb you and use it as a learning opportunity. Important things to clarify are:

- When and where were they diagnosed?
- Who do they see for follow-up?
- Have they been admitted to hospital before with their respiratory disease?
- If so, did they have to attend the intensive therapy unit and, if so, were they ventilated?
- If they have medication they can use as required, have they been using more recently, e.g., inhalers or COPD rescue packs?
- If they use regular inhaled steroids or immunosuppressive treatment, how often do they miss a dose in an average week or month?
- How many courses of oral steroids have they had in the past year?
- Do they use oxygen at home?
- Do they have a history of childhood infections such as pneumonia or whooping cough or measles as these could have resulted in bronchiectasis?
- Always ask about previous infections with or exposure to TB.
- Enquire about vaccination history – the elderly, young and those with chronic illnesses are often eligible for seasonal influenza and pneumococcal vaccines in the United Kingdom.
- Enquire about low mood and depression and how their illness affects their quality of life.

## Drug history

Make a comprehensive list of medications the patient is taking, along with doses. If the patient is unsure, then you can make a quick call to their GP or review their online records if available. Be sure to ask specifically about over-the-counter medications, and contraceptives in women. Also note whether the patient uses any inhaler regimens, noting if these have changed recently and remember to check their inhaler technique (see Chapter 7: Pharmacology).

Ensure patients know what each of their medications is for and check their compliance – a surprising number of patients do not use their medications regularly or correctly. If you identify the reasons why you can look for alternative treatments.

Always ask about *allergies*!

## Family history

A specific knowledge of respiratory disorders that run in the family can be useful in aiding diagnosis of atopic disorders such as asthma, but also rarer conditions such as cystic fibrosis and $\alpha_1$-antitrypsin deficiency. A significant history of cardiac risk factors or death at a young age may be relevant.

## Social history

Understanding a patient's social situation is of utmost importance in respiratory medicine. You are able to assess specific risk factors for diseases and understand the burden their illness has on their daily lives.

Always ask about smoking and quantify the amount smoked – how long have they smoked for and how many cigarettes a day (see Box 8.1: Clinical notes: Pack-years). Ask about passive smoking. Occupation is often important – always ask about current or previous jobs to gain clues of exposure to hazardous materials. For example, mining (and type of material mined, e.g., coal, metals such as beryllium), building/plumbing (often asbestos exposure risks), road-work (silica or dust exposure) or bartending (high passive smoking rates) are just some of many occupations relevant to respiratory disease. Ask specifically about previous asbestos exposure – patients may or may not be aware of occupational or incidental contact. Other important exposures include pets (both the patient's own and those in close contact) and travel history (consider infectious diseases endemic to an area and long-haul flight risks). Has the patient ever lived abroad for a significant period of time or been away in the last 12 months?

Next consider how the patient lives with their symptoms. Establish who is at home, whether they live in a house with stairs or in a bungalow and whether they live independently or require assistance with daily activities such as cooking, cleaning and getting dressed. Ask about mobility and quantify the distances they can mobilize before having to stop, both on the flat and stairs, and if walking aids are needed. Are they housebound or can they walk long distances; how do they manage shopping?

---

**BOX 8.1 CLINICAL NOTES**

### Pack-years
This is a simple and useful method of quantifying cigarette smoking.

Number of pack-years = (packs smoked per day) × (years as a smoker).

## Addressing patient's concerns

One of the most important aspects to building a therapeutic relationship is understanding the patient's perspective of their illness. Explore the patient's ideas, concerns and expectations by asking them what they think is wrong. Empower the patient to ask questions and address any concerns that they raise.

### SUMMARY

It is good practice to summarize things briefly back to the patient, cementing the story in your own mind as well as giving the patient a chance to correct unclear points or expand on any unresolved issues.

### ● Chapter Summary

You should now be able to:

- Describe the most common presentations of respiratory disease.
- Give nonrespiratory differential diagnoses for symptoms such as cough, chest pain and breathlessness.
- Identify the symptoms and signs that indicate serious pathology.
- Be comfortable with the structure and content of a respiratory history.

**MLA Conditions**

Acute bronchitis
COVID-19
Lower respiratory tract infection
Upper respiratory tract infection

**MLA Presentations**

Breathlessness
Chest pain
Fever
Haemoptysis
Hoarseness and voice change
Stridor
Wheeze

## INTRODUCTION

As with any examination, it is important that you:

- Introduce yourself to the patient
- Explain to the patient the purpose of the examination and gain consent
- Wash your hands before you begin and when you finish the examination
- Ask the patient if they are in any pain or discomfort, adjusting your examination accordingly.

For a respiratory examination, patients should be fully exposed to the waist, comfortable and sitting at a 45-degree angle, with their hands by their sides. The structure of the respiratory examination is always:

- Inspection
- Palpation
- Percussion
- Auscultation.

## PERIPHERAL EXAMINATION

### General inspection

The purpose of general inspection is to gain as much information about the patient as possible before you begin examination. It is an important skill to learn as a doctor, as this will often decide how sick a patient is, which will then guide whether you do a thorough history and examination or begin emergency management.

General inspection is hugely important in respiratory examination as a large amount of information can be learnt about the patient by simply observing from the bedside. When inspecting the patient, you should ask yourself the following questions:

- Is this patient in respiratory distress (Fig. 9.1)?
- What is the patient's respiratory rate (Table 9.1)?
- Can the patient talk to me in full sentences without becoming breathless?
- Is the patient's breathing noisy (is there wheeze or stridor?)?
- What is the patient's pattern of breathing (Table 9.2)?
- Are there inhalers, sputum pots or oxygen around the bedside?
- Is there any hint as to the underlying cause of the respiratory disease, e.g., cachexia in lung cancer or classic features of scleroderma in lung fibrosis?
- Is there any evidence of potential side effects of respiratory medications, i.e., signs of use of corticosteroids (Fig. 9.2) or tremor with salbutamol excess?

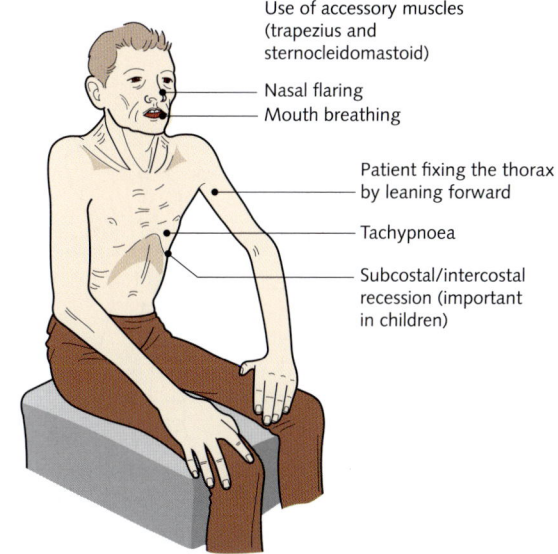

Use of accessory muscles (trapezius and sternocleidomastoid)

Nasal flaring
Mouth breathing

Patient fixing the thorax by leaning forward

Tachypnoea

Subcostal/intercostal recession (important in children)

**Fig. 9.1** Features of respiratory distress. The clinical findings shown are important signs of respiratory distress – with these features the patient will require urgent attention.

**Table 9.1** Respiratory rate

| Normal respiratory rate | 12–20 breaths/min |
|---|---|
| Tachypnoea | >20 breaths/min |
| Bradypnoea | <12 breaths/min |

**Table 9.2** Abnormal breathing patterns

| Breathing pattern | Causes |
|---|---|
| Kussmaul respiration (hyperventilation with deep sighing respirations) | Diabetic ketoacidosis Aspirin overdose Acute massive pulmonary embolism |
| Cheyne–Stokes respiration (increased rate and volume of respiration followed by periods of apnoea) | Terminal disease Increased intracranial pressure |
| Prolongation of expiration | Airflow limitation |
| Pursed-lip breathing | Air trapping |
| Agonal breathing (not getting enough oxygen so gasping for air) | Cardiac arrest Stroke |

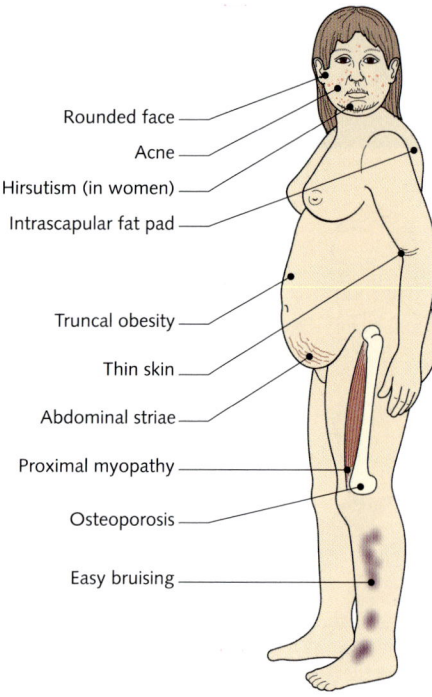

Rounded face
Acne
Hirsutism (in women)
Intrascapular fat pad

Truncal obesity
Thin skin
Abdominal striae
Proximal myopathy
Osteoporosis
Easy bruising

**Fig. 9.2** Side effects of long-term steroid treatment.

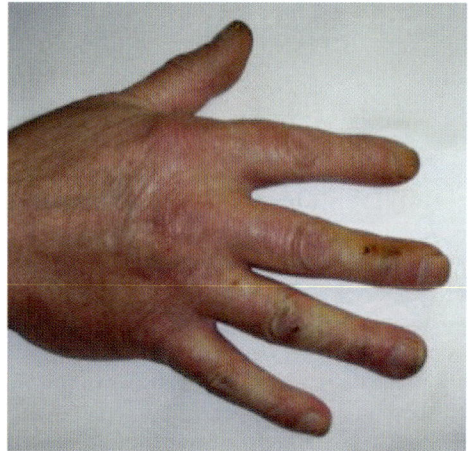

**Fig. 9.3** Tar staining. (From Devereux G, Douglas G. The respiratory system. In: Douglas G, Nicol EF, Robertson C, Macleod J., eds. *Macleod's clinical examination*. 13th ed. London: Elsevier; 2013.)

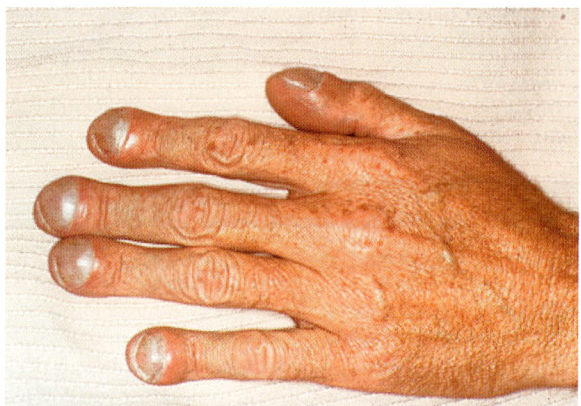

**Fig. 9.4** Clubbing. (From Little JW, Falace DA, Miller CS, et al. Patient evaluation and risk assessment. In: Little JW, ed. *Little and Falace's dental management of the medically compromised patient*. 8th ed. St. Louis: Elsevier; 2013.)

## Hands

Examination of the hands is a key stage in the respiratory examination as there are many important peripheral manifestations of respiratory disease. Ask patients to place their hands in front of them and carefully inspect for the following features:

- Tar staining
- Clubbing
- Peripheral cyanosis
- Carbon dioxide retention
- Tremor
- Muscle wasting
- Rheumatoid arthritis.

### Tar staining

Tar staining is an important clinical feature to note as smoking is an important risk factor for many lung diseases, including chronic obstructive pulmonary disease (COPD) and lung cancer. Tar staining is a yellow discoloration of the fingers and is usually most notable around the fingertips (Fig. 9.3).

### Clubbing

Clubbing is a painless, bulbous enlargement of the distal fingers, which is accompanied by softening of the nail bed and loss of nail bed angle (Fig. 9.4). One method of detecting clubbing is to look

for Schamroth sign (Fig. 9.5). The respiratory causes of clubbing include the following:

- Congenital illness
- Cystic fibrosis
- Bronchial carcinoma
- Mesothelioma
- Pulmonary metastases
- Empyema
- Bronchiectasis
- Lung fibrosis.

There are other, nonrespiratory, causes, which include inflammatory bowel disease, liver cirrhosis, congenital cyanotic heart disease, infective endocarditis and hyperthyroidism (thyroid acropachy).

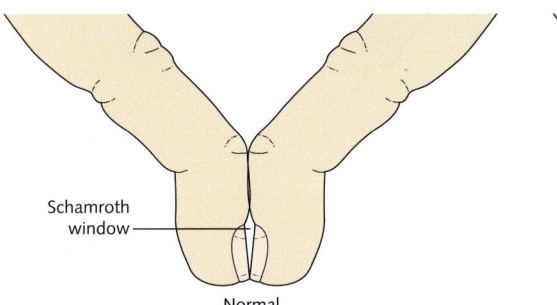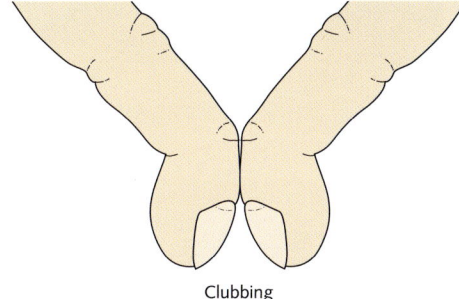

Schamroth window ── Normal

Clubbing

**Fig. 9.5** Schamroth sign (finger clubbing). (Based on Schamroth L. Personal experience. *S Afr Med J*. 1976;50(9):297–300.)

---

**COMMON PITFALLS**

Note chronic obstructive pulmonary disease (COPD) is NOT a cause of clubbing. If a patient with COPD is seen with clubbing, a diagnosis of lung cancer must be excluded. Bronchiectasis, however, is a common differential.

---

## Peripheral cyanosis

Peripheral cyanosis is bluish discoloration of the skin, particularly the fingers. In lung disease this is caused by inadequate oxygenation and warrants further investigation; however, this change may reflect circulatory disorders or cold peripheries.

## Carbon dioxide retention

There are several signs of carbon dioxide retention that can be detected in the hands:

- Warm, well-perfused hands
- Palmar erythema (reddening of the palms)
- Bounding radial pulse
- Carbon dioxide retention flap.

The carbon dioxide retention flap is elicited by asking patients to hold their arms outstretched and to extend their wrists fully. Patients should remain in this position for 30 seconds; in the presence of carbon dioxide retention, they will develop a coarse, irregular tremor as their fingers 'flap' backwards and forwards.

## Tremor

It is common for respiratory patients using $\beta_2$-agonists (i.e., salbutamol) to develop a fine resting tremor. This tremor is again assessed by asking patients to hold their arms outstretched. Unlike carbon dioxide retention, this tremor is very fine and regular and can be exaggerated by laying a piece of paper over the patient's hands.

## Muscle wasting and bony deformities of the hands

These signs are often indirectly related to lung disease and thus are not essential to detect in the respiratory examination. However, if they are detected, they can provide useful information as to the underlying pathology of lung disease. Unilateral muscle wasting

of the hands (particularly in T1 distribution) may hint at the presence of a Pancoast tumour. Another important differential of this pattern of muscle wasting is motor neurone disease, with later stages affecting respiratory muscles causing difficulty in breathing and respiratory failure. Patients with rheumatoid arthritis have classical hand deformities (Fig. 9.6): this autoimmune condition is associated with lung fibrosis. Other rheumatological diseases with pulmonary manifestations may be present, such as sclerodactyly (hard thickening of the skin of the fingers) in systemic sclerosis.

## Radial pulse

A normal resting pulse in an adult is 60–100 beats per minute (bpm). Bradycardia is defined as a pulse rate of less than 60 bpm and tachycardia of greater than 100 bpm. Palpate the radial pulse and count for 15 seconds, then multiply by four to give a rate per minute. Is the pulse regular (Table 9.3)?

The radial pulse can also be assessed for the presence of pulsus paradoxus. In normal individuals, the pulse decreases slightly in volume on inspiration and systolic blood pressure falls by 3–5 mmHg. In severe obstructive diseases (e.g., severe asthma), the contractile force of respiratory muscles is so great that there is a marked fall in systolic pressure on inspiration. A fall of greater than 10 mmHg is pathological.

---

**HINTS AND TIPS**

You will gain marks if your examination looks fluent and professional. It is easy to move smoothly from introducing yourself and shaking the patient's hand, to examination of the hands, to testing the radial pulse. You can then discreetly test for respiratory rate without patients realizing and altering their breathing.

---

## Head and neck

### Examination of the face

First, observe the face generally. You may notice:

- Signs of superior vena cava obstruction (Fig. 9.7)
- Cushingoid features (see Fig. 9.2).

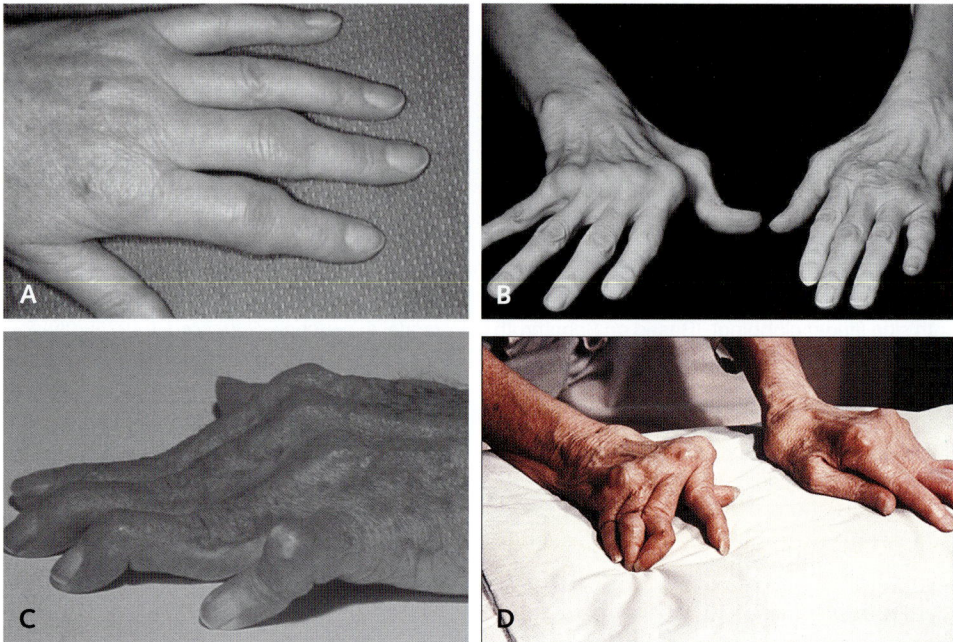

**Fig. 9.6** Rheumatoid hands showing (A) boutonnière deformity (B) ulnar deviation (C) swan neck and (D) Z thumbs.

| Table 9.3 Radial pulse | |
| --- | --- |
| Rate < 100 bpm | Normal |
| Rate > 100 bpm (tachycardia) | Pain |
| | Shock |
| | Infection |
| | Thyrotoxicosis |
| | Pulmonary embolism |
| | Drugs, e.g., salbutamol |
| Full, exaggerated arterial pulsation (bounding pulse) | CO$_2$ retention |
| | Thyrotoxicosis |
| | Fever |
| | Anaemia |
| | Hyperkinetic states |

Look at the mouth for signs of:

- *Candida* infection – white coating on tongue, often seen after steroids or antibiotics
- Central cyanosis.

Central cyanosis is blue discoloration of the mucous membranes of the mouth and represents >5 g/dL of haemoglobin in its reduced form. With normal haemoglobin concentrations, true cyanosis roughly corresponds to a fall in arterial oxygen saturation of <90% or $P_aO_2$ of <8 kPa. In anaemia or hypovolaemia, this sign will only present at lower oxygen concentrations. In lung

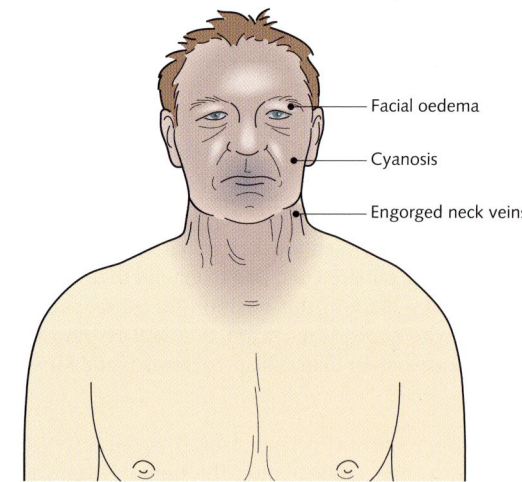

**Fig. 9.7** Superior vena cava obstruction. This can occur in patients with an apical lung tumour.

disease, this is caused by inadequate oxygenation, i.e., in asthma, COPD or pulmonary embolism.

## Eyes

Examine the eyes for evidence of anaemia by asking the patient to look up while pulling down (gently) one lower eyelid. A pale conjunctiva is indicative of anaemia.

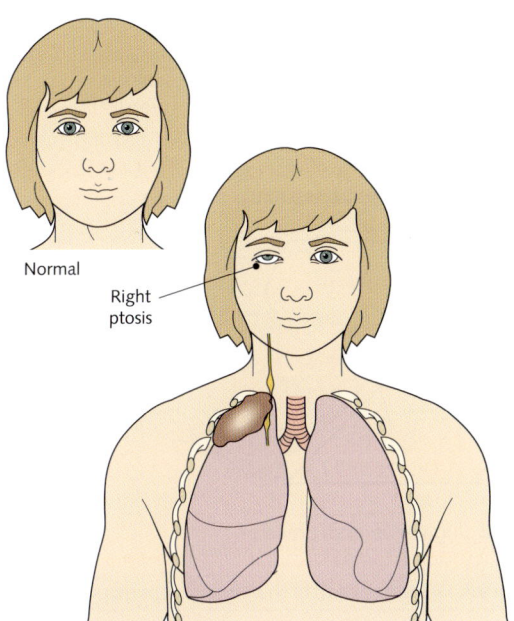

**Fig. 9.8** Horner syndrome.

Examine the eyes carefully, looking for evidence of Horner syndrome (Fig. 9.8), which is characterized by:

- Partial ptosis (drooping of the eyelid)
- Miosis (small pupil)
- Anhydrosis (lack of sweating)
- Enophthalmos (sunken eyeball, not always present).

In respiratory medicine, Horner syndrome can be caused by a Pancoast tumour (see Chapter 17), which is an apical lung tumour. This tumour can press on the sympathetic chain as it ascends in the neck, causing Horner syndrome.

## Examination of the neck

In the neck it is important to examine:

- Trachea (Fig. 9.9) and cricosternal distance (Fig. 9.10)
- Jugular venous pressure (JVP)
- Lymph nodes (Fig. 9.11).

Develop a set system of palpating the lymph nodes of the neck. Sit the patient up and examine from behind with both hands (see Fig. 9.11).

When examining the JVP, ensure the patient is sitting at a 45-degree angle and ask the patient to turn their head to the left (Fig. 9.12). A normal JVP is visible just above the clavicle in between the two heads of the sternocleidomastoid. The JVP can be difficult to see and so it can be accentuated by the hepatojugular reflux (i.e., press down gently over the liver; this increases venous return to the heart and thus increases the JVP). Once found, the height of the JVP should be measured from the sternal notch. If this is >4 cm, the JVP is said to be raised (Table 9.4).

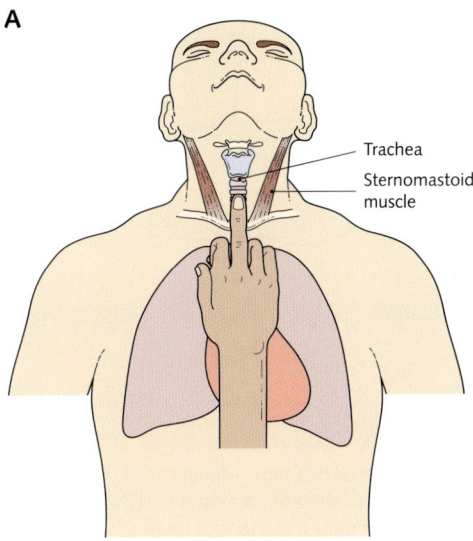

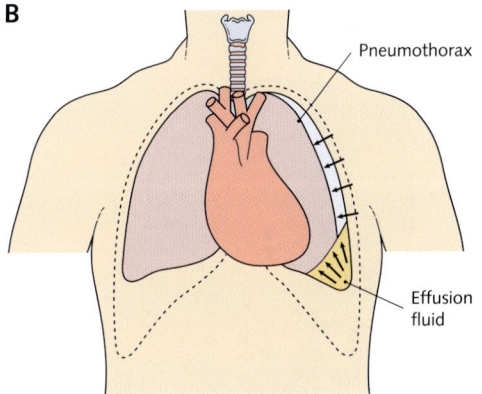

**Fig. 9.9** Tracheal deviation. (A) Tracheal deviation is measured by placing the index and ring fingers on either head of the clavicle. The middle finger is then placed gently on the trachea. In normal patients the trachea will be equidistant between the two heads of the clavicle, i.e., your middle finger will be the same distance from index and ring fingers. (B) In the presence of a tension pneumothorax on the left, the pressure of air in the pleural space causes the trachea to shift to the right. On clinical examination, the trachea would be closer to the right clavicular head than the left.

## The chest

### General inspection of the chest

When undertaking a close inspection of the chest, it is important to pay specific attention to:

- Chest wall deformities (Fig. 9.13)
- Abnormalities of the spine (Fig. 9.14)
- Surgical thoracic incisions (Fig. 9.15)
- Radiotherapy tattoos.

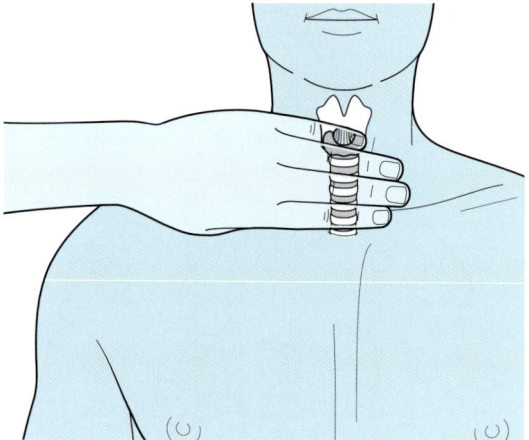

**Fig. 9.10** Cricosternal distance. Measure the distance (using your fingers) between the sternal notch and the cricoid cartilage. This distance is normally three to four fingers. Less than three fingers are indicative of airflow limitation (common in chronic obstructive pulmonary disease).

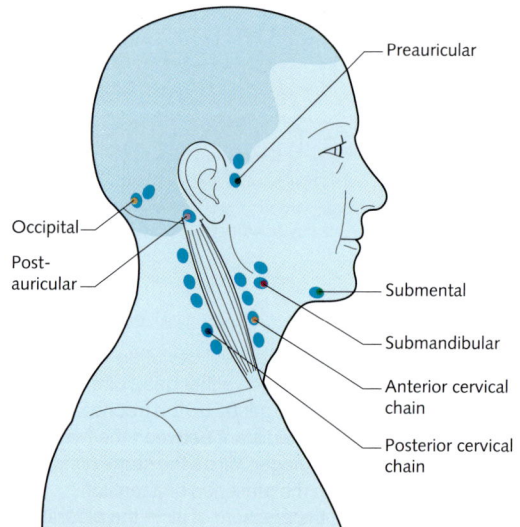

**Fig. 9.11** Anatomy of cervical lymph nodes.

Deformities of the chest wall and spine are clinically important as they can restrict the ventilatory capacity of the lungs.

---

**COMMON PITFALLS**

Remember to look at the front, back and sides of the patient, as key signs may be hidden on initial inspection.

---

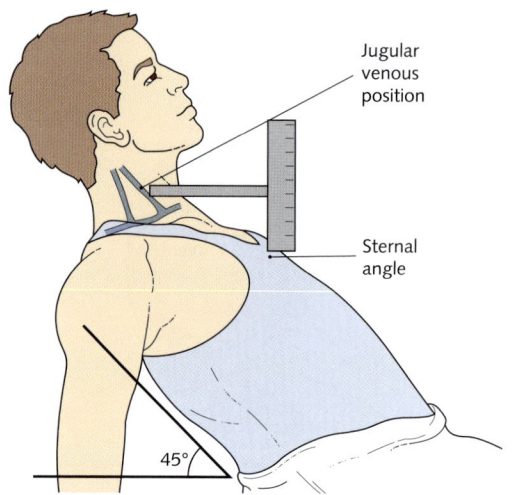

**Fig. 9.12** Jugular venous pressure.

**Table 9.4** Abnormalities of the jugular venous pressure

| Abnormality | Cause |
| --- | --- |
| Raised with normal waveform | Cor pulmonale Fluid overload |
| Raised with absent waveform | Superior vena cava obstruction |
| Absent | Dehydration, shock |

## Palpation

Palpation in the respiratory examination primarily involves assessing chest expansion both anteroposteriorly (AP) and laterally (Fig. 9.16). When testing chest expansion in the AP direction, place the palms of both hands on the pectoral region and ask the patient to take a deep breath. The chest should expand symmetrically. Any asymmetry suggests pathology on the side that fails to expand adequately. Testing lateral expansion of the chest involves gripping the chest (Fig. 9.16) between both hands and then asking the patient to take a deep breath while observing the movement of your own thumbs. Again, the movement of your thumbs should be symmetrical and any asymmetry suggests pathology on the side of the chest that does not expand fully.

Next, examine for the position of the apex beat of the heart by moving your hand inwards from the lateral chest until you feel the pulsation. The apex beat should be in the fifth intercostal space at the midclavicular line. Displacement of the apex beat normally signifies cardiomegaly, but other respiratory conditions may cause the apex beat to become displaced, including:

- Pulmonary fibrosis
- Bronchiectasis
- Pleural effusions
- Pneumothoraces.

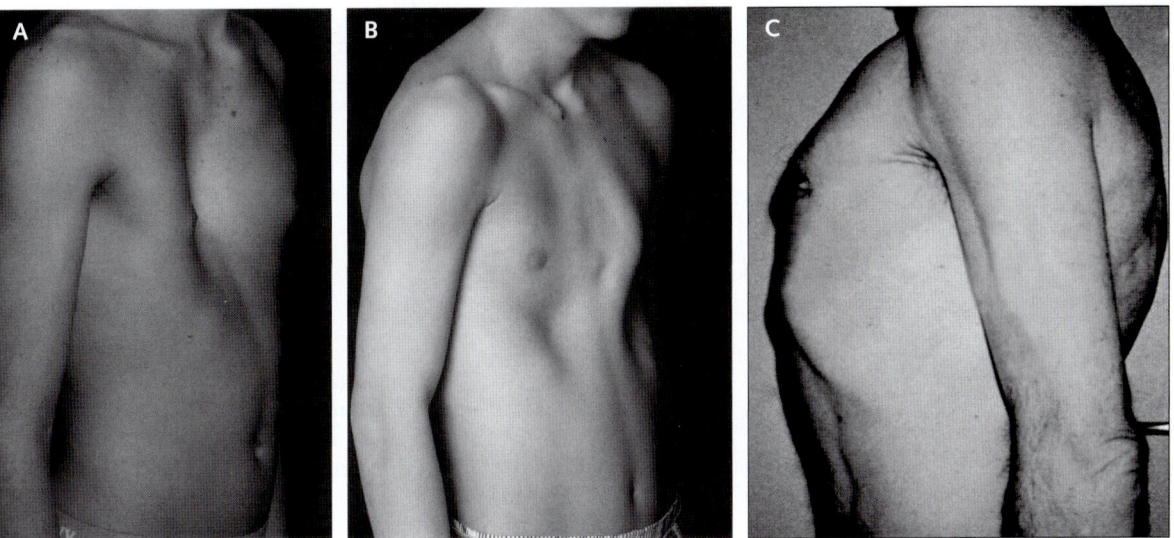

**Fig. 9.13** Chest wall deformities. (A) Pectus excavatum: a benign condition whereby the sternum is depressed in relation to the ribs. (B) Pectus carinatum (pigeon chest): the sternum is more prominent in comparison to the ribs – often caused by severe childhood asthma. (C) Barrel chest: the anteroposterior diameter of the chest is greater than the lateral diameter. Caused by hyperinflation of the lungs.

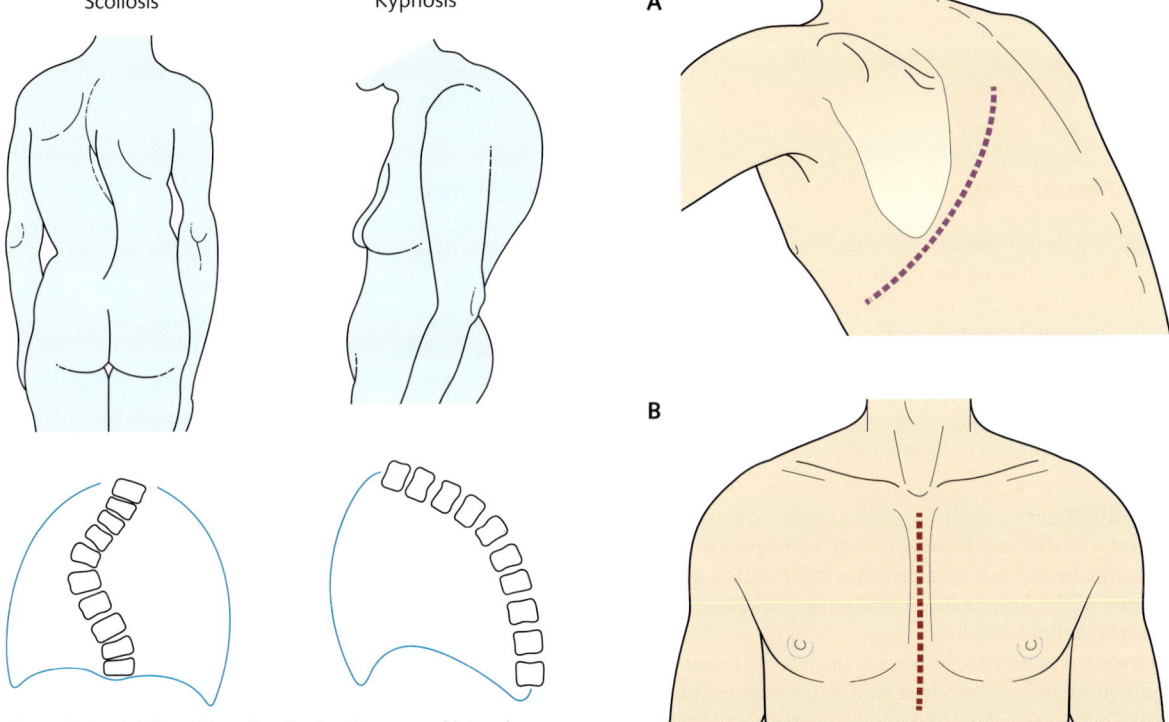

**Fig. 9.14** Spinal deformities. Scoliosis – increased lateral curvature of the spine. Kyphosis – increased forward curvature of the spine (osteoporosis/ankylosing spondylitis). Both cause ventilatory defects and can cause respiratory failure.

**Fig. 9.15** Common thoracic surgical incisions. (A) Lateral thoracotomy; (B) midline sternotomy.

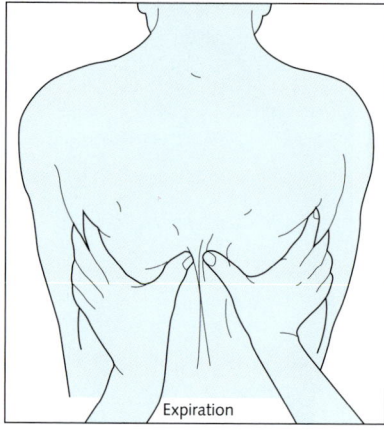

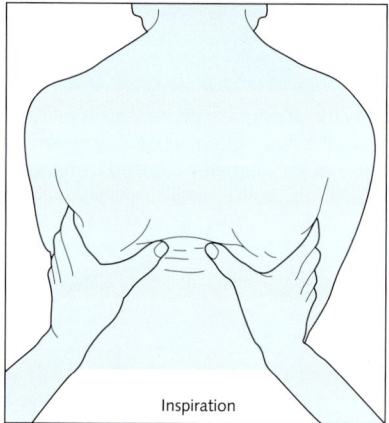

**Fig. 9.16** Chest expansion.

Finally, in palpation you may find it useful to perform tactile vocal fremitus by placing the ulnar edge of your hand on the chest wall while asking the patient to say '99' repeatedly. This is repeated throughout the chest, both front and back, comparing opposite zones. The vibrations produced by this manoeuvre are transmitted through the lung parenchyma and felt by the hand. Tactile vocal fremitus is increased by consolidation of the lungs and decreased by pleural effusions and pleural thickening.

## Percussion

Percussion is an extremely useful tool in the respiratory examination, as the percussion note provides information about the consistency of the lung matter underlying the chest wall, i.e., whether it is air, fluid or solid.

Percussion is performed by placing the middle finger of your nondominant hand on the chest wall palm downwards in an intercostal space. You then strike this finger with the terminal phalanx (fingertip) of the middle finger of your dominant hand. To achieve a good percussion note, the striking finger should be partially flexed and struck at right angles to the other finger.

| Table 9.5 Abnormalities of percussion | |
|---|---|
| **Percussion note** | **Pathology** |
| Hyperresonant | Pneumothorax |
| | Emphysema with large bullae |
| Dull | Consolidation |
| | Fibrosis |
| | Pleural thickening |
| | Collapse |
| | Infection |
| Stony dull | Pleural effusion |

Percuss in a logical order. Begin percussion at the apices by percussing (gently) onto the clavicles directly and then move down the chest wall, remembering to compare both sides directly. A normal percussion note is described as resonant; in the presence of lung pathology, the percussion note may be described as dull, stony dull or hyperresonant (Table 9.5).

Map out any abnormality you find but do not confuse the cardiac borders or liver edge with lung pathology; they will sound dull normally. The note also sounds muffled in a very muscular or obese patient.

**HINTS AND TIPS**

When percussing, remember that the upper lobe predominates anteriorly and the lower lobe predominates posteriorly.

## Auscultation

Normal breath sounds are described as vesicular and have a rustling quality heard in inspiration and the first part of expiration. Listen to the patient's chest:

- Using the bell of the stethoscope in the apices (supraclavicular area)
- Using the diaphragm of the stethoscope elsewhere on the chest.

Auscultate in a logical order, comparing the two sides (as for percussion) and ask the patient to breathe through an open mouth. You should be listening for:

- Diminished breath sounds
- Bronchial breathing
- Added sounds, such as wheezes or stridor, crackles or pleural rubs. Crackles are characterized by their timing: fine crackles usually indicate an interstitial process and may be in early or late inspiration (early indicates pulmonary oedema, late inspiratory indicates pulmonary fibrosis). Coarse crackles usually indicate an airway disease such as bronchiectasis and are in early inspiration.

It is important to remember that added sounds that disappear when the patient coughs are not significant (Table 9.6).

**Table 9.6** Abnormal breath sounds

| Abnormality | Definition | Associated with: |
|---|---|---|
| Diminished vesicular breath sounds | Reduced breath sounds | Airway obstruction |
| | | Asthma |
| | | COPD |
| Bronchial breathing | Harsh breath sounds whereby inspiration and expiration are of equal duration | Consolidation |
| | | Pneumonia |
| | | Empyema |
| **Added sounds** | | |
| Monophonic wheeze | Prolonged musical sound (expiratory) | Large-airway obstruction |
| Polyphonic wheeze | Prolonged musical sound – many notes (expiratory) | Small-airway obstruction |
| | | Asthma |
| | | COPD |
| Coarse crackles | Nonmusical uninterrupted sounds (inspiratory) | Consolidation |
| | | COPD |
| | | Bronchiectasis |
| | | BB |
| Fine crackles | Nonmusical uninterrupted sounds (inspiratory) like Velcro | Early inspiration |
| | | Pulmonary oedema |
| | | Late inspiration |
| | | Fibrosis |
| Pleural rub | Pneumonia | Pulmonary embolism |
| | | Pleurisy |

*BB, Bronchial breathing; COPD, chronic obstructive pulmonary disease.*

## Vocal resonance

Vocal resonance is the auscultatory equivalent of tactile vocal fremitus. It is performed using the diaphragm of the stethoscope on the chest and asking the patient to say '99'. Vocal resonance is increased by consolidation and reduced by conditions such as pleural effusion and pneumothoraces.

## Whispering pectoriloquy

Whispering pectoriloquy is a variation of vocal resonance that can be used to confirm the presence of consolidation. The patient is asked to whisper '99'. In normal lungs, this cannot be heard by auscultation. However, solid lung conducts sound better than normal aerated lung and thus in patients with areas of consolidation the words are clear and seem to be spoken into the examiner's ear.

# Examination summary

Once you have finished your examination, summarize your findings in a clear and concise manner. Give an overview of the patient's general condition and present your positive examination findings, as well as relevant negatives. Based on your examination findings, you should give a differential diagnosis and explain the relevant next investigation steps to confirm this. Normally, to complete the respiratory examination you would inform the examiner that you would like to:

- View the patient's observations, including temperature and oxygen saturations
- Take a peak flow reading
- Examine a sputum pot and send samples for MCS
- Perform relevant blood tests
- Consider an erect chest X-ray.

Table 9.7 summarizes the common clinical findings for the most common respiratory conditions.

**Table 9.7** Summary of signs found on examination of the respiratory system

| | Consolidation | Pneumothorax | Pleural effusion | Lobar collapse | Pleural thickening |
|---|---|---|---|---|---|
| Chest radiograph | | | | | |
| Mediastinal shift and trachea | None | None (simple), away (tension) | None or away | Towards the affected side | None |
| Chest wall excursion | Normal or decreased on the affected side | Normal or decreased on the affected side | Decreased on the affected side | Decreased | Decreased |
| Percussion note | Dull | Hyperresonant | Stony dull | Dull | Dull |
| Breath sounds | Increased (bronchial) | Decreased | Decreased | Decreased | Decreased |
| Added sounds | Crackles | Click (occasional) | Rub (occasional) | None | None |
| Tactile vocal fremitus or vocal resonance | Increased | Decreased | Decreased | Decreased | Decreased |

## Chapter Summary

- A full respiratory examination comprises inspection, palpation, percussion and auscultation.
- Features of respiratory distress seen on inspection determine whether urgent intervention is needed.
- Differences in percussion and auscultation allow you to differentiate between pleural effusion, consolidation and pneumothorax.
- Advanced examination techniques such as tactile vocal fremitus and whispering pectoriloquy distinguish finer examination points.
- Giving a clear summary of relevant examination findings allows you to form a differential diagnosis. This can be used to guide next steps for investigation and treatment.

### MLA Conditions

Asthma
Bronchiectasis
COPD
Diabetic ketoacidosis
Motor neurone disease
Pleural effusion
Pneumonia
Pneumothorax
Pulmonary embolism

### MLA Presentations

Breathlessness
Ptosis
Stridor
Tremor
Wheeze

# The respiratory patient: clinical investigations  10

## INTRODUCTION

There are a large number of investigations used in respiratory medicine, ranging from basic bedside tests to more invasive procedures such as bronchoscopy. As you read this chapter, you should bear in mind that some of the investigations detailed are performed only rarely in specialized pulmonary laboratories, while others are performed by patients at home every day. The investigations that are most commonly performed, and of which you should have a thorough knowledge, include:

- Arterial blood gas (ABG) analysis
- Sputum examination
- Basic tests of pulmonary function
- Bronchoscopy
- Chest radiographs (chest X-rays).

Other, less commonly performed, investigations will be discussed in less detail in this chapter.

## ROUTINE INVESTIGATIONS

### Blood tests

In the associated figures, you will find some of the commonly performed haematological tests:

- Full blood count (Table 10.1)
- Differential white blood cell count (Table 10.2).

## Clinical chemistry

The commonly performed biochemical tests include:

- Renal function – baseline important prior to imaging with contrast or when prescribing medications.
- Calcium levels – may be raised in metastatic disease, paraneoplastic syndromes or sarcoidosis.
- Liver function tests – may be abnormal in malignancy.
- C-reactive protein (CRP) – inflammatory marker useful in acute and chronic infections.

In addition, endocrine tests should be performed for paraneoplastic manifestations, such as syndrome of inappropriate antidiuretic hormone, if clinically appropriate (see Chapter 17 for more detail).

## Measures of oxygenations

### Pulse oximetry

This is a simple, noninvasive method of monitoring the percentage of haemoglobin that is saturated with oxygen. The patient wears a probe on a finger or earlobe linked to a unit which displays the readings. The unit can be set to sound an alarm when saturation drops below a certain level (usually 90%). The pulse oximeter works by calculating the absorption of light by haemoglobin, which alters depending on whether it is saturated with oxygen or desaturated. A number of factors may lead to inaccurate oximeter readings. These include:

- Poor peripheral perfusion, such as in hypothermia or Raynaud disease

**Table 10.1** Full blood count

| Test | Normal values | Increased values | Decreased values | Diagnostic inference |
|------|---------------|-------------------|------------------|----------------------|
| Haemoglobin (g/dL) | Male: 13–18 Female: 11.5–16.5 | Increased in chronic respiratory disease such as COPD, as part of a secondary polycythaemia due to longstanding hypoxia | | Decreased in anaemia (look at MCV for further information); a normal MCV (i.e., normocytic anaemia) is common in chronic disease |
| MCV (fL) | 76–98 | Macrocytosis (vitamin $B_{12}$ or folate deficiency, etc.) | | Microcytosis (common in iron-deficiency anaemia and thalassaemias) |
| Red blood cells (× $10^9$/L) | Male: 4.5–6.5 Female: 3.8–5.8 | Polycythaemia; may be secondary to chronic lung disease, smoking, altitude | | |

*COPD, Chronic obstructive pulmonary disease; MCV, mean cell volume.*

**Table 10.2** Differential white blood cell count

| Cell type | Normal values | Diagnostic inference | |
|---|---|---|---|
| | | **Increased values** | **Decreased values** |
| White blood cell | $4–11 \times 10^9$/L | Bacterial infections<br>Malignancy<br>Pregnancy<br>Long-term steroids | Viral infections<br>Drugs<br>Systemic lupus erythematosus<br>Overwhelming bacterial infection |
| Neutrophil | $2.5–7.5 \times 10^9$/L, 60%–70% | Bacterial infections<br>Malignancy<br>Pregnancy<br>Steroid treatment | Viral infections<br>Drugs<br>Systemic lupus erythematosus<br>Overwhelming bacterial infection |
| Eosinophil | $0.04–0.44 \times 10^9$/L, 1%–4% | Allergic reactions<br>Asthma<br>Sarcoidosis<br>Pneumonia<br>Eosinophilic granulomatosis | Steroid therapy |
| Monocyte | $0.2–0.8 \times 10^9$/L, 5%–10% | Tuberculosis | Chronic infection |
| Lymphocyte | $1.5–4.0 \times 10^9$/L, 25%–30% | Infection<br>Cytomegalovirus infection<br>Toxoplasmosis<br>Tuberculosis | Tuberculosis |

- Carbon monoxide poisoning
- Skin pigmentation
- Nail varnish
- Dirty hands.

A more accurate assessment of oxygen saturation, if necessary, can be obtained by ABG analysis.

## Arterial blood gas analysis

In Chapter 5 we learnt about the role of the lungs in acid–base balance. Analysis of an ABG sample tells us about the patient's gas exchange and their acid–base status. Consider performing an ABG in all acutely unwell patients. If possible, the analysis should be performed initially on room air and then repeated soon after starting oxygen therapy to assess response to treatment; however, in the acutely unwell, this may not be appropriate.

An ABG sample is normally taken from a patient's radial artery using a heparinized syringe. The radial artery is preferred to other sites (e.g., brachial or femoral arteries) because it is easily accessed on the radial aspect of a patient's wrist. It is palpable as it is relatively superficial and it has collateral blood supply to the hand via the ulnar artery. However, in about 3% of people, the blood running through the ulnar artery is not enough to adequately perfuse the hand. In rare instances, an ABG could lead to a potential occlusion of the radial artery due to clot formation and therefore prior to performing this test, an Allen test should be performed. The Allen test is performed by asking the patient to first elevate both arms for 30 seconds; next the patient makes a tight fist and the examiner occludes the ulnar artery. The patient then opens their hands rapidly. The initial pallor should be replaced with normal colour. The test is then repeated with the

**Table 10.3** Arterial blood gas normal values

| Test | Normal value |
|---|---|
| pH | 7.35–7.45 |
| $P_aO_2$ | >10 kPa |
| $P_aCO_2$ | 4.6–6.0 kPa |
| Base excess | +/−2 mmol/L |
| Bicarbonate | 22–26 mmol/L |
| Lactate | <2 mmol/L |

*The normal values presented here are internationally accepted values, however, the reference ranges may vary slightly based on the laboratory that they are being conducted in.*

radial artery occluded. Persistent pallor on occlusion of the radial artery suggests inadequate collateral blood flow. In this instance an ABG should be performed from a different site. The ABG sample should be tested immediately using a standard automated machine, which measures:

- $P_aO_2$
- $P_aCO_2$
- pH.

Bicarbonate, oxygen saturations and base excess are derived by the analyzer from the above measurements and given on the standard readout, along with other values including electrolytes, glucose and lactate.

The patient's results are compared with the normal ranges (Table 10.3) and assessed in two parts:

- Oxygenation and ventilation – is the patient hypoxic? Is the patient hypercapnic?
  - Type I respiratory failure – $P_aO_2 < 8$ kPa and $P_aCO_2 \leq 6$ kPa

**Table 10.4** Summary of arterial blood gas findings

| pH | $P_aCO_2$ | Bicarbonate | Summary | Causes |
|---|---|---|---|---|
| <7.35 | Normal/low (respiratory compensation) | Low | Metabolic acidosis | Lactic acid Uraemia Ketones Toxins |
| <7.35 | High | May be raised if chronic type II respiratory failure | Respiratory acidosis | Decompensated type II respiratory failure |
| 7.35–7.45 | Normal | Normal | Normal | Healthy patient |
| >7.45 | Low | Normal | Respiratory alkalosis | Hyperventilation: intracranial causes, e.g., stroke Pulmonary embolism Anxiety |
| >7.45 | Normal/high (respiratory compensation) | Raised | Metabolic alkalosis | Vomiting Burns |

- Type II respiratory failure – $P_aO_2 < 8\,kPa$ and $P_aCO_2 > 6\,kPa$
- Acid–base balance disturbances – is the patient acidotic or alkalotic? What is the cause for this disturbance? Look at the $P_aCO_2$ and bicarbonate levels.

ABG results should always be interpreted within the clinical picture. Different underlying pathologies will cause different patterns in the ABG. It is important to remember that a metabolic disturbance (such as high lactate from shock) can be partially or completely compensated for by the respiratory system, which may be seen clinically as an increased respiratory rate and will be demonstrated in the ABG result by a low $P_aCO_2$. Table 10.4 shows a summary of ABG findings and their possible underlying pathologies. An approach to interpreting a blood gas can be found in Chapter 12.

# Microbiology

Microbiological examination is possible with samples of sputum, bronchial aspirate, pleural aspirate, throat swabs and blood. The aim of examination is to identify bacteria, viruses or fungi.

Tests to request are microscopy, culture and antibiotic sensitivity (M, C & S). The microbiological findings should be interpreted in view of the whole clinical picture.

## Sputum culture

Testing of sputum for the presence of bacteria is the most common microbiological test performed. If the patient is expectorating, obtain a sample of sputum, preferably before antibiotic treatment is started. Collect in a sterile container, inspect the sample and send it to the laboratory.

A sputum sample is valuable in diagnosing the causative organism in severe pneumonia or when mycobacterial or fungal infection is suspected. Failure to isolate an organism from the sputum is not uncommon. As antimicrobial resistance is increasing if an organism is isolated, sensitivity to antibiotics should be checked to guide antibacterial treatment choice. If tuberculosis (TB) is suspected, samples should be sent for Ziehl–Neelsen staining to look for acid–fast bacilli – further information can be found in Chapter 18: Respiratory infections.

If the patient is unable to expectorate sputum, a physiotherapist can help to obtain induced sputum using nebulized hypertonic saline. If chronic infection is present or an atypical pathogen is suspected, bronchoscopy may be required to obtain bronchial washings for microbiological analysis.

## Blood culture

Blood cultures identify systemic bacterial and fungal infections. Results may be positive while sputum culture is negative. It is important to collect at least one set of cultures before starting antibiotic therapy. A blood culture should always be performed in patients with fever and signs of a lower respiratory tract infection, or if a patient meets sepsis criteria as defined by the National Institute for Clinical Excellence Sepsis Guideline 2016.

When collecting blood cultures, it is important to clean the skin site thoroughly prior to taking blood, using 2% chlorhexidine in 70% isopropyl alcohol to disinfect the skin. Using a sterile nontouch technique and a blood-sampling device with blood culture adapter, collect 10 mL of blood into both the aerobic and anaerobic culture bottles. Ideally, two sets of blood cultures should be taken within the first hour.

## Viral tests

Testing for viruses has changed from traditional viral culture and serology techniques to molecular diagnostics, including viral polymerase chain reaction (PCR) tests. Molecular diagnostics are much faster and often give results within 24 hours. This can help guide patient management and is also useful when monitoring for viral epidemics. A throat swab can be sent for viral PCR testing if a patient has signs suggesting a viral respiratory tract

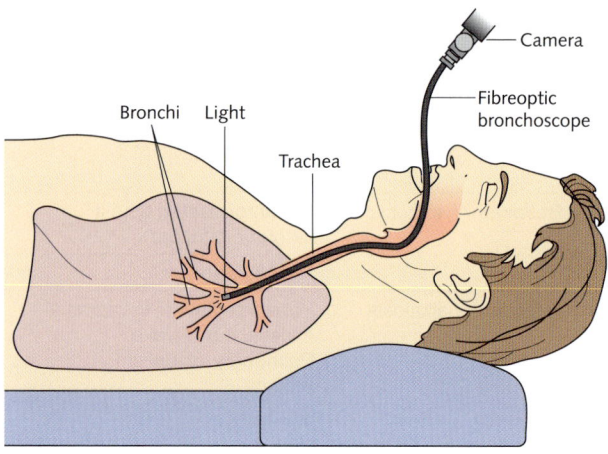

**Fig. 10.1** Bronchoscopy.

infection. Viral testing of sputum samples or bronchial washings may be considered in immunocompromised or very sick patients with suspected viral pneumonia.

## INVASIVE PROCEDURES

## Bronchoscopy

Bronchoscopy is the passing of a telescope via the nose or mouth into the trachea to inspect the large and medium-sized airways via visualization with a camera (Fig. 10.1). It can be used to sample tissues via brushings, lavage or biopsy. Two types of bronchoscope are used:

- Flexible fibreoptic bronchoscope – used by respiratory physicians normally under light sedation to reduce anxiety and suppress cough mechanisms. Topical lidocaine is used as a local anaesthetic to numb the pharynx, vocal cords and bronchial tree.
- Rigid bronchoscope – used by thoracic surgeons in theatre with the patient under general anaesthetic.

Flexible bronchoscopy is most commonly used. The main indications for bronchoscopy are:

- Diagnosis and staging of lung cancer – if the diagnosis is suspected following symptoms or suspicious imaging.
- Diagnosis of infections – especially useful in immunocompromised patients and those with atypical infections or suspected TB.
- Diagnosis of interstitial lung disease (ILD) – transbronchial biopsy may be required.
- Removal of suspected proximal foreign body, e.g., an inhaled pea.
- Investigating unexplained haemoptysis.

Flexible bronchoscopy is generally a safe procedure with very low mortality rates but complications include respiratory depression, laryngospasm and haemorrhage following scope trauma. It usually takes place as a day case procedure. Relative contraindications to performing the procedure include low oxygen levels at rest (<90%) and clotting abnormalities or a low platelet count (<50,000/mm$^3$).

## Bronchoalveolar lavage

Sterile saline (usually around 100 mL) is infused down the flexible bronchoscope into the bronchioles and then aspirated. This technique is commonly used to look for evidence of neoplasms or opportunistic infections in immunocompromised patients. If this is done in the acute setting and the patient is unwell, a smaller volume of saline (usually around 10–20 mL) is used to avoid airway compromise, known as bronchial washing.

## Transbronchial biopsy

Transbronchial biopsy provides samples from outside the airways, e.g., of parenchymal tissue. The technique is performed using biopsy forceps fed through a flexible bronchoscope. The bronchoscopist cannot directly visualize the biopsy site ('blind' biopsy) as the biopsy forceps are passed down to the terminal bronchus out of sight of the scope. There is an increased risk of haemorrhage and pneumothorax with this procedure and therefore a chest X-ray should be performed as routine following the bronchoscopy.

## Endobronchial ultrasound

Endobronchial ultrasound (EBUS) is a technique in which an ultrasound probe is placed down the bronchoscope, allowing real-time visualization of deeper structures through the bronchial wall, such as lymph nodes, major vessels and paratracheal masses. This allows image-guided transbronchial needle aspiration (TBNA) of lymph nodes and is therefore very useful in both diagnosing and staging lung cancer.

## Lung biopsy

### Percutaneous fine-needle aspiration

This technique is used to sample lung lesions under the guidance of radiography. It is commonly performed by interventional radiologists under computed tomography guidance. Complications include pneumothorax post biopsy which may require a chest drain.

## Surgical lung biopsy

In some cases of diffuse lung disease, or where a lesion cannot easily be reached, a more extensive lung biopsy is required for diagnosis. Surgical lung biopsy can be performed using video-assisted thoracoscopic surgery (VATS) techniques or via open-lung biopsy. Both surgical interventions require general anaesthesia; however, VATS is less invasive as it does not require thoracotomy. Surgical techniques allow therapeutic intervention at the same time as biopsy.

## Pleural procedures

Details on pleural aspiration and interpretation of results can be found in Chapter 20: Pleural disease.

### Thoracoscopy

Respiratory physicians perform medical thoracoscopy under local anaesthetic and light sedation. The procedure allows the examination and biopsy of the pleura, the drainage of fluid from the pleural space and, if indicated, chemical pleurodesis. The main indication for the procedure is to investigate the cause of an exudative pleural effusion and diagnose diseases such as cancer or TB. The pleural effusion is first identified using pleural ultrasound, and then the port is inserted through an intercostal space via blunt dissection through which the fluid is drained and an iatrogenic pneumothorax is created. A rigid thoracoscope with a camera is then passed into the pleural space and the pleura can be inspected and biopsied. If the appearance is consistent with malignancy, 4 g of sterile talc may be inserted into the pleural space to irritate the pleural surface and try to achieve pleurodesis (the visceral and parietal pleura to 'stick' together) and prevent fluid reaccumulation. At the end of the procedure, a chest drain is inserted down the tract made by the port to allow drainage of the pneumothorax. The patient normally requires an overnight stay in hospital, but can be discharged once the lung has reinflated and the chest drain is removed.

## INVESTIGATIONS OF PULMONARY FUNCTION

Tests of pulmonary function are used in:

- Diagnosis of lung disease
- Monitoring disease progression
- Assessing patient response to treatment.

## Tests of ventilation

Ventilation can be impaired in two basic ways:

- The airways become narrowed (obstructive disorders)
- Expansion of the lungs is reduced (restrictive disorders).

These two types of disorder have characteristic patterns of lung function which can be measured using the tests below.

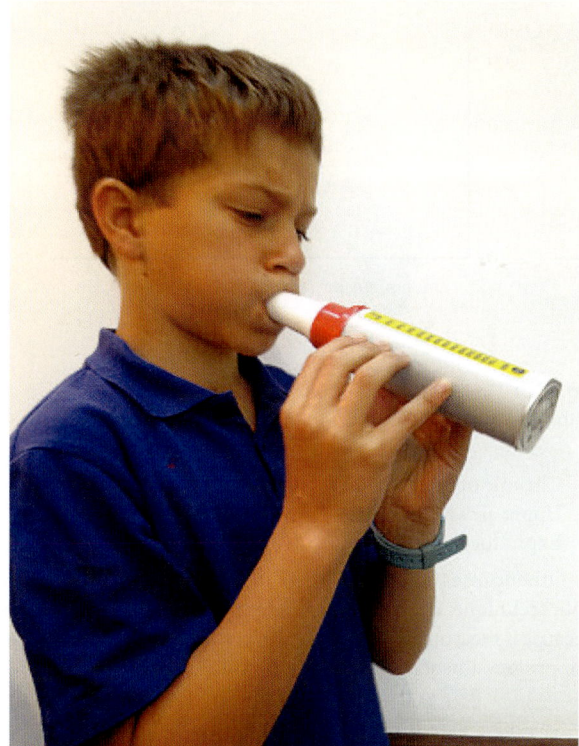

**Fig. 10.2** Peak flow meter. (From Lissauer T, Carroll W. *Illustrated Textbook of Paediatrics*. 5th ed. Elsevier; 2018.)

## Peak expiratory flow rate

Peak expiratory flow rate (PEFR) is a simple and cheap test that uses a peak flow meter (Fig. 10.2) to measure a person's maximum speed of expiration. Peak flow meters can be issued on prescription and used at home by patients to monitor their lung function.

Before measuring PEFR, the practitioner should instruct the patient to:

- Take a full inspiration to maximum lung capacity.
- Seal the lips tightly around the mouthpiece.
- Blow out forcefully into the peak flow meter, which is held horizontally.

The best of three measurements is recorded and plotted on the appropriate graph. Normal PEFR is 400–650 L/min in healthy adults. At least two recordings per day are required to obtain an accurate pattern. A patient would normally be asked to do this for a couple of weeks in order to obtain a peak flow diary, which could then be analyzed to look at the type of airways disease.

PEFR is reduced in conditions that cause airway obstruction:

- Asthma, where there is wide diurnal variation in PEFR, known as 'morning dipping' (Fig. 10.3)

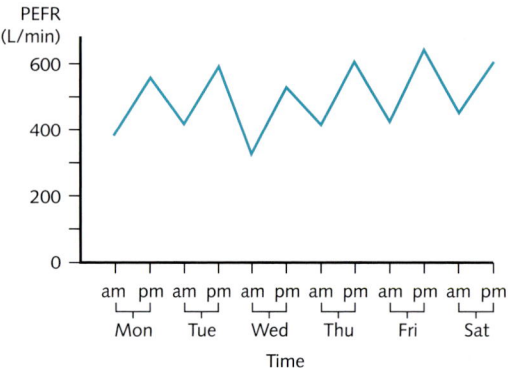

**Fig. 10.3** Typical peak expiratory flow rate graph for an asthmatic patient.

- Chronic obstructive pulmonary disease (COPD)
- Upper airway tumours
- Expiratory muscle weakness.

Other causes of reduced PEFR include inadequate effort and poor technique. PEFR is not a good measure of airflow limitation because it measures only initial expiration; it is best used to monitor progression of disease and response to treatment.

---

**CLINICAL NOTES**

In asthma, regular home monitoring of peak expiratory flow rate with a home device can be useful for predicting the onset and severity of an exacerbation. Asthma patients are issued with a personalized asthma action plan telling them what to do if their peak flow is lower than normal, depending on how severe the reduction is. By increasing treatment earlier can help reduce the severity and length of exacerbations and also ensures that the sickest patients seek medical help sooner.

---

# Spirometry

The forced expiratory volume in 1 second ($FEV_1$) and the forced vital capacity (FVC) are measured using a spirometer. The spirometer works by converting volumes of inspiration and expiration into a single line trace. Spirometry is now performed using electronic devices with a mouthpiece into which the subject breathes. In addition to producing $FEV_1$ and FVC readings, some spirometers produce flow–volume loops and calculate the results as a percentage of the normal predicted value for the patient. The test should be performed with the patient seated and with a nose clip in place. To obtain an $FEV_1$ measurement, the patient should take a full breath in and blow out into the

mouthpiece forcibly, as hard and fast as possible, for as long as possible. The test should be repeated three times to achieve at least two comparable readings.

---

**HINTS AND TIPS**

**PULMONARY FUNCTION TESTS**

Pulmonary function tests can seem confusing, but there are just three basic questions that most tests aim to answer:

- Are the airways narrowed? (PEFR, $FEV_1$, $FEV_1$:FVC, flow–volume loops)
- Are the lungs a normal size? (TLC, RV and FRC)
- Is gas uptake normal? ($T_LCO$ and KCO).

So, as a minimum, make sure you have a good understanding of peak flow monitoring and spirometry and know how you would measure RV, FRC and gas transfer.

*$FEV_1$,* Forced expiratory volume in 1 second; *FRC,* functional residual capacity; *FVC,* forced vital capacity; *KCO,* transfer coefficient; *PEFR,* peak expiratory flow rate; *RV,* residual volume; *TLC,* total lung capacity; *$T_LCO$,* transfer factor.

---

## $FEV_1$ and FVC

$FEV_1$ and FVC are related to the height, age and sex of the patient. $FEV_1$ is the volume of air expelled in the first second of a forced expiration, starting from full inspiration. FVC is a measure of total lung volume exhaled; the patient is asked to exhale with maximal effort after a full inspiration.

## $FEV_1$:FVC ratio

The $FEV_1$:FVC ratio is a more useful measurement than $FEV_1$ or FVC alone. $FEV_1$ is 80% of FVC in normal subjects. The $FEV_1$:FVC ratio is an excellent measure of airway limitation and allows us to differentiate obstructive from restrictive lung disease.

In restrictive disease:

- Both $FEV_1$ and FVC are reduced, often in proportion to each other
- $FEV_1$:FVC ratio is normal or increased (>80%)

whereas in obstructive diseases:

- High intrathoracic pressures generated by forced expiration cause premature closure of the airways with trapping of air in the chest
- $FEV_1$ is reduced much more than FVC
- $FEV_1$:FVC ratio is reduced (<70%).

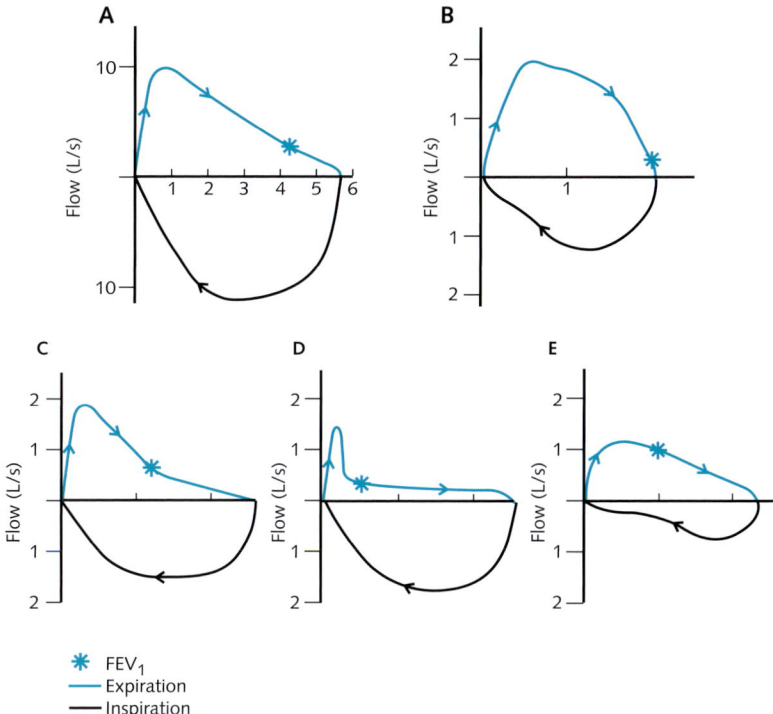

**Fig. 10.4** Typical flow–volume loops. (A) Normal. (B) Restrictive defect (phrenic palsy). (C) Volume-dependent obstruction (e.g., asthma). (D) Pressure-dependent obstruction (e.g., severe emphysema). (E) Rigid obstruction (e.g., tracheal stenosis). *FEV₁*, Forced expiratory volume in 1 second.

## Flow–volume loops

Flow–volume loops are graphs constructed from maximal expiratory and inspiratory manoeuvres performed on a spirometer. The loop is made up of two halves: above the $x$-axis is the flow of air out of the mouth on expiration, and below the $x$-axis, flow into the mouth on inspiration. The loop shape can identify the type and distribution of airway obstruction. After a small amount of gas has been exhaled, flow is limited by:

- Elastic recoil force of the lung
- Resistance of airways upstream of collapse.

When looking at flow–volume loops, look for a normal-shaped loop (Fig. 10.4): a triangular expiratory curve created by an initially fast expiration of air, slowing down as total lung capacity (TLC) is reached, and a semicircular inspiratory curve. Any deviation away from this triangle and semicircle pattern suggests pathology. Additionally, read off the $FEV_1$ (marked by a star) from the $x$-axis. Reduced $FEV_1$ suggests an obstructive airway disease.

Flow–volume loops are useful in diagnosing upper airway obstruction, restrictive and obstructive disease (Fig. 10.4).

In restrictive diseases:

- Maximum flow rate is reduced (read from $y$-axis).
- Total volume exhaled is reduced (read from $x$-axis).
- Flow rate is high during the latter part of expiration because of increased lung recoil.

In obstructive diseases:

- Flow rate is low in relation to lung volume.
- Expiration ends prematurely because of early airway closure, most easily spotted by a scooped-out appearance after the point of maximum flow rather than the triangular-shaped expiratory curve seen in healthy lungs.

## Tests of diffusion

Oxygen and carbon dioxide pass by diffusion between the alveoli and pulmonary capillary blood. The diffusing capacity of carbon monoxide measures the ability of gas to diffuse from inspired air to capillary blood, and also reflects the uptake of oxygen from the alveolus into the red blood cells. Carbon monoxide (CO) is used because:

- It is highly soluble.
- It combines rapidly with haemoglobin.

The single-breath test is the test most commonly used to determine diffusing capacity.

## Single-breath test

The patient takes a single breath from residual volume (RV) to TLC. The inhaled gas contains 0.28% CO and 13.5% helium. The patient is instructed to hold the breath for 10 seconds before expiring. The concentration of helium and carbon monoxide in the final part of the expired gas mixture is measured and the diffusing capacity of carbon monoxide is calculated. You need to know the haemoglobin level before the test as the amount of CO transferred will drop with a lower Hb. This test allows measurement of:

1. TLCO (transfer factor/diffusing capacity of the lungs for carbon monoxide [DLCO]) – the total amount of CO transferred by the lung per minute, corrected for the concentration gradient of CO across the alveolar–capillary membrane.
2. kCO (transfer coefficient) – the gas transfer per unit lung volume. This is calculated by dividing the TLCO by the total lung volume during breath hold.

## Transfer factor in lung disease

Measurement of the diffusing capacity of the lungs is used in the evaluation of dyspnoea and hypoxia, diagnosis and monitoring of ILD and detection of pulmonary vascular disease. $T_LCO$ and KCO may be reduced in:

- Emphysema following destruction of the alveoli.
- ILDs, owing to a thickened alveolar capillary membrane.

The causes of a low TLCO can be seen in Table 10.5. The TLCO may be raised following pulmonary haemorrhage (e.g., in vasculitis) as the extra red cells in the lungs absorb CO and falsely elevate the TLCO.

## Tests of lung volumes

The amount of gas in the lungs can be thought of as being split into subdivisions, with disease processes altering these volumes in specific ways (see Chapter 4 and Fig. 4.1). In measuring tidal volume and vital capacity, we use spirometry; alternative techniques are needed for the other volumes.

**Table 10.5** Causes of low TLCO

| Normal spirometry | Obstructive spirometry | Restrictive spirometry |
|---|---|---|
| Pulmonary vascular disease Early interstitial lung disease Anaemia | Emphysema | Interstitial lung disease |

*TLCO, Transfer factor of the lung for carbon monoxide.*

## Residual volume and functional residual capacity

One important lung volume, RV, is not measured in simple spirometry, because gas remains in the lungs at the end of each breath (otherwise the lungs would collapse). Without a measure for RV, we cannot calculate FRC or TLC.

RV is a useful measure in assessing obstructive disease. In a healthy subject, RV is approximately 30% of TLC. In obstructive diseases such as COPD, the lungs are hyperinflated with 'air trapping' so that RV is greatly increased and the ratio of RV:TLC is also increased. There are three methods of measuring RV: helium dilution, plethysmography and nitrogen washout.

## Helium dilution

The patient is connected to a spirometer containing a mixture of 10% helium in air. Helium does not cross the alveolar–capillary membrane into the bloodstream and so, after several breaths, the helium concentration in the spirometer and lung becomes equal. TLC can be calculated from the difference in helium concentration at the start of the test and at equilibrium; then RV can be calculated by subtracting vital capacity from TLC.

This method only measures gas that is in communication with the airways and therefore can underestimate the TLC in lower airway obstruction.

## Body plethysmography

Plethysmography determines changes in lung volume by recording changes in pressure. The patient sits in a large airtight box and breathes through a mouthpiece (Fig. 10.5). At the end of a

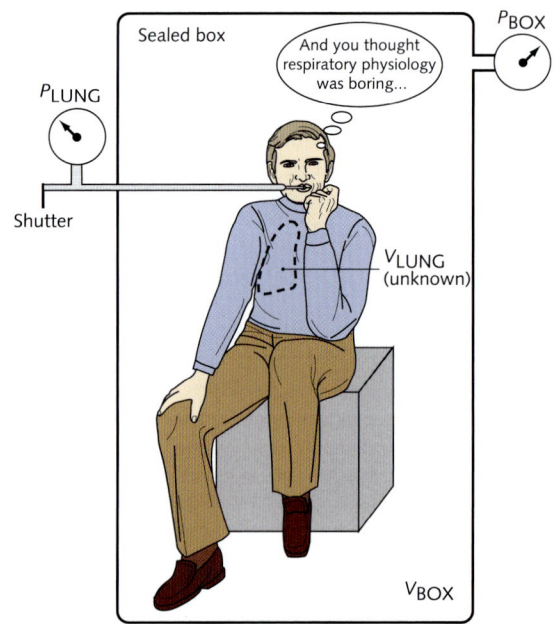

**Fig. 10.5** Plethysmography. This assumes pressure at the mouth is the pressure within the lung. *P*, pressure; *V*, volume.

normal expiration, a shutter closes the mouthpiece and the patient is asked to make respiratory efforts. As the patient tries to inhale, box pressure increases. Using Boyle's law, lung volume can be calculated.

In contrast to the helium dilution method, body plethysmography measures all intrathoracic gas, including cysts, bullae and pneumothoraces, i.e., noncommunicating air spaces. This is important in patients with emphysema who have bullae, in whom helium dilution underestimates RV.

This technique tends to be performed in specialized respiratory centres in respiratory function laboratories.

## Nitrogen washout

Following a normal expiration, the patient breathes 100% oxygen. This 'washes out' the nitrogen in the lungs. The gas exhaled subsequently is collected and its total volume and the concentration of nitrogen are measured. The concentration of nitrogen in the lung before washout is 80%. The concentration of nitrogen left in the lung can be measured by a nitrogen meter at the lips, measuring end-expiration gas. Assuming no net change in the amount of nitrogen (it does not participate in gas exchange), it is possible to estimate the FRC.

## Exercise testing

Exercise testing is primarily used to:

- Diagnose unexplained breathlessness that is minimal at rest.
- Assess the extent of lung disease, by stressing the system.
- Determine the level of impairment in disability testing.
- Assist in differential diagnosis (e.g., when it is not known whether a patient is limited by cardiac or lung disease).
- Test the effects of therapy on exercise capacity.
- Prescribe a safe and effective exercise regime.

There are a number of established tests, including the shuttle test, and a progressive exercise test, which is commonly performed on a cycle ergometer.

## Shuttle test

This is a standardized test in which the patient walks up and down a 10-metre course, marked by cones, in a set time interval. The time intervals are indicated by bleeps played from a tape recorder

**Table 10.6** Medical Research Council Dyspnoea Scale

| Grade | Degree of breathlessness related to activities |
|---|---|
| 1 | Not troubled by breathlessness except on strenuous exercise |
| 2 | Short of breath when hurrying or walking up a slight hill |
| 3 | Walks slower than contemporaries on level ground because of breathlessness, or has to stop for breath when walking at own pace |
| 4 | Stops for breath after walking about 100 metres or after a few minutes on level ground |
| 5 | Too breathless to leave the house, or breathless when dressing or undressing |

and become progressively shorter. The test is stopped if patients become too breathless or if they cannot reach the cone in the time allowed. Usually, oxygen saturations, heart rate and breathlessness (using the Medical Research Council Dyspnoea Scale: Table 10.6) are measured at the beginning and the end to provide objective and subjective measures of the level of dyspnoea.

## Cardiopulmonary exercise testing

This is performed in a laboratory and stresses the patient to a predetermined level based on heart rate. It is usually performed on a cycle ergometer. It is useful for preoperative assessment to assess suitability for anaesthetic and surgery and also in the diagnosis of the cause of exercise limitation (either cardiac or respiratory). A number of tests are performed as the patient exercises, including:

- Electrocardiograph
- Volume of gas exhaled
- Concentration of oxygen and carbon dioxide in exhaled gas.

The volume of gas exhaled per minute (Minute ventilate $V_E$ L/min), oxygen consumption ($VO_2$ L/min) and carbon dioxide output ($VCO_2$ L/min) are calculated both at rest and throughout exercise. The ventilatory threshold marks the onset of anaerobic respiration and can be determined during the test. The test indicates whether exercise tolerance is limited by the cardiovascular or respiratory system and assesses increases in heart rate and ventilation against a known oxygen uptake.

● **Chapter Summary**

- Investigations in respiratory medicine range from simple bedside tests such as peak flow monitoring to invasive procedures including bronchoscopy and thoracoscopy.
- Arterial blood gas sampling is useful in determining if a patient has type I or II respiratory failure and assessing their acid–base status.
- Flexible bronchoscopy is commonly used in respiratory medicine to aid in the diagnosis of suspected lung cancer, chronic or atypical infections and interstitial lung diseases.
- Bedside spirometry and flow–volume loops may reveal an obstructive or restrictive airflow pattern and may indicate the underlying diagnosis.
- The TLCO is a measure of diffusion and represents the total amount of carbon monoxide transferred by the lung per minute. It measures the ability of the lungs to transfer inhaled air to the red blood cells in the pulmonary capillaries. It is decreased in diseases such as interstitial lung disease.
- Cardiopulmonary exercise testing is a useful test when trying to differentiate exercise limitation caused by respiratory disease from that caused by cardiac disease. It is also used as a preoperative assessment tool.

**MLA Conditions**
Acid–base abnormalities
Fibrotic lung disease
Respiratory failure

**MLA Presentations**
Breathlessness
Chest pain
Cough

## INTRODUCTION

Imaging is one of the most important components of modern respiratory medicine. It is used to confirm diagnosis, guide treatment and monitor treatment response in a variety of conditions. Owing to technological advances and a greater number of detailed imaging modalities, respiratory imaging has improved significantly in the last 20 years, including the use of bedside testing and interventional procedures.

## PLAIN RADIOGRAPHY

The plain film radiograph is of paramount importance in the evaluation of pulmonary disease. The standard radiographic examinations of the chest are described below.

### Posteroanterior erect chest radiograph

In the posteroanterior (PA) erect radiograph, X-rays travel from the posterior of the patient to the film, which is held against the front of the patient (Fig. 11.1). The scapula can be rotated out of the way, and accurate assessment of cardiac size is possible. The radiograph is performed in the erect position because:

- Gas passes upwards, making the detection of pneumothorax easier.
- Fluid passes downwards, making pleural effusions easier to diagnose.
- Blood vessels in mediastinum and lung are represented accurately.

### Anteroposterior chest radiograph

As the name suggests, the anteroposterior chest radiograph (AP chest) is performed in the opposite way to a PA chest film, with X-rays travelling anterior to posterior before being captured on film. Owing to the differing angle of projection, the cardiac shadow is superficially enlarged and cannot be commented on, which, coupled with increasing projection of the scapulae, makes this an inferior method of imaging. The significant advantage to AP chest imaging is that it can be performed with a portable machine and in patients too breathless to comply with an erect PA film. It is therefore often done in the critically unwell patient as a secondary format where PA film is not possible.

### Lateral radiograph

Largely a historic modality, lateral films have now become largely superseded by computed tomography (CT) imaging. Lateral views help to localize lesions seen in PA views, as well as giving views of the mediastinum and thoracic vertebrae (Fig. 11.2).

In women of reproductive age, radiography should be performed only following a negative pregnancy test.

### Reporting a chest X-ray

While images used to be reported on viewing boxes, the advance of digital imaging is such that most reporting is performed on a high-resolution digital screen. Always follow a set routine for reporting plain films. If possible, compare with the patient's previous films.

### Clinical data

Take down the following details:

- Patient's name
- Age and sex
- Clinical problem
- Date of radiography.

### Technical qualities

Note that radiographs contain right- or left-side markers. With good penetration of X-rays, you should just be able to see the vertebral bodies through the cardiac shadow. In overpenetration, the lung fields appear too black. Conversely, in underpenetration, the lung fields appear too white. These settings can often be adjusted on a digital image.

Note the projection (AP, PA or lateral; erect or supine). This can give a good indication of the overall health of the patient, e.g., an erect PA film suggests the patient could sit or stand unaided, whereas a supine AP film suggests the patient was too unwell to move at all. To deduce whether the patient was straight or rotated, compare the sternal ends of both clavicles.

With adequate inspiration, you should be able to count six ribs anterior to the diaphragm. Make sure that the whole lung field is included.

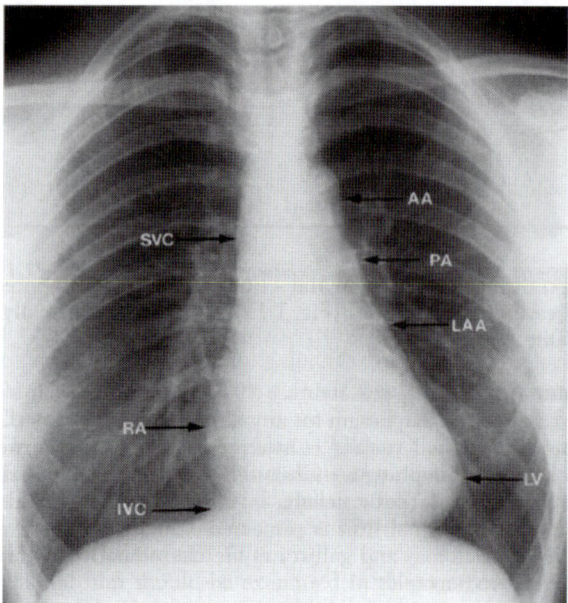

**Fig. 11.1** Normal posteroanterior chest radiograph. The lungs are equally transradiant; the pulmonary vascular pattern is symmetrical. *AA,* Aortic arch; *IVC,* inferior vena cava. *LAA,* left atrial appendage; *LV,* left ventricle; *PA,* pulmonary artery; *RA,* right atrium; *SVC,* superior vena cava. (Courtesy Dr D Sutton and Dr JWR Young.)

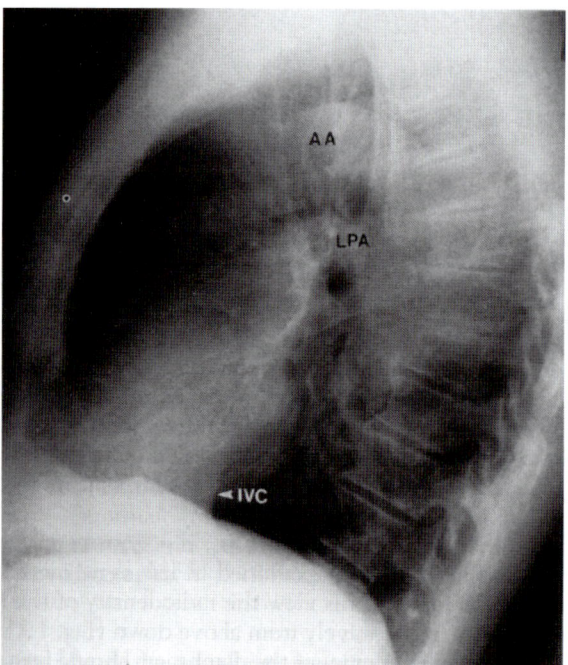

**Fig. 11.2** Normal lateral chest radiograph. *AA,* Aortic arch; *IVC,* inferior vena cava; *LPA,* left pulmonary artery. (Courtesy Dr D Sutton and Dr JWR Young.)

Also note any foreign bodies, such as endotracheal tubes, electrocardiograph leads or pacemakers. These can point towards the overall state of the patient, as well as possible comorbidities.

## Lungs

The lung fields should look symmetrical, with fine lung markings throughout. It is easiest when describing an abnormality to divide the lung into approximate upper, middle and lower zones, rather than trying to guess a lobe. If the lung fields are asymmetrical, combine with clinical findings to determine which is the abnormal side. If the lung fields look symmetrical but abnormal, think of a pathology that would affect both lungs.

Some examples of common findings include:

- Reduced lung markings in one lung only – you should always rule out a pneumothorax. Look for a lung edge and tracheal deviation away from the affected side.
- Reduced lung markings in both lungs – think of destructive parenchymal disease such as emphysema.
- Patchy change in one lung – most likely an infectious process, such as bacterial pneumonia. If it is in the apex, consider tuberculosis.
- Patchy change in both lungs – consider parenchymal disease such as pulmonary fibrosis. Also consider nonrespiratory causes, such as cardiogenic pulmonary oedema. This would be made more likely by a large heart shadow.
- Dense shadowing on one or both sides with a meniscus (air–fluid level) – likely a pleural effusion.
- Dense shadowing on one or both sides without a meniscus – could be consolidation, secondary to infection. If there is a complete 'white-out' of one lung, consider severe infection. Also check the history and make sure the patient hasn't had a pneumonectomy!
- Well-demarcated, round patches of shadowing – the most important thing to rule out here is malignancy. Further imaging and, if possible, a biopsy are needed. If the clinical findings are suggestive of infection, it could be an abscess – look for an air–fluid level.

## Heart and mediastinum

When examining the cardiac shadow, observe the position, size and shape of the heart. It is important to note that, owing to the projection of the X-rays in an AP film, you cannot accurately assess heart size, as it will always look bigger than it actually is. This can only be done on a PA film. A normal-size heart should be less than 50% of the width of the whole thorax. You must also assess if the cardiac borders are clearly visible. If they are not, this may indicate consolidation of the lung immediately next to them, which will be of similar density and will blur the border.

Note whether the trachea is central or deviated to either side. This information should be combined with findings in the lung fields. If the trachea is moving away from a lung field which has very few lung markings and looks very dark, think of a pneumo-thorax. If it is moving towards a lung field which has increased lung markings and shadowing, consider lobar collapse. Identify blood vessels and each hilum. Very prominent blood vessels may be a sign of pulmonary hypertension.

## Other

Note the following points:

- Diaphragm – visible behind the heart; costophrenic angles are acute and sharp. An erect chest X-ray can also be used by surgeons to rule out bowel perforation. If this is the case, air can be seen under the diaphragm (pneumoperitoneum).
- Bones – ribs, clavicles, sternum, thoracic vertebrae.
- Finally, recheck the apices, behind the heart, and hilar and retrodiaphragmatic regions.

## Lateral radiograph

On a lateral radiograph, note the following:

- Diaphragm – right hemidiaphragm seen passing through the heart border.
- Lungs – divide lungs into area in front, behind and above the heart.
- Retrosternal space – an anterior mass will cause this space to be white.
- Fissures – horizontal fissure (faint white line that passes from midpoint of hilum to anterior chest wall); oblique fissure (passes from T4/5 through hilum to the anterior third of the diaphragm).
- Hilum.
- Bones – check vertebral bodies for shape, size and density; check sternum.

## Interpreting abnormalities

Once you have completed your overall review of the film, return to any areas of abnormal lucency or opacity and assess them according to:

- Number – single or multiple
- Position and distribution (lobar, etc.)
- Size, shape and contour
- Texture (homogeneous, calcified, etc.).

The radiological features of common lung conditions are described below.

## Collapse

Atelectasis (collapse) is loss of volume of a lung, lobe or segment for any cause. The most important mechanism is obstruction of a major bronchus by tumour, foreign body or bronchial plug.

A new collapse with no clear cause is considered tumour until proven otherwise and requires CT imaging to further assess.

**Table 11.1** The silhouette sign

| Nonaerated area of lung | Border that is obscured |
| --- | --- |
| Right upper lobe | Right border of ascending aorta |
| Right middle lobe | Right heart border |
| Right lower lobe | Right diaphragm |
| Left upper lobe | Aortic knuckle and upper left cardiac border |
| Lingula of left lung | Left heart border |
| Left lower lobe | Left diaphragm |

Compare with old films where available. The silhouette sign can help localize the lesion (Table 11.1).

**HINTS AND TIPS**

The lateral borders of the mediastinum are silhouetted against the air-filled lung that lies underneath. This silhouette is lost if there is consolidation in the underlying lung.

### Signs of lobar collapse

Signs of lobar collapse are:

- Decreased lung volume.
- Displacement of pulmonary fissures.
- Compensatory hyperinflation of remaining part of the ipsilateral lung.
- Elevation of hemidiaphragm on ipsilateral side.
- Mediastinal and hilar displacement; trachea pulled to side of collapse.
- Radiopacity (white lung).
- Absence of air bronchogram.

Some signs are specific to lobe involvement.

In upper-lobe collapse of the right lung, a PA film is most valuable in making the diagnosis; the collapsed lobe lies adjacent to the mediastinum and there is elevation of the right hilum (Fig. 11.3A). In the lateral film, the lobe can be seen to collapse superomedially and anteriorly (Fig. 11.3B).

Left upper lobe collapse can be more difficult to appreciate on a PA film with the signs being more challenging to identify. The left hilum is pulled upwards resulting in a horizontal course of the left main bronchus.

Right middle lobe collapse results in obstruction of the right heart border and the horizontal border is no longer visible.

Lower lobe collapse of the right lung leads to a triangular opacity in the right lower zone and an elevated right hemidiaphragm. There is inferior displacement of the horizontal fissure.

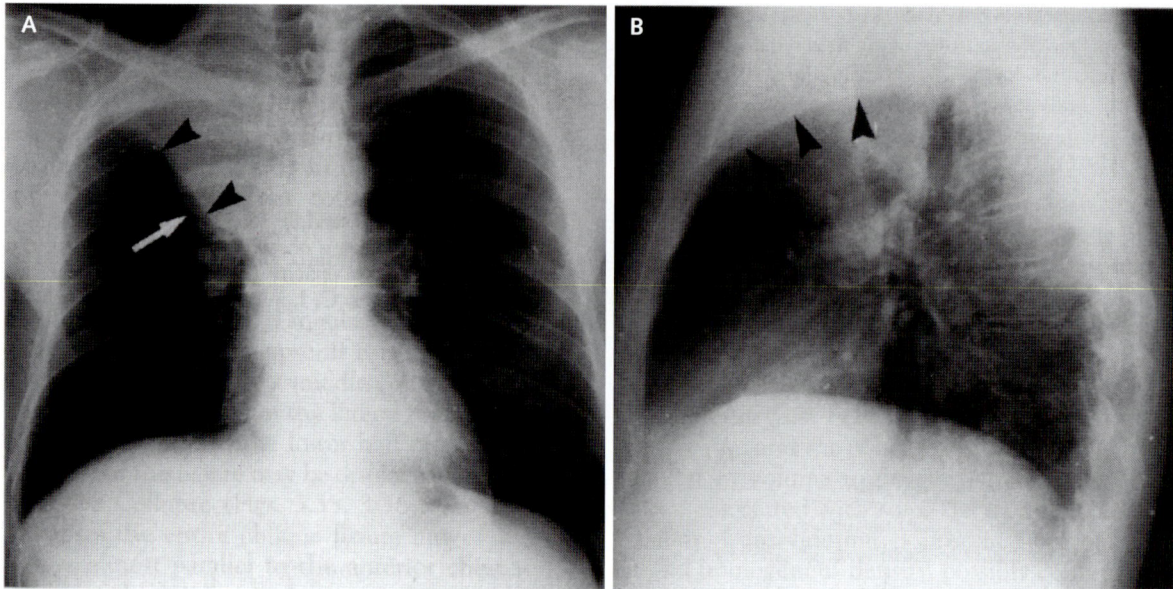

**Fig. 11.3** (A and B) Right upper-lobe collapse. The horizontal and oblique fissures (*black arrowheads*) are displaced. There is a mass (*white arrow*) at the right hilum. (Courtesy Dr D Sutton and Dr JWR Young.)

Left lower lobe collapse results in a triangular opacity in the lower zone, flattening of the left heart border and inferior displacement of the oblique fissure.

## Consolidation

Consolidation is seen as an area of white lung and represents fluid or cellular matter where there would normally be air (Table 11.2 and Fig. 11.4). There are many causes of consolidation, including:

- Pneumonia
- Pulmonary oedema
- Pulmonary haemorrhage.

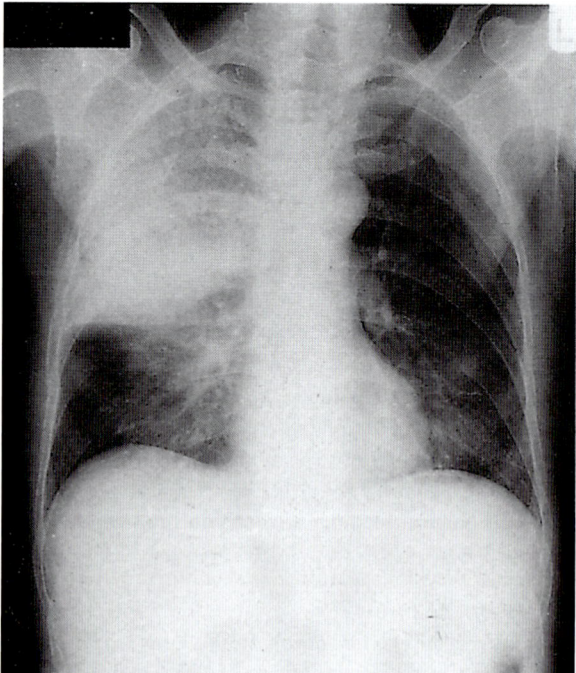

**Fig. 11.4** Consolidation of the right upper lobe. (Courtesy Professor CD Forbes and Dr WF Jackson.)

**Table 11.2** Radiological distribution of alveolar processes

| Segmental pattern | Bat-wing pattern | |
| | Acute | Chronic |
|---|---|---|
| Pneumonia | Pulmonary oedema | Atypical pneumonia |
| Pulmonary infarct | Pneumonia | Lymphoma |
| Segmental collapse | Pulmonary haemorrhage | Sarcoidosis |
| Alveolar cell carcinoma | | Pulmonary alveolar proteinosis |
| Alveolar cell carcinoma | | |

106

In contrast to collapse:

- The shadowing is typically heterogeneous (i.e., not uniform)
- The border is ill defined
- Fissures retain their normal position.

There are two patterns of distribution:

- Segmental or lobar distribution
- Bat-wing distribution.

Peripheral lung fields may be spared (e.g., in pulmonary oedema). Air bronchograms may be seen, because they are delineated by surrounding consolidated lung.

**CLINICAL NOTES**

An elderly woman presented to her general practitioner with fever, a productive cough and general malaise. A chest X-ray showed left lower-lobe consolidation with air bronchograms. Air bronchograms are mostly seen in infection, when consolidated alveoli are lying adjacent to air-filled small and medium bronchioles. These radiographic features suggested a left lower-lobe pneumonia, for which she was treated accordingly.

## Interstitial patterns

Three types of interstitial patterns exist (linear, nodular and honeycomb), and overlap may occur.

## Linear pattern

A linear pattern is seen as a network of fine lines running throughout the lungs. These lines represent thickened connective tissue and are termed Kerley A and B lines:

**HINTS AND TIPS**

Kerley B lines can help to limit the possible diagnoses. They are caused by increased fluid between alveoli, in the interlobular septa. They are seen in pulmonary oedema and malignant lymphatic infiltration.

## Nodular pattern

This pattern is seen as numerous well-defined small nodules (1–5 mm) evenly distributed throughout the lung. Causes include miliary tuberculosis and chickenpox pneumonia.

## Honeycomb pattern

A honeycomb pattern indicates extensive destruction of lung tissue, with lung parenchyma replaced by thin-walled cysts.

Pneumothorax may be present. Normal pulmonary vasculature is absent. Pulmonary fibrosis leads to a honeycomb pattern. This must be quite severe to be seen on chest X-ray. It is more commonly identified on CT scan.

## Pulmonary nodules

### Solitary nodules

The finding of a solitary pulmonary nodule on a plain chest radiograph is not an uncommon event. The nodule, which is commonly referred to as a coin lesion, is usually well circumscribed, less than 3 cm in diameter, lying within the lung. The rest of the lung appears normal and the patient is often asymptomatic.

A solitary nodule on a chest radiograph may be an artefact or it may be owing to:

- Malignant tumour – bronchial carcinoma or secondary deposits.
- Infection – tuberculosis (Fig. 11.5), abscess or aspergilloma.
- Benign tumour – hamartoma.

The presence of a suspicious-looking nodule, particularly where malignancy is considered, should be further investigated with CT imaging rather than plain radiography alone. If the patient is older than 35 years of age, malignancy should be at the top of the list of differential diagnoses. If the lesion is static for a

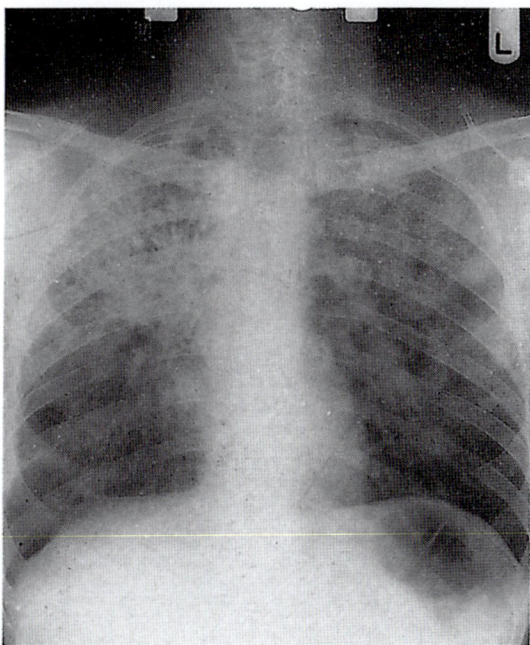

**Fig. 11.5** Tuberculosis in a Greek immigrant to the UK. The film shows multiple areas of shadowing, especially in the upper lobes, and several lesions have started to cavitate. (Courtesy Professor CD Forbes and Dr WF Jackson.)

long period of time, as determined by reviewing previous images, then it is likely to be a benign lesion. However, a slow-growing nodule in an elderly patient is likely to be malignant.

It is important to take into account clinical history and compare with a past chest image if available. You should be able to distinguish carcinoma from other causes:

- Size of lesion – if lesion is >3 cm diameter, be suspicious of malignancy.
- Margin – an ill-defined margin suggests malignancy.
- Cavitation indicates infection or malignancy.
- Calcification – unlikely to be malignancy.
- Presence of air bronchogram – sign of consolidation, not malignancy.

If the lesion is too small to biopsy but is considered to look suspicious for malignancy, a repeat image should be performed to compare the nodule, known as an interval scan. Time intervals depend on the nature of the lesion, but are typically between 3 and 6 months apart. See Chapter 17, Lung cancer, for more information.

## Multiple nodules

Metastases are usually seen as well-defined nodules varying in size, which are more common at the periphery of lower lobes (Fig. 11.6) – they are also known as cannonball metastases;

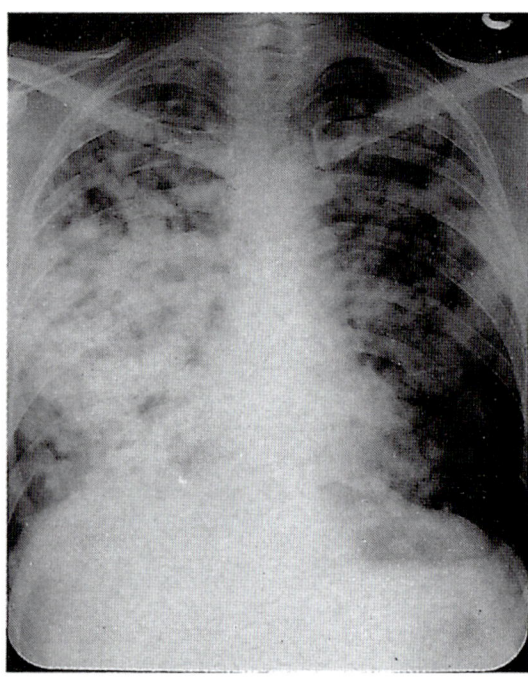

**Fig. 11.6** Snowstorm mottling in both lung fields. In this case, the underlying diagnosis was testicular seminoma, with disseminated haematogenous metastases. (Courtesy Professor CD Forbes and Dr WF Jackson.)

**Table 11.3** Causes of hilar enlargement

| Unilateral enlargement | Bilateral enlargement | |
| | Enlarged lymph nodes | Enlarged vessels |
| --- | --- | --- |
| Bronchial carcinoma | Lymphomas | Left-to-right cardiac shunts |
| Metastatic malignancy | Sarcoidosis | Pulmonary arterial hypertension |
| Lymphomas | Cystic fibrosis | Chronic obstructive pulmonary disease |
| Primary tuberculosis | Infectious mononucleosis | Left heart failure |
| Sarcoidosis | Leukaemia | Pulmonary embolism |

cavitation may be present. Abscesses are cavitated with a thick and irregular wall. Cysts are often large.

Other nodules include:

- Rheumatoid nodules
- Granulomatosis with polyangiitis (formerly Wegener granulomatosis)
- Multiple arteriovenous malformations
- Tuberculosis
- Sarcoidosis.

## Hilar masses

Normal hilar complex includes:

- Proximal pulmonary arteries and bifurcations
- Bronchus
- Pulmonary veins
- Lymph nodes, not seen unless enlarged.

Hilar size varies from person to person, so enlargement is difficult to diagnose (Table 11.3). Radiological features of the hilum are:

- Concave lateral margin
- Equal radiopacity
- Left hilum lies higher than right.

**CLINICAL NOTES**

Sarcoidosis commonly presents as an incidental finding of bilateral hilar lymphadenopathy on chest radiography.

PA films are most valuable in assessing hilar shadow, but to accurately view the area, CT imaging is necessary. In chest radiography, technical qualities of the film need to be adequately

**Table 11.4** Mediastinal masses

| Anterior masses | Middle masses | Posterior masses |
|---|---|---|
| Retrosternal thyroid | Bronchial carcinoma | Neurogenic tumour |
| Thymic mass | Lymphoma | Paravertebral abscess |
| Dermoid cyst | Sarcoidosis | Oesophageal lesions |
| Lymphomas | Primary tuberculosis | Aortic aneurysm |
| Aortic aneurysm | Bronchogenic cyst | — |

assessed before conclusions can be made, because patient rotation commonly mimics hilar enlargement.

## Mediastinal masses

A mediastinal mass typically has a sharp, concave margin, visible because of the silhouette sign. Lateral films may be particularly useful. Mediastinal masses are frequently asymptomatic and are grouped according to their anatomical position (Table 11.4). CT is advised where there is doubt as to the nature of the lesion.

### Anterior mediastinal masses
Characteristics of anterior mediastinal masses:

- Hilar structures still visible
- Mass merges with the cardiac border
- A mass passing into the neck is not seen above the clavicles
- Small anterior mediastinal masses are difficult to see on PA films.

### Middle mediastinal masses
- A middle mediastinal mass merges with hila and cardiac borders
- The majority are caused by enlarged lymph nodes.

### Posterior mediastinal masses
In posterior mediastinal masses, the cardiac border and hila are seen but the posterior aorta is obscured. Vertebral changes may be present.

---

**CLINICAL NOTES**

Tension pneumothorax is seen as a displacement of the mediastinum and trachea to the contralateral side, depressed ipsilateral diaphragm and increased space between the ribs.

---

## Pleural lesions

### Pneumothorax
Pneumothorax is usually obvious on normal inspiratory PA films. Look carefully at upper zones, because air accumulates first here; you will see an area devoid of lung markings (black lung), with the lung edge outlined by air in the pleural space. Small pneumothoraces can be identified on the expiratory film and may be missed in the supine film.

**Tension pneumothorax**
Tension pneumothorax is a medical emergency. You should never see a chest X-ray of a tension pneumothorax, as it is life-threatening. If you suspect your patient has one and he or she is increasingly dyspnoeic, you must treat the condition immediately.

### Pleural effusions
PA erect radiography is performed. Classically, there is a radiopaque mass at the base of the lung and blunting of the costophrenic angle, with the pleural meniscus higher laterally than medially. Large effusions can displace the mediastinum contralaterally.

A horizontal upper border implies that a pneumothorax is also present. An effusion has a more homogeneous texture than consolidation and air bronchograms are absent.

### Mesothelioma
Mesothelioma is a malignant tumour of the pleura, which may present as discrete pleural deposits or as a localized lesion.

On chest X-ray, thickened pleura is seen; in 50% of cases the pleural plaques lie on the medial pleura, causing the medial margin to be irregular. Pleural effusions are common, usually containing blood (Fig. 11.7). Rib destruction is uncommon.

## Vascular patterns

### Normal vascular pattern
Lung markings are vascular in nature. Arteries branch vertically to upper and lower lobes. On erect films, upper-lobe vessels are smaller than lower-lobe vessels. It is difficult to see vessels in the peripheral one-third of lung fields.

### Pulmonary venous hypertension
On erect films, upper-lobe vessels are larger than lower-lobe vessels. Pulmonary venous hypertension is associated with oedema and pleural effusions.

### Pulmonary arterial hypertension
Pulmonary arterial hypertension is seen as bilateral hilar enlargement associated with long-standing pulmonary disease.

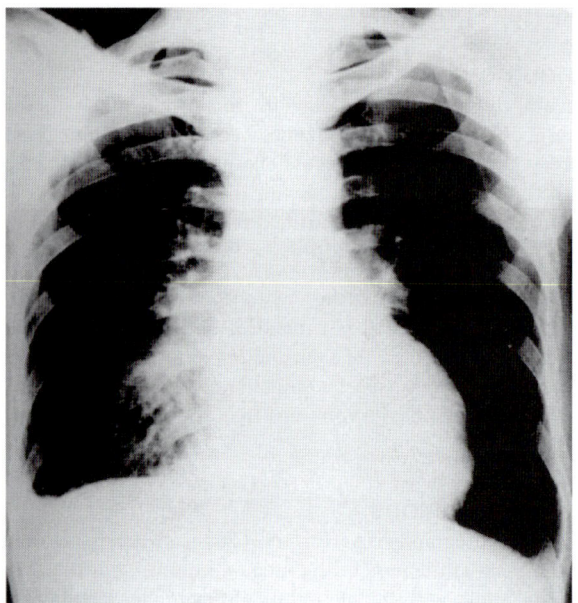

**Fig. 11.7** Small pleural effusions. Both costophrenic angles are blunted. (Courtesy Dr D Sutton and Dr JWR Young.)

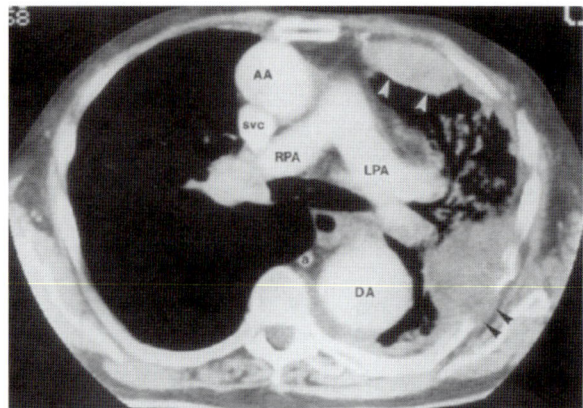

**Fig. 11.8** Computed tomography (CT) scan of a pleural mass. Enhanced CT scan at level of bifurcation of main pulmonary artery. The left lung is surrounded by pleural masses *(arrowheads)*, and the posterior mass is invading the chest wall. The vascular anatomy of the mediastinum is well shown. *a,* Azygos vein (left of descending aorta); *AA,* ascending aorta; *DA,* descending aorta; *LPA,* left pulmonary artery; *RPA,* right pulmonary artery; *SVC,* superior vena cava. (Courtesy Dr D Sutton and Dr JWR Young.)

# Computed tomography

CT is the imaging modality of choice for mediastinal and many pulmonary conditions. CT scans provide detailed cross-sectional images of the thorax. The images can be electronically modified to display different tissues (e.g., by using a bone setting compared with a soft tissue setting).

The patient passes through a rotating gantry which has X-ray tubes on one side and a set of detectors on the other. Information from the detectors is analyzed and displayed as a two-dimensional image on visual display units, recorded as slices.

The frequency and definition of the slices determine the type of CT performed. A standard CT performs slices at frequent intervals and averages the information between slices which are roughly 5 mm thick (volume averaging), meaning small masses are better detected but the definition if each image is less fine. This modality is better looking for small nodules such as in lung cancer. A high-resolution CT image gives a very detailed single-resolution slice (<1.5 mm) but at wider intervals (1–2 cm) and without volume averaging, meaning a small mass may be missed between slices. This modality is better for looking at the texture of the lung itself (for interstitial lung disease). A greater number of advanced CT techniques exist, which can be used for a variety of conditions.

Typically, CT chest imaging gives a dose of radiation approximately 100 times that of a standard plain film chest radiograph.

## Applications of computed tomography

### Detection of pulmonary nodules

CT can evaluate the presence of metastases in a patient with known malignancy; however, it cannot definitively distinguish between benign and malignant masses. It can also be a useful imaging modality for biopsy of these lesions through interventional radiology, typically performed for lesions located more peripherally that cannot be accessed via bronchoscopy.

### Mediastinal masses

CT is a useful technique in searching for lymphadenopathy in a person with primary lung carcinoma.

### Carcinoma of the lung

CT can evaluate the size of a lung carcinoma, and detect mediastinal extension and staging, including the detection of metastases in other organs. A typical lung cancer staging CT will include the liver and adrenal glands in the abdomen, as these are typical sites of metastases (see Chapter 17 for more information).

### Pleural lesions

CT is effective at detecting small pleural effusions and identifying pleural plaques (Fig. 11.8).

### Vascular lesions

Contrast studies allow imaging of vascular lesions (e.g., aortic aneurysms or aortic dissection). Contrast is injected intravenously, which highlights the vascular structures. The timing of the contrast injection is synchronized to whether the arterial or

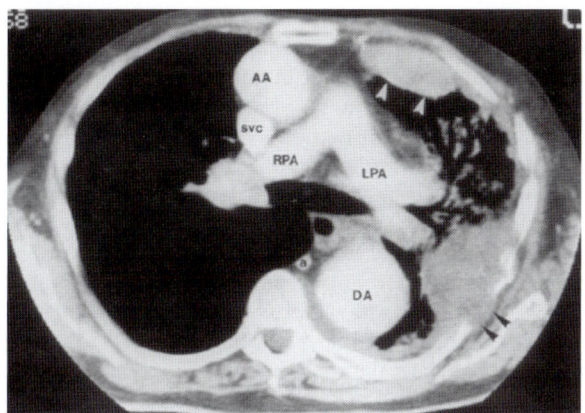

**Fig. 11.9** Technical differences between computed tomography (CT) and high-resolution CT (HRCT).

venous system is being imaged, and so it is important to state the type of abnormality you are suspecting.

## Application of high-resolution computed tomography

High-resolution CT is useful in imaging diffuse lung disease: thinner sections of <1.5 mm show greater lung detail (Fig. 11.9).

### Bronchiectasis
High-resolution CT is used for the diagnosis of bronchiectasis, demonstrating characteristic dilated bronchi. Other features include:

- Collapse
- Scarring
- Consolidation.

### Interstitial lung disease
High-resolution CT is more specific than plain film radiography. Disorders that have specific appearances on high-resolution CT include sarcoidosis, occupational lung disease and interstitial pneumonia. A prone CT scan is also helpful in this condition as it eliminates changes due to dependency or gravity. Thus useful in basal predominant disease.

High-resolution CT can be used for biopsy guidance.

### Atypical infections
High-resolution CT provides diagnosis earlier than plain chest radiography and is useful in monitoring disease and response to treatment. It also provides good delineation of disease activity and destruction.

High-resolution CT is used in imaging of patients with acquired immunodeficiency syndrome (e.g., *Pneumocystis jirovecii* pneumonia).

### Lymphangitis carcinomatosis
High-resolution CT can be used in the diagnosis of lymphangitis carcinomatosis, a condition of inflammation of the lymph vessels caused by malignancy.

### Chronic obstructive pulmonary disease
High-resolution CT can be used to measure small-airways thickening, gas trapping and emphysema found in chronic obstructive pulmonary disease (COPD).

## Computed pulmonary angiogram

A special type of CT scan called a CT pulmonary angiogram (CTPA) is a noninvasive and accurate method of detecting blood clots in the lungs or pulmonary embolism (PE). It is a contrast study performed by injecting dye intravenously in a peripheral cannula in order to image the pulmonary vasculature. Filling defects of the pulmonary arterial tree are seen demonstrating pulmonary emboli. In massive PE, there may be signs of right heart strain also seen on CT imaging. CTPA has replaced pulmonary angiography (an invasive test where a catheter is inserted into the main pulmonary artery) as the gold standard for PE diagnosis.

There are problems with CTPA. There is a radiation dose to consider, particularly important in pregnant women, both for the developing baby and the patient's breast tissue, carrying an increase in risk of breast cancer. Contrast allergies can produce anaphylactic reactions, while the contrast dye can be nephrotoxic and should only be used with suitable renal function. In cases where complication risks are high, other imaging techniques such as ventilation:perfusion (*V/Q*) scans may be performed, discussed below.

## Ventilation:perfusion scans

*V/Q* relationships are measured by means of isotope scans (also known as *V/Q* scans).

## Ventilation scans

Ventilation is detected by inhalation of a gas or aerosol labelled with the radioisotope Xe. The patient breathes and rebreathes the gas until it comes into equilibrium with other gases in the lung.

### Inequality of ventilation
In diseases such as asthma or COPD, the lungs may be unevenly ventilated. Inequality of ventilation is measured using the single-breath nitrogen test, similar to the method for measuring anatomical dead space, described previously.

## Perfusion scans

Radioactive particles larger than the diameter of the pulmonary capillaries are injected intravenously, where they remain for several hours. $^{99m}$Tc-labelled macroaggregated albumin (MAA) is used. A gamma camera is then used to detect the position of the MAA particles. The pattern indicates the distribution of pulmonary blood flow.

### Inequality of perfusion

This occurs in conditions such as a pulmonary embolus, where there is good ventilation of the lung but poor perfusion owing to venous thrombosis.

## Ventilation:perfusion scans

*V/Q* scans are primarily used to detect pulmonary emboli. The principle is that a pulmonary embolus produces a defect on the perfusion scan (a filling defect) that is not matched by a defect on the ventilation scan, i.e., there is an area of the lung that is ventilated but not perfused. As the clot itself is not visualized, small emboli may be missed, and other lung conditions affecting ventilation may mask areas of poor perfusion on the scan. As a result, *V/Q* scans are less sensitive than CTPA scans for diagnosis of PE, but do not carry the same radiation and contrast risks. They are therefore preferred in select clinical circumstances. The advantage of *V/Q* scans is they are better for quantifying clot burden and so useful in patients with chronic thromboembolic pulmonary disease.

## ULTRASOUND

Ultrasound uses high-frequency sound waves to image internal structures. A transducer probe is pressed against the patient with a gel used to provide optimum contact. The transducer emits pulses of ultrasound waves into the body. Different structures in the body have different acoustic impedances, meaning some waves can travel further than others before being reflected back to the transducer. The reflected waves are processed and combined to generate an image. Ultrasound is safe, portable and fast; it can be used at the bedside and is increasingly used in modern clinical practice.

In respiratory medicine the technique is primarily used in the investigation of pleural effusions and empyemas. Ultrasound can differentiate between consolidation and effusion, or localize an effusion before it is drained by thoracentesis.

Ultrasound imaging can assess whether the effusion is simple or loculated – meaning separated into multiple different pockets by fibrotic scar tissue, and can, in experienced hands, even differentiate fluid densities to suggest empyema, haemothorax or transudate effusions. Ultrasound is so effective that British thoracic guidelines currently state that thoracentesis for pleural effusions should always be performed with bedside ultrasound guidance.

A variation on this technique, Doppler ultrasound, is a noninvasive method for detecting deep vein thrombosis. It is used in investigating patients with suspected pulmonary thromboembolism. The technique examines blood flow and can detect thrombus in the veins above the popliteal fossa.

## Positron emission tomography

Positron emission tomography (PET) scanning is used for the staging of lung cancer and assessing unknown lesions previously detected on CT. Malignant cells have a higher metabolic uptake of glucose than nonmalignant cells. A positron-emitting glucose analogue is injected into the patient and then detected by the scanner, with suspicious lesions lighting up on PET scan. False positives can occur in other metabolically active nodules such as in tuberculosis or sarcoidosis, while false negatives can occur if the lesion is small (<1 cm).

## MAGNETIC RESONANCE IMAGING

Magnetic resonance imaging (MRI) uses the magnetic properties of the hydrogen atom to produce images. MRI gives excellent imaging of soft tissues and the heart and its role in respiratory disease is increasing. It was initially not used much because air does not generate a signal on an MRI scan. However, it is being developed as a technique to obtain dynamic images of the lungs, through the inhalation of hyperpolarized inert gases such as xenon and helium. Flowing blood does not provide a signal for MRI, and vascular structures appear as hollow tubes. MRI can be used to differentiate masses around the aorta or in the hilar regions. It has the advantage of not using ionizing radiation, making it safer to use than a CT scan. However, scans require the patient to lie flat for 30–60 minutes, which can be difficult for a breathless patient.

● **Chapter Summary**

- Posteroanterior (PA) plain film chest radiograph remains one of the most important imaging techniques in respiratory medicine.
- Based on plain film appearance, it is possible in many cases to differentiate between collapse, consolidation and effusion.
- Ultrasound is useful to differentiate simple and complex effusions from consolidation and guide interventions such as thoracentesis.
- Computed tomography (CT) is the main investigation for further imaging of the chest. Depending on the pathology suspected, the most appropriate CT can be ordered, differentiating between plain CT, high-resolution CT and CT pulmonary angiogram (CTPA).
- There remains a role in certain clinical circumstances for ventilation:perfusion (*V/Q*) scanning in the investigation of pulmonary embolism, although CTPA is often the preferred modality where possible.

**MLA Conditions**
Fibrotic lung disease
Metastatic disease
Pleural effusion
Pneumothorax
Pulmonary embolism

**MLA Presentations**
Breathlessness
Chest pain
Cough
Haemoptysis

# Section 3

# RESPIRATORY CONDITIONS

# Acute respiratory failure

## INTRODUCTION

Acute respiratory failure is a life-threatening consequence of many disease processes and is the most common emergency presentation of respiratory medicine. The incidence is approximately 80 people in every 100,000, with around 4000 patients per year managed in the intensive care unit. It requires early recognition and correction, or it can be fatal. We will describe the assessment of the critically ill patient in respiratory medicine, then discuss the different types of respiratory failure and how to manage them.

## INITIAL ASSESSMENT OF THE ACUTELY BREATHLESS PATIENT

When you are called to see a patient who is acutely unwell, it is important to be able to make a rapid assessment of the patient's condition before starting a more thorough examination. The method used by all doctors is very easy to remember, it is as easy as 'ABC'.

### ABCDE assessment

This is a common tool for assessing any unwell patient. Work through the sequence and whenever you encounter a problem, correct it where you can before moving to the next step. As a junior doctor, if you are worried about a patient and feel you need more support, always ask for senior help.

## A – airway

- Is your patient's airway patent? Determine this by asking the patient a question. If the patient replies, then their airway is patent.
- Listen for added sounds, such as stridor (a high-pitched wheezing noise) or gurgling, which may indicate upper airway obstruction. If this is the case, tilt the patient's head and lift the chin, or thrusting the jaw forward, to open up the upper airways.
- If this does not improve, insert an airway adjunct such as a nasopharyngeal or oropharyngeal airway.
- More complex adjuncts, such as a laryngeal mask airway or even an endotracheal tube, may be necessary to obtain a definitive patent airway. In reality, only those trained to do so (such as anaesthetists) should intubate a patient.

## B – breathing

- Once you have established a patent airway, the next assessment is breathing.
- Patients with a respiratory emergency will need supplemental oxygen.
- Oxygen can be delivered via nasal cannulae, or controlled oxygen via a Venturi mask (which ensures only a specific percentage of oxygen is delivered) or a nonrebreather mask (Fig. 12.1).
- In an emergency setting, a nonrebreather mask is the most effective, as it delivers high oxygen volumes in a ward setting.

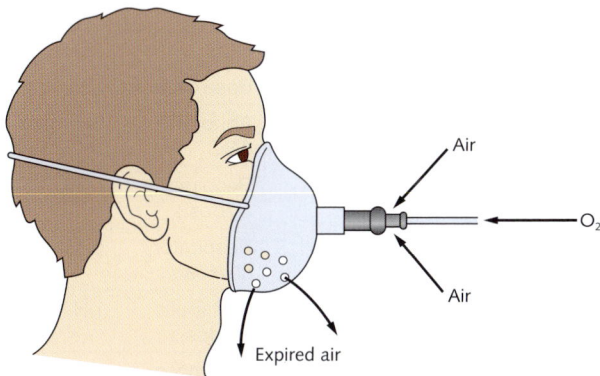

Air

$O_2$

Air

Expired air

**Fig. 12.1** Venturi and nonrebreather masks.

– What is the patient's respiratory rate? A normal respiratory rate is between 12 and 16 breaths per minute. If the patient is talking to you, can they talk in full sentences or do they need to stop after every couple of words?
– Use a finger probe to measure oxygen saturation. In a healthy person at rest, it should be 94%–98%. However, in someone with chronic airways disease [such as chronic obstructive pulmonary disease (COPD)], individuals may have oxygen saturations as low as 88% on air.
– Examine the chest, including inspection, percussion and auscultation. In this crucial initial assessment, you can omit parts of the respiratory examination, such as examining the hands, as this can be done later and any signs will not be immediately lifesaving.
– An arterial blood gas (ABG) test and chest radiograph are pertinent investigations at this stage.

## C – circulation

– If you feel the patient's breathing is satisfactory, move on to assess the circulation.
– What is the patient's pulse and blood pressure? Feel for a central and peripheral pulse and check capillary refill.
– Establish intravenous (IV) access and insert one cannula in each arm, using as large a size as possible.
– Intravenous fluids may be appropriate, given as a bolus to assess response.
– An electrocardiogram should be performed to detect any underlying arrhythmias or cardiac ischaemia.
– Also, think about appropriate and relevant blood tests necessary at this stage.

## D – disability

– Further assessments give vital clues to the underlying diagnosis or how unwell the patient is.
– Assessing consciousness level, either using the AVPU scale (alert, responds to voice, responds to pain, unconscious) or the Glasgow Coma Scale can give you information on how well the patient can protect their own airway. Even subtle signs such as new confusion can indicate an underlying sepsis.
– -Also, always check the blood glucose to rule out hypo- or hyperglycaemia.

## E – exposure (and everything else)

– Have a look at the rest of the patient from top to toe. Always lift up the covers – a swollen leg demonstrating a deep vein thrombosis may give a vital clue to the cause of the patient's respiratory failure [pulmonary embolism (PE)]. Examine the abdomen and other relevant areas.

– Once you have completed your assessment, think about the underlying diagnosis, as well as assessing response to your given treatment. For example, if you are suspecting a chest infection, antibiotics may be appropriate.
– The ABC approach involves constant reassessment and is a continuous loop. Also, you must never move on to the next step before you are completely satisfied with the current one. There is no point administering oxygen to a patient who does not have a patent airway!

## HOW TO READ AN ARTERIAL BLOOD GAS RESULT

ABG analysis is a definitive method for assessing respiratory failure and should be performed in patients requiring oxygen therapy. It gives vital information allowing differentiation between type I and type II respiratory failure, as well as providing information on many other metabolic parameters. Performing and interpreting the test is discussed in Chapter 10, while Table 12.1 demonstrates a brief guide to interpreting an ABG result and gives examples of both respiratory and metabolic acidosis and alkalosis.

1. Always know the clinical context. Why was the test performed and why is the patient unwell? Is the patient on oxygen; if so, how much?
2. Look at the $PO_2$ (normal range 10–14 kPa) – is the patient in respiratory failure ($P_aO_2 < 8$ kPa)? Remember to consider the inspired $O_2$. If the patient is on high-flow oxygen, is the $PO_2$ appropriate?

Table 12.1 Example normal ranges for arterial blood gas analysis

| Parameter | Normal range |
|---|---|
| pH | 7.35–7.45 |
| $PO_2$ | 10–14 kPa |
| $PCO_2$ | 4.5–6 kPa |
| $HCO_3$ | 22–26 mmol/L |
| Base excess | –2 to 2 mmol/L |
| Abnormal ABG | Example |
| Respiratory acidosis | pH 7.27, $PO_2$ 7.3, $PCO_2$ 6.8, $HCO_3$ 29, BE +2 |
| Respiratory alkalosis | pH 7.49, $PO_2$ 13.9, $PCO_2$ 3.5, $HCO_3$ 22, BE +2 |
| Metabolic acidosis | pH 7.25, $PO_2$ 11.1, $PCO_2$ 4.5, $HCO_3$ 11, BE –8 |
| Metabolic alkalosis | pH 7.56, $PO_2$ 10.7, $PCO_2$ 5.0, $HCO_3$ 31, BE +5 |

3. Look at the pH (normal range 7.35–7.45) – is the patient acidaemic or alkalaemic (pH < 7.35 or > 7.45, respectively)? If so, the next steps will help you work out the underlying cause (metabolic versus respiratory).
4. Look at the $PCO_2$ (normal range 4.5–6.0 kPa) – raised $PCO_2$ may be causing a respiratory acidosis, while a low $PCO_2$ could reflect the respiratory compensation of a metabolic acidosis. Remember respiratory compensation can begin quickly while metabolic compensation takes days to occur.
5. Look at the $HCO_3$ (normal range 22–26 mmol/L) and base excess (−2 to +2 mmol/L) – low bicarbonate may demonstrate underlying metabolic acidosis, while a raised bicarbonate can demonstrate chronic compensation of respiratory acidosis secondary to $CO_2$ retention.
6. Is there compensation? Remember the body will never overcompensate an acidosis or alkalosis.
7. Look at all additional tests performed by the blood gas analyzer, such as electrolytes, lactate and glucose.

### HINTS AND TIPS

Arterial blood gas (ABG) analysis is a common topic for exam questions, and its interpretation is a useful skill in clinical practice. It can be difficult and is often confused. Everyone develops their own way of reading ABG results; find a system you like, stick to it and keep practising.

## RESPIRATORY FAILURE

### Definition

Respiratory failure is defined as a failure to maintain adequate gas exchange, with a $P_aO_2 < 8$ kPa by blood gas analysis. Respiratory failure can be further subdivided into type I or type II, depending on $P_aCO_2$ level.

- Type I respiratory failure – $P_aO_2 < 8$ kPa with a low or normal $P_aCO_2$.
- Type II respiratory failure – $P_aO_2 < 8$ kPa with a raised $P_aCO_2$ of ≥6 kPa.

Respiratory failure is not a presentation seen in isolation, but an outcome of many different respiratory diseases. The respiratory pump is comprised of the chest wall, the muscles of respiration as well as the central and peripheral nervous systems. During the initial stages of lung disease, the body maintains adequate oxygenation by adapting to meet an increased ventilatory demand. However, if one of the components of the respiratory pump fails, this causes an inability to ventilate the lung adequately and impairs gas exchange.

### Type I respiratory failure
- Acute hypoxaemia: $P_aO_2$ low (<8 kPa)
- $P_aCO_2$ is normal or low.

Type I respiratory failure is primarily caused by ventilation: perfusion ($V/Q$) mismatch.

Common causes include:

- Severe acute asthma
- Pneumonia
- PE
- Pulmonary oedema.

### Type II respiratory failure
- Low $P_aO_2 < 8$ kPa.
- High $P_aCO_2 > 6.0$ kPa.

Type II respiratory failure is also known as ventilatory failure; the rise in $P_aCO_2$ is no longer matched by an increase in alveolar ventilation. This can be because:

- Ventilatory drive is insufficient
- The work of breathing is excessive
- The lungs are unable to pump air in and out efficiently.

As a result, patients are unable to 'blow off' the excess $CO_2$ causing $P_aCO_2$ levels to rise. In the acute setting, this can lead to a respiratory acidosis, as the excess $CO_2$ is converted to carbonic acid in the bloodstream.

$$\underset{\text{carbon dioxide + water}}{CO_2 + H_2O} \rightleftarrows \underset{\text{carbonic acid}}{H_2CO_3} \rightleftarrows \underset{\text{bicarbonate + hydrogen ion}}{HCO_3^- + H^+}$$

In chronic type II respiratory failure, the patient may be able to metabolically compensate with a gradual rise in serum bicarbonate preventing acidaemia.

Common causes are displayed in Table 12.2. The commonest cause is an acute exacerbation of COPD. Patients with COPD can be hypoxaemic +/− hypercapnic for many years, with daytime somnolence and morning headache symptoms of a raised $P_aCO_2$. An acute exacerbation (e.g., precipitated by respiratory infection) further increases the work of breathing, leading to 'acute-on-chronic' respiratory failure.

### Clinical features

Depending on the type of respiratory failure, patients will demonstrate features of hypoxia ± hypercapnia (Table 12.3). The most common feature is breathlessness, and in any breathless patient, respiratory failure should be suspected.

### Investigations

Investigations used to confirm respiratory failure include an initial peripheral oxygen saturation reading, then an ABG as the definitive test. Further investigations should primarily focus on

119

**Table 12.2** Common causes of respiratory failure divided into categories of aetiology

| Pulmonary | Reduced respiratory drive | Neuromuscular |
|---|---|---|
| Disorders of airways: Asthma, Chronic obstructive pulmonary disease, Bronchiectasis, Cystic fibrosis | Primary CNS injury – brainstem trauma | Spinal cord: Motor neurone disease (MND), Multiple sclerosis, Injury of the spinal cord, Tetanus, Neoplasm, Amyotrophic lateral sclerosis, Spinal muscular atrophy |
| Infections: Viral, Bacterial pneumonia | Sedative drugs | Anterior horn cell: Post-polio syndrome |
| Disorders of lung parenchyma: Interstitial Lung Disease, Sarcoidosis | Stroke | Peripheral nerve: Guillain-Barré syndrome |
| Chest trauma: Flail chest | Overdose of sedative or opioid | Neuromuscular junction: Myasthenia gravis, toxins (botulism) <br> Drugs: Corticosteroids, Anticholinesterase inhibitors |
| Disorders of thoracic cage with increased chest wall stiffness: Kyphoscoliosis, Obesity hypoventilation syndrome | | Myopathies: Duchenne muscular dystrophy, muscular dystrophy (Congenital, Limb-girdle muscular dystrophy), Myotonic dystrophies, Mitochondrial disease |

**Table 12.3** Symptoms of hypoxia and hypercapnia

| Hypoxia (type I and II respiratory failure) | Hypercapnia (type I respiratory failure only) |
|---|---|
| Dyspnoea | Headaches |
| Restlessness and agitation | Drowsiness |
| Confusion | Confusion |
| Cyanosis (peripheral and central) | Tachycardia with a bounding pulse |
| | $CO_2$ retention hand flap |
| | Peripheral vasodilation |
| | Papilloedema |

**Table 12.4** Common respiratory presentations causing acute respiratory failure

| Emergency presentation | Chapter |
|---|---|
| Anaphylaxis | 13 |
| Foreign body aspiration | 13 |
| Asthma exacerbation | 14 |
| Chronic obstructive pulmonary disease exacerbation | 15 |
| Pneumonia | 18 |
| Infective exacerbation of bronchiectasis | 19 |
| Empyema | 20 |
| Pneumothorax | 20 |
| Pulmonary embolism | 21 |

determining the underlying cause of respiratory failure. Some useful investigations include:

- Blood tests and blood cultures
- Chest radiograph
- Sputum culture
- Bedside spirometry testing.

Once initial investigations are complete, more specialist tests can be used if the diagnosis is not yet confirmed. For example, a pulmonary embolus may require computed tomography pulmonary angiogram (CTPA) imaging to confirm, while specialist serological or high-resolution computed tomography CT may be required if a particular infection is suspected.

## Management

Ultimately, management is dependent on the underlying cause of respiratory failure (Table 12.4). However, adequate oxygenation and respiratory support are often needed while the diagnosis is confirmed and the treatment has time to take effect.

Respiratory support can be divided into three broad categories – oxygen delivery, noninvasive ventilation and invasive ventilation. The type of support required depends on the type and severity of the respiratory failure. The goal of respiratory support is to provide adequate oxygenation, with effective removal of carbon dioxide.

Special care should be taken in patients at risk of type II respiratory failure, such as those with severe COPD. Overoxygenation can lead to many mechanisms that suppress ventilation; these may include the abolition of a hypoxic drive which stimulates ventilation, loss of hypoxic vasoconstriction and lastly absorption atelectasis leading to an increase in dead-space ventilation and Haldane effect. If $P_aCO_2$ continues to rise rather than fall, a respiratory acidosis can lead to decompensated type II respiratory failure. In such patients, controlled oxygen therapy with target saturations of 88%–92% is preferred to standard targets of 94%–98%.

# OXYGEN DELIVERY AND VENTILATION

## Oxygen delivery

Oxygen delivery can be provided in a variety of forms, depending on the severity of the hypoxia. In the initial assessment of a critically unwell patient, delivery of high-flow oxygen is recommended until further investigations can be performed, as hypoxia is often the most imminent threat to the patient. Once the patient is stabilized, oxygen can be stepped down and delivered in a controlled manner where appropriate, via a number of devices and at different rates, providing varying oxygen concentrations (Table 12.5):

Nasal cannulae – used for low-flow oxygen delivery, comfortable and easily administered.

Simple oxygen mask – used for medium-concentration oxygen delivery. Can be delivered with humidification if required to prevent mouth drying.

Venturi mask – provides fixed oxygen delivery using separate adapters for different oxygen concentrations. Good for giving reliable controlled oxygen at medium concentration. Comes in different colours to guide use.

Nonrebreather mask – has a reservoir bag attached which is filled prior to use, meaning patients are only able to breathe in the concentrated oxygen. Delivers the highest concentrated oxygen available in a nonspecialist ward setting.

High-flow nasal oxygen – an oxygen supply system capable of delivering up to 100% humidified and heated oxygen at a flow rate of up to 60 L per minute.

## Continuous positive airway pressure

Continuous positive airway pressure (CPAP) provides oxygen delivery plus added fixed positive pressure throughout the respiratory cycle. CPAP is used for patients with type I respiratory failure to correct hypoxaemia and, while the strongest evidence for successful use is in those with cardiogenic pulmonary oedema, it is used in a variety of settings for critically unwell patients, with specialist advice. In the nonemergency setting, CPAP is used for obstructive sleep apnoea (see Chapter 22). The continuous airway pressure is used to stent open the small airways and minimize alveolar collapse. This aims to reduce the work of breathing and improve any existing ventilation:perfusion mismatching.

CPAP can be delivered either nasally or via a tight-fitting mask. The pressure delivered can vary from 5 to 15 $cmH_2O$ (higher in specialist cases) and oxygen can be delivered in higher concentrations than standard oxygen mask therapy.

CPAP should be delivered with trained staff who know how to fit the mask and set up the equipment required. The patient should be alert and cooperative, and without any facial trauma that prevents the mask from being fitted. The pressure can be uncomfortable and some patients may not be able to tolerate the device.

## Noninvasive ventilation

While CPAP provides a continuous pressure, noninvasive ventilation (NIV) varies this airway pressure to provide ventilation support, rather than simply supplying maximum oxygen concentrations to treat hypoxaemia (Fig. 12.2).

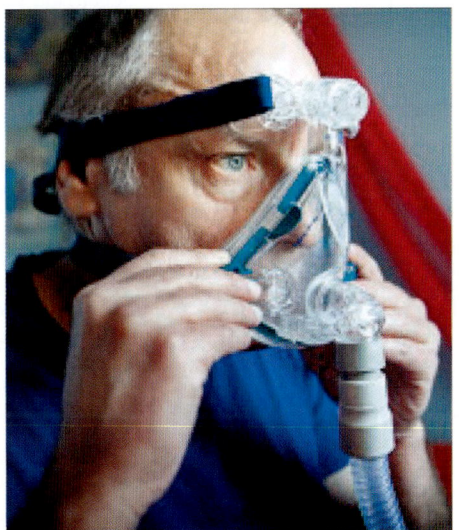

**Fig. 12.2** Patient wearing a noninvasive ventilation mask. (From Smith TA, Davidson PM, Jenkins CR, Ingham JM. Life behind the mask: the patient experience of NIV. *Lancet Respir Med*. 2015;3:1.)

| Table 12.5 Oxygen delivery devices | | |
|---|---|---|
| Type of device | Flow rate of oxygen (L/min) | Estimated % oxygen delivered |
| Nasal cannulae | 1 | 25 |
| | 2 | 28 |
| | 4 | 36 |
| Simple face mask | 6 | 35 |
| | 8 | 47 |
| | 10 | 60 |
| Venturi mask | Blue | 24 |
| | White | 28 |
| | Yellow | 35 |
| | Red | 40 |
| | Green | 60 |
| Nonrebreather | 15 | 85 |
| High-flow nasal oxygen | 60 | 100 |

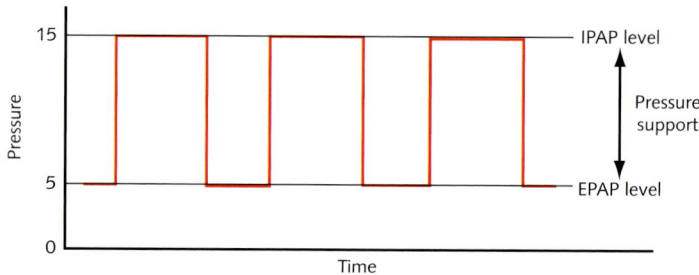

**Fig. 12.3** Pressure differences in bilevel positive airway pressure (BiPAP). BiPAP provides two fixed levels of positive airway pressure. The difference between the inspiratory positive airway pressure (IPAP) and expiratory positive airway pressure (EPAP) is known as pressure support, and can be varied to increase the expulsion of excess $CO_2$. (Modified from Kato T, Suda S, Kasai T. Positive airway pressure therapy for heart failure. *World J Cardiol.* 2015;6:11.)

Although different methods of NIV exist, the most common form is bilevel positive airway pressure (BiPAP), which will be discussed here. Again, a mask is attached to the patient's face with a tight seal to prevent oxygen escaping and pressure changing. The machine recognizes the patient's breathing pattern and aims to synchronize support within both inspiration and expiration. As the patient breathes in, air at a higher pressure is delivered, opening the airways to promote a strong inspiratory phase and aiding oxygenation [inspiratory positive airway pressure (IPAP)]. As the patient breathes out, this is again detected by the machine and the pressure drops, aiding expiration and promoting the expulsion of carbon dioxide, while still providing enough pressure to splint open the small airways and maximize efficient gas exchange [expiratory positive airway pressure (EPAP)]. This variation of pressure (pressure support) acts to aid ventilation and is used in type II respiratory failure, promoting not only oxygenation but adequate expulsion of $CO_2$ (Fig. 12.3).

The use of NIV has strict criteria for use, set out in Table 12.6. It should not be used in situations where invasive ventilation is more appropriate, but is often preferred initially, as a trial in circumstances where it is thought that reversing respiratory failure is possible with noninvasive techniques alone. It requires ABG analysis before treatment, 1 hour following initiation to ensure improvement and further ABGs to assess for improvement as needed or to guide subsequent adjustments to therapy. Where ventilation support alone is not sufficient to maintain oxygenation, supplemental oxygen can be delivered through the device. Given the high levels of monitoring required, NIV should be delivered only on a specialist ward with trained staff, typically a high dependency unit or specialist respiratory ward.

**Table 12.6** Noninvasive ventilation: Indications for acute NIV and contraindications

| |
|---|
| **Indications for noninvasive ventilation** |
| Exacerbation of chronic obstructive airway disease where respiratory acidosis (pH < 7.35, $pCO_2$ > 6) persists despite maximum medical treatment and controlled oxygen therapy |
| Acute-on-chronic hypercapnic respiratory failure secondary to neuromuscular disease or chest wall deformity (pH < 7.35, $pCO_2$ > 6 or if $pCO_2$ > 6 or if vital capacity < 1 L) |
| Obesity (pH < 7.35, $pCO_2$ > 6), or daytime $pCO_2$ > 6 and somnolent |
| Weaning from invasive ventilation in intensive care settings where traditional weaning methods have failed |
| Use with a view to progress to invasive ventilation if fails in type II respiratory failure under specialist advise in an intensive care setting |
| **Contraindications to noninvasive ventilation** |
| Facial trauma, deformity, burns or upper airway obstruction |
| Inability to protect the upper airway, e.g., reduced consciousness (relative) |
| Inability to tolerate, e.g., confusion or agitation (relative) |
| Pneumothorax without the insertion of an intercostal drain (relative) |
| Severe life-threatening hypoxaemia |

## ETHICS

For any patient who is critically unwell and potentially requiring ventilatory support, consideration should be made about what level of treatment is suitable. Some patients with severe, irreversible lung disease, or other significant comorbidities such as cardiac failure, do not have the physiological reserve to survive intensive ventilation or be weaned off a ventilator which can lead to an undignified, protracted and difficult death. For other patients, ventilation may be the only chance of survival. Some patients do not wish to be ventilated and may have advanced directive decisions on the matter.

Decisions about ventilation are complex and should be made by senior clinicians and intensive care specialists. It is important to establish the ceiling of treatment before starting noninvasive treatments, and to involve the patient and family in the decision-making process.

## Invasive ventilation

Invasive ventilation occurs when a patient has an endotracheal or tracheostomy tube in place. It aims to optimize oxygenation, remove carbon dioxide and decrease the work of breathing. The ventilator can be adjusted to provide different inspiratory and expiratory pressures, depending on the patient's needs.

Broadly, mechanical ventilation is used for patients who are unable to maintain their own airway or for those in respiratory failure unresponsive to less invasive measures. Objective criteria for ventilation include a pH < 7.3, $P_aO_2$ < 8 kPa or $P_aCO_2$ > 6 kPa, but these need to be used in combination with clinical features such as apnoea or respiratory distress with altered mental state.

Ventilated patients are managed on intensive care units, as they almost always need further invasive monitoring and treatment. Once the reversible cause of the respiratory failure is treated, the patient can be weaned off the ventilator machine and extubated. This process can take a long time, as patients become physically deconditioned during the weaning process. Complications of mechanical ventilation include airway damage, haemodynamic instability, barotrauma and ventilator-acquired pneumonias.

## USEFUL LINKS

Davidson AC, Banham S, Elliott M, et al. BTS/ICS guideline for the ventilatory management of acute hypercapnic respiratory failure in adults. *Thorax*. 2016;71(Suppl 2):ii1–35.

https://www.resus.org.uk/resuscitation-guidelines/abcde-approach/.

https://www.brit-thoracic.org.uk/document-library/clinical-information/niv/niv-guidelines/btsrcpics-guideline-on-niv-in-copd/.

## ● Chapter Summary

- An acutely unwell patient should be assessed using the ABCDE approach, correcting adverse features as you progress through each step.
- Arterial blood gas interpretation is vital in the management of respiratory failure. Having a systematic approach ensures reliable interpretation and management.
- Type I respiratory failure is defined as $P_aO_2$ < 8 kPa with a low or normal $P_aCO_2$. This represents a ventilation:perfusion mismatch.
- Type II respiratory failure is defined as $P_aO_2$ < 8 kPa with a raised $P_aCO_2$. This represents a failure of ventilation.
- Respiratory failure is managed with oxygen support +/– ventilator support, with immediate attention to the underlying cause of the respiratory failure.
- Endotracheal intubation and mechanical ventilation are employed when less invasive manoeuvres have failed or there is airway compromise. Patients must be fit enough to tolerate invasive ventilation.

**MLA Conditions**
Cardiorespiratory arrest
Respiratory arrest
Respiratory failure

**MLA Presentations**
Cyanosis
Shock

## INTRODUCTION

The upper respiratory tract comprises the nose and nasal passages, the sinuses, pharynx and the part of the larynx above the vocal cords. While much upper respiratory tract pathology is managed by ear, nose and throat (ENT) specialists, in modern practice a number of conditions overlap into respiratory medicine. We will outline some of these conditions, beginning with the emergency presentations of upper airway pathology.

## EMERGENCY PRESENTATIONS OF THE UPPER RESPIRATORY TRACT

### Anaphylaxis

Anaphylaxis is a serious allergic reaction that is potentially life-threatening.

#### Pathogenesis
Anaphylaxis is an immune-mediated systemic reaction to a particular pathogen. It is an acute type 1 immune reaction mediated by IgE and mast cells, which release a wide variety of cytokines and inflammatory mediators such as histamine. This causes constriction of bronchial smooth muscle and vascular leakage throughout the body.

#### Aetiology
Various foodstuffs and environmental agents can provoke an anaphylactic reaction. Common agents include nuts, bee stings and drugs such as penicillin. The incidence of anaphylaxis is higher in those with other allergic diseases such as asthma or hay fever.

#### Clinical features
- Rash
- Generalized itchiness
- Wheeze and stridor
- Shortness of breath
- Tachycardia
- Hypotension
- Gastrointestinal symptoms such as nausea and diarrhoea.

#### Investigations
- The diagnosis of anaphylaxis is clinical.
- Mast cell tryptase is an enzyme that serves as a marker for mast cell activation. It is used to confirm whether a reaction is anaphylactic in suspected cases and to differentiate between pseudoallergic or anaphylactoid reactions. Blood tests for mast cell tryptase should be taken as soon as possible after resuscitation, at 1 hour and at 24 hours post event. Note that measurements should never delay acute management.

#### Management
- Resuscitation with intravenous (IV) fluids and oxygen.
- Intramuscular (IM) adrenaline 0.5 mL of 1:1000 which is equal to 500 micrograms.
- Chlorphenamine (an antihistamine) 10 mg IM or slow IV infusion.
- Hydrocortisone 200 mg IM or slow IV infusion.

Note that the above doses are for adults and children over the age of 12 years. Specific doses should be sought for children under the age of 12 years.

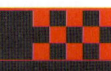

**RED FLAG**

**UPPER AIRWAY COMPROMISE**

Any upper airway compromise is an emergency. The presence of stridor, tachypnoea, cyanosis and respiratory distress in the setting of airway compromise may require advanced airway management techniques such as intubation. In the emergency setting, this is only performed by trained individuals such as anaesthetists or emergency doctors. In severe cases where intubation is not possible, emergency tracheotomy may be required. In any airway compromise, call for help early.

### Foreign body aspiration

Aspiration of a foreign body can be life-threatening. It is most commonly seen in children but can occur at any age. The most serious cases are those where the foreign body lodges in the larynx or trachea, as this causes complete airway obstruction. If the object tracks down to below the carina (more commonly to the right main bronchus as it has a more vertical position), it can often go unnoticed for some time, with only mild symptoms.

#### Prevalence
The prevalence of foreign body aspiration is variable depending on age group. It is most common in the very young and very old.

## Aetiology

Foreign bodies encompass a wide variety of objects. In young children, these tend to be toys and small household objects, which are put in the mouth out of curiosity. However, in the older population, aspiration may occur in those who have a poor swallow (such as following a stroke).

## Clinical features

In upper airways:

- Stridor
- Respiratory distress
- Cyanosis
- Respiratory arrest

Beyond the carina:

- Recurrent cough
- Pneumonia
- Shortness of breath
- Haemoptysis

## Investigations

- Blood tests – may demonstrate an inflammatory response.
- Chest X-ray – will show up any radiopaque objects and may also demonstrate pneumonia.
- Bronchoscopy – direct visualization of the object.

## Management

- Management depends on the severity and location of the obstruction. In mild cases, encourage coughing.
- If the object is in the proximal airways and the symptoms are severe or coughing alone is not working, try simple techniques such as five back slaps and then five abdominal thrusts (the Heimlich manoeuvre).
- Airway suction.
- If the object is further down the airways, remove it at bronchoscopy.
- Antibiotics to prevent/treat pneumonia. If secondary to aspiration of gastric contents, antibiotics need to cover anaerobic gut bacteria.

## DISORDERS OF THE NOSE

## Infectious rhinitis (acute coryza or common cold)

Rhinitis is inflammation of the mucosal membrane lining the nose. Inflammation seen in the common cold is caused by a number of viral infections:

- Rhinovirus (commonest cause)
- Coronavirus (seasonal and COVID-19)

- Adenovirus
- Parainfluenza virus
- Respiratory syncytial virus.

The common cold is a highly contagious, self-limiting condition, with the highest incidence in children. Symptoms are nasal obstruction, rhinorrhoea (runny nose) and sneezing. Complications include sinusitis, otitis media and lower respiratory tract infections.

## Pathology

There is acute inflammation with oedema, glandular hypersecretion and loss of surface epithelium.

## Treatment

Infections with such viruses are self-limiting and no medical treatment is required. Analgesia and nasal decongestants can be used to relieve symptoms.

# Chronic rhinitis

Chronic rhinitis may develop following an acute inflammatory episode. Predisposing factors such as inadequate drainage of sinuses, nasal obstruction caused by polyps and enlargement of the adenoids increase the risk of developing chronic rhinitis.

# Allergic rhinitis

Allergic rhinitis is an inflammatory condition of the nasal mucosa caused by an IgE-mediated response to common environmental allergens.

## Epidemiology

Allergic rhinitis is a common condition: prevalence has been estimated to be 15%–20%. Symptoms of allergic rhinitis are most commonly present in childhood and adolescence; it is estimated that 80% of people with the condition develop symptoms before the age of 20 years.

The prevalence of allergic rhinitis is equal in men and women; however, the age at which men and women develop symptoms differs. Men are more likely to develop allergic rhinitis in childhood, whereas the peak incidence in women occurs during adolescence. There is a geographical variation in the prevalence of allergic rhinitis – it is much more common in developed countries than in developing countries.

## Aetiology

The development of allergic rhinitis cannot be attributed to one single genetic or environmental factor. It is likely to arise as a result of interaction between multiple genes and specific environmental variables (Fig. 13.1).

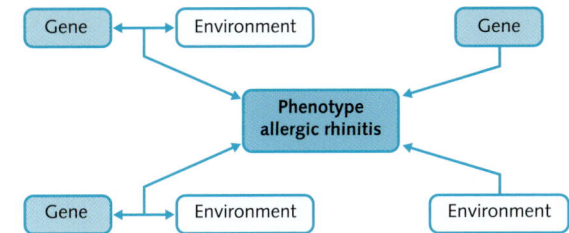

**Fig. 13.1** Polygenic inheritance of allergic rhinitis.

A family history of atopy is an important risk factor for developing allergic rhinitis. Studies have suggested that the risk of developing atopic disease in the absence of parental family history is only 13%. This risk increases to 47% if both parents are atopic and 72% if both parents have the same atopic manifestation.

Environmental factors also play a large role in the development of allergic rhinitis; many believe the 'hygiene hypothesis' can account for the increasing prevalence of allergic rhinitis in the Western world. The hygiene hypothesis suggests that lack of exposure to bacteria and microorganisms in childhood (i.e., our environment is too clean) increases the risk of developing allergic rhinitis and other atopic diseases (Fig. 13.2).

## Pathology
Symptoms are caused by a type 1 IgE-mediated hypersensitivity reaction. IgE fixes on to mast cells in nasal mucous membranes. Upon re-exposure to allergen, cross-linking of the IgE receptor occurs on the surface of the mast cells, leading to mast cell degranulation and release of histamine and leukotrienes (Fig. 13.3).

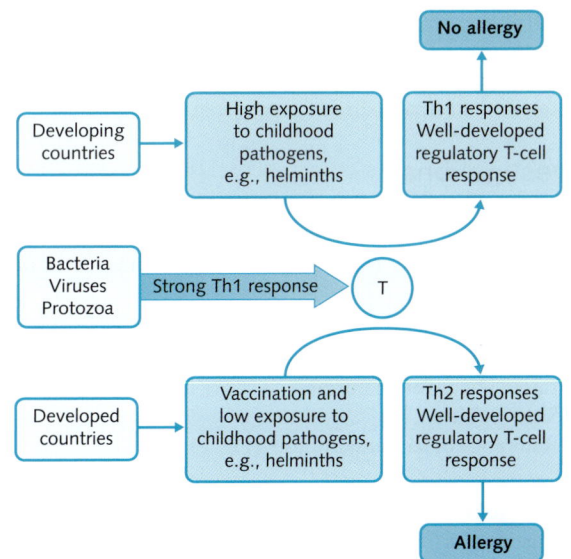

**Fig. 13.2** Hygiene hypothesis. *T*, thymus

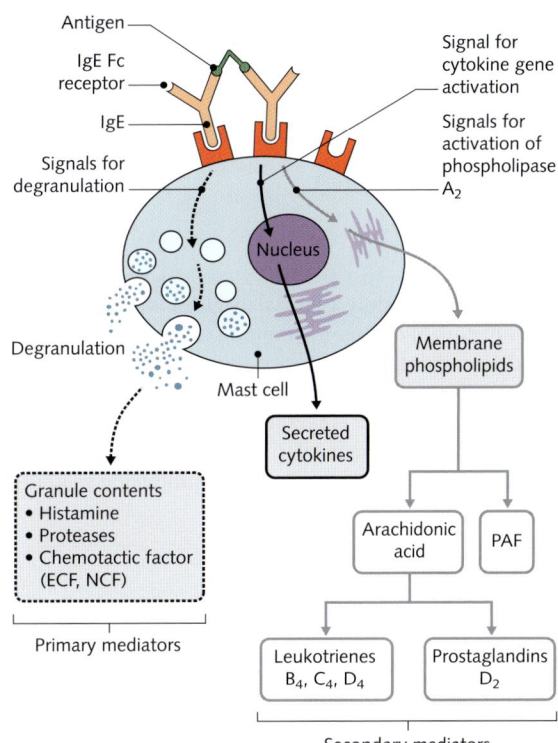

**Fig. 13.3** Type 1 hypersensitivity reactions. *ECF,* Eosinophil chemotactic factor; *Fc,* Fc receptor; *IgE Fc,* immunoglobulin E; *NCF,* neutrophil chemotactic factor; *PAF,* platelet-activating factor.

## Classification
Allergic rhinitis can be classified into seasonal or perennial rhinitis, depending on whether a patient is allergic to pollens (seasonal, also known as hay fever) or allergens that are present year-round, such as house dust mites, pets and moulds.

However, it is much more useful clinically to classify allergic rhinitis in terms of severity and the impact on a patient's quality of life (Table 13.1).

**Table 13.1** Classification of allergic rhinitis

**Mild**

None of the following items are present:
- Sleep disturbance
- Impairment of daily activities, leisure and/or sport
- Impairment of school or work
- Troublesome symptoms

**Moderate/severe**

One or more of the following items are present:
- Sleep disturbance
- Impairment of daily activities, leisure and/or sport
- Impairment of school or work
- Troublesome symptoms

## Symptoms

The common symptoms of allergic rhinitis include:

- Nasal congestion
- Rhinorrhoea
- Sneezing
- Itching (eyes/nose/throat)
- Fatigue.

## Investigation

Allergic rhinitis is mainly a clinical diagnosis based on taking an accurate history of common symptoms and identifying risk factors and potential allergens.

Skin prick testing can be undertaken to identify specific allergens to which the patient is allergic; however, in clinical practice, a diagnosis is usually made by treating empirically, with trial of antihistamines and nasal corticosteroids producing an improvement in a patient's symptoms.

## Management

Management of allergic rhinitis largely depends on the frequency and severity of a patient's symptoms and the extent to which they impact on the patient's life. Table 13.2 provides broad guidance for the management of allergic rhinitis.

# Acute sinusitis

Sinusitis is an inflammatory process involving the lining of paranasal sinuses (Fig. 13.4). The maxillary sinus is most commonly clinically infected. The majority of infections are rhinogenic in origin and are classified as either acute or chronic.

## Aetiology

The common causes of acute sinusitis are:

- Secondary bacterial infection (by *Streptococcus pneumoniae* or *Haemophilus influenzae*), often following an upper respiratory tract viral infection.
- Dental extraction or infection.
- Swimming and diving.
- Fractures involving sinuses.

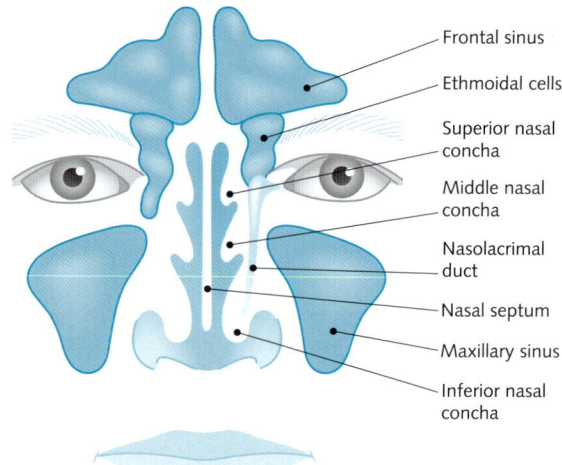

**Fig. 13.4** Anatomy of the sinuses.

## Pathology

Hyperaemia and oedema of the mucosa occur. Blockage of sinus ostia and mucus production increases. The cilia lining the paranasal sinuses stop beating efficiently, leading to stasis of secretions causing secondary infection.

## Clinical features

Symptoms occur over several days:

- Purulent nasal discharge
- Malaise
- Sinus tenderness
- Disturbed sense of smell.

There may be fullness and pain over the cheeks, a maxillary toothache or a frontal headache. Pain is classically worse on leaning forward. Postnasal discharge may lead to cough.

## Investigations

Sinusitis is like allergic rhinitis – a clinical diagnosis is based on an accurate history. The following investigations may be useful in particularly severe or recurrent cases but are not essential in the majority of cases:

- Blood tests – white cell count and inflammatory markers (erythrocyte sedimentation rate/C-reactive protein) may be raised but are often normal.
- Sinus culture.
- Radiology of paranasal sinuses (Fig. 13.5).

## Management

Management is mainly symptomatic with:

- Analgesia
- Nasal decongestants

| Table 13.2 Management of allergic rhinitis | |
|---|---|
| Mild intermittent symptoms | Allergen avoidance<br>Oral antihistamine |
| Mild persistent symptoms or moderate to severe intermittent symptoms | Allergen avoidance<br>Oral antihistamine<br>Intranasal corticosteroid |
| Moderate to severe persistent symptoms | Allergen avoidance<br>Oral antihistamine<br>Intranasal corticosteroid ± oral corticosteroid |

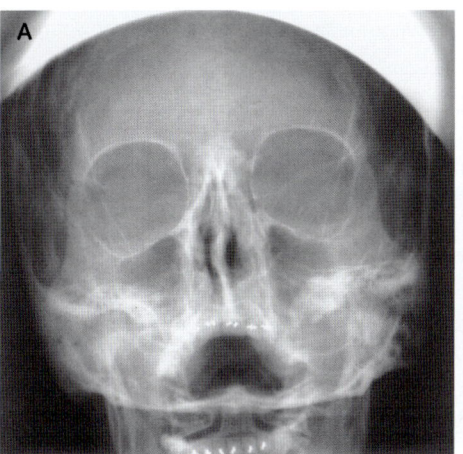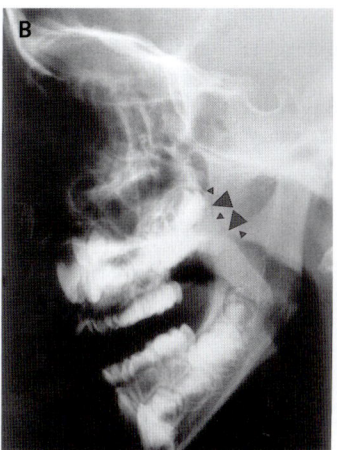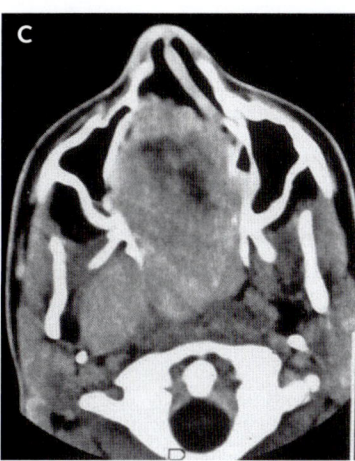

**Fig. 13.5** Radiology of the paranasal sinuses. (A) The most commonly used imaging modality in sinusitis is X-ray, which may show an air–fluid level in the affected sinus. (B) Lateral X-rays are useful in children with recurrent sinusitis as they can reveal enlarged adenoids which predispose. (C) Computed tomography scans are useful for assessing the extent of disease and identifying unusual anatomy of the sinuses, which also predisposes to sinusitis.

- Saline nasal rinse
- Intranasal steroids in some cases

Where the sinusitis is suspected to be bacterial in origin (a persistent pyrexia and very purulent discharge), patients should be managed with antibiotics. In patients who are immunocompromised, there should be a very low threshold for treating with antibiotics.

A referral to an ENT specialist is warranted in patients with unresolving or recurring symptoms.

## Chronic sinusitis

Chronic sinusitis is an inflammation of the sinuses which has been present for more than 4 weeks. It usually occurs after recurrent acute sinusitis and is common in patients who are heavy smokers or who work in dusty environments.

### Clinical features
Clinical features are similar to those of acute sinusitis but are typically less severe.

### Pathology
Prolonged infection leads to irreversible changes in the sinus cavity, including:

- An increase in vascular permeability
- Oedema and hypertrophy of the mucosa
- Goblet cell hyperplasia
- Chronic cellular infiltrate
- Ulceration of the epithelium, resulting in granulated tissue formation.

### Investigations
Investigations are through sinus radiographs, high-definition coronal section computed tomography (CT) and diagnostic endoscopy.

### Treatment
This condition is difficult to treat. Treatments are:

- Medical – broad-acting antibiotics and decongestants.
- Surgical – antral lavage, inferior meatal intranasal antrostomy and functional endoscopic sinus surgery.

> **CLINICAL NOTES**
>
> **KARTAGENER SYNDROME**
>
> Rarely, recurrent sinusitis may be caused by Kartagener syndrome, a congenital mucociliary disorder caused by the absence of the ciliary protein dynein. It is characterized by sinusitis, bronchiectasis, otitis media, situs invertus and infertility.

# DISORDERS OF THE LARYNX

## Laryngitis

Laryngitis is an inflammatory condition of the larynx. It is extremely common and usually caused by viral infection.

### Epidemiology

The true incidence of laryngitis is hard to quantify as symptoms often go unreported, although the Royal College of General Practitioners in the UK reported a peak average incidence of laryngitis as 23 cases per 100,000 population per week, at all ages, over the period from 1999 to 2005. There is,

129

as expected, a seasonal variation in laryngitis, with peaks in viral laryngitis in autumn and spring (rhinovirus) and in winter (influenza).

The incidence of bacterial laryngitis has reduced significantly since the introduction of the *H. influenzae* type B (Hib) vaccine.

## Aetiology

Laryngitis is most commonly caused by a viral infection, that is, rhinovirus. Other infectious causes include:

- Bacterial (diphtheria, *Haemophilus* in unvaccinated children)
- Tuberculosis
- *Candida* (particularly in immunosuppressed patients).

## Symptoms

- Dysphagia
- Hoarseness
- Odynophagia
- Cough.

## Investigation and management

Laryngitis is a clinical diagnosis based on accurate history and examination findings. Management is usually supportive with analgesia, and viral infections are self-limiting. Bacterial infections will require treatment with a course of antibiotics. Recurrent laryngitis may warrant referral to an ENT surgeon.

## Chronic laryngitis

Chronic laryngitis is inflammation of the larynx and trachea associated with excessive smoking, continued vocal abuse and excessive alcohol.

The mucous glands are swollen and the epithelium is hypertrophied. Heavy smoking leads to squamous metaplasia of the larynx. Biopsy is mandatory to rule out malignancy. Management is directed at avoidance of aetiological factors.

## Laryngotracheobronchitis (croup) versus acute epiglottitis

Laryngotracheobronchitis (croup) is an extremely common condition in paediatrics, particularly during the winter months, and is caused by a viral infection (Table 13.3). In clinical practice, it is vitally important to make the distinction between children presenting with croup and those presenting with acute epiglottitis, which is a medical emergency.

The clinical features of these conditions are shown in Table 13.3. The incidence of epiglottitis has dramatically fallen, owing to the introduction of the Hib vaccine.

**Table 13.3** Laryngotracheobronchitis (croup) and acute epiglottitis

|  | Croup | Epiglottitis |
|---|---|---|
| **Aetiology** | Viral | Bacterial |
| **Organism** | Parainfluenza, respiratory syncytial virus | Group B *Haemophilus influenzae* |
| **Age range** | 6 months to 3 years | 3–7 years |
| **Onset** | Gradual over days | Sudden over hours |
| **Cough** | Severe barking | Minimal |
| **Temperature** | Pyrexia < 38.5°C | Pyrexia > 38.5°C |
| **Stridor** | Harsh | Soft |
| **Drooling** | No | Yes |
| **Voice** | Hoarse | Reluctant to speak |
| **Able to drink** | Yes | No |
| **Active** | Yes | No, completely still |
| **Mortality** | Low | High |

## Pathology

In epiglottitis, there is necrosis of epithelium and formation of an extensive fibrous membrane on the trachea and main bronchi. Oedema of the subglottic area occurs, with subsequent danger of laryngeal obstruction.

In croup, there is an acute inflammatory oedema and infiltration by neutrophil polymorphs. No mucosal ulceration occurs.

## Treatment

To treat laryngotracheobronchitis, keep the patient calm and hydrated. Nurse in a warm room in an upright position. Drug treatment, if required, includes steroids (oral dexamethasone), oxygen and nebulized adrenaline (epinephrine).

### CASE STUDY

Lucy, a 2-year-old girl, came into the accident and emergency unit with a cough, difficulty breathing and a sore throat. Her mother said that she had had a cold for the past week. Closer examination revealed that Lucy had a hoarse voice and a cough that sounded like a bark. There was some sternal recession and discomfort when lying down. Lucy was diagnosed as having croup.

She had moderate-to-severe croup and was treated with 100% oxygen, nebulized adrenaline (epinephrine) and budesonide, as well as oral dexamethasone.

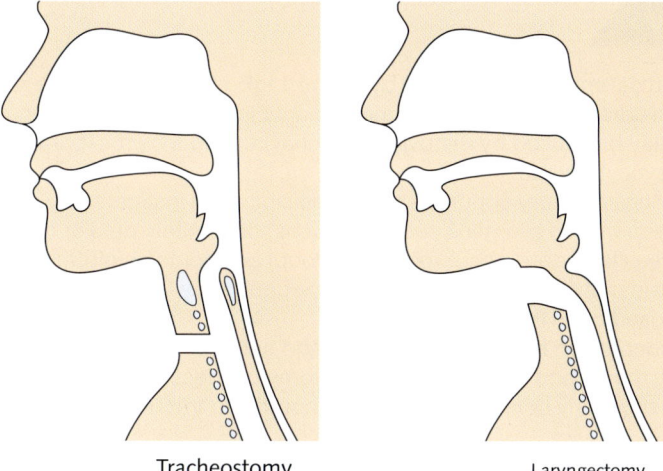

Tracheostomy

Laryngectomy

**Fig. 13.6** Tracheostomy and laryngectomy.

Acute epiglottitis is a medical emergency. Call for the anaesthetist, ENT surgeon and, if appropriate, the paediatric team. Never attempt to visualize the epiglottis. Keep calm and reassure the patient. Never leave the patient alone. As with other serious *H. influenzae* infections, prophylactic treatment with rifampicin is offered to the close contacts.

## Reactive nodules

Reactive nodules are common, small inflammatory polyps, usually measuring less than 10 mm in diameter. They are also known as singer's nodules. They present in patients aged 40–50 years and are more common in men. Reactive nodules are caused by excessive untrained use of vocal cords. Patients present with hoarseness of the voice.

### Pathology

Keratosis develops at the junction of the anterior and middle thirds of the vocal cord on each side. Oedematous myxoid connective tissue is covered by squamous epithelium. The reactive nodules may become painful because of ulceration.

## TRACHEOSTOMY AND LARYNGECTOMY

A tracheostomy is a connection between the trachea and the anterior aspect of the neck to allow patients to breathe without the use of the nose or mouth, with a tracheal tube inserted to keep the connection open. It can be inserted for a number of different reasons, including the use of long-term mechanical ventilation (e.g., with a prolonged intensive care stay) and head and neck surgery for cancers, or it may be inserted in the acute setting for severe angioedema or upper airway obstruction. As patients breathe through the stoma, air bypasses the vocal cords and so they cannot speak while the tracheostomy is open. As there is still a connection, air can pass if the stoma is blocked, meaning speaking valves can also be used to temporarily block off the valve.

Care of the tracheostomy is important. As the patient bypasses the filtering mechanisms of the nasal passages and upper airways, they are more susceptible to chest infections. Likewise, the stoma can easily block off with thick secretions. The tracheostomy often requires suction in infective episodes to prevent plugging off, often supervised by critical care staff (Fig. 13.6).

Laryngectomy is a surgical procedure performed primarily for laryngeal cancers. It involves the removal of the larynx, leaving a connection between the mouth and oesophagus, plus a separate distinct connection between trachea and upper neck. The stoma in laryngectomy typically does not require a tracheostomy tube to keep it open, although a humidification device may appear similar. Laryngectomy patients cannot talk nor receive airway treatments through the mouth or nose, which is particularly important in resuscitation. Similar care techniques apply to manage the airway in terms of suction to clear secretions. Differentiating between tracheostomy and laryngectomy can be done on clinical examination if no history is available. There is a significant psychosocial impact of either procedure, which should also be considered when managing these patients.

## ● Chapter Summary

- Anaphylaxis is a medical emergency caused by a type 1 IgE-mediated immune response and is managed with adrenaline, hydrocortisone and antihistamines in the first instance.
- The common cold may be caused by rhinovirus, coronavirus, adenovirus, parainfluenza virus or respiratory syncytial virus.
- Allergic rhinitis is an inflammatory condition of the nasal mucosa instigated by an IgE-mediated immune response to allergens such as pollens, dust mites, pets or moulds.
- Distinguishing between laryngotracheobronchitis (croup) and acute epiglottitis in paediatrics is vital to identifying an acute medical emergency (the latter may require intubation and is caused by *H. influenzae*).
- Tracheostomy is a connection between the trachea and anterior neck wall with a patent connection between mouth and trachea. A laryngectomy connects the trachea and anterior neck wall without any connection between mouth and trachea.

| MLA Conditions | MLA Presentations |
|---|---|
| Allergic disorder | Allergies |
| Anaphylaxis | Anaphylaxis |
| Rhinosinusitis | Hoarseness and voice change |
| Tonsillitis | Sore throat |
| Upper respiratory tract infection | Stridor |

## Further reading

Resuscitation Council (UK). Anaphylaxis UK resuscitation guidelines. https://www.resus.org.uk/anaphylaxis/emergency-treatment-of-anaphylactic-reactions/.

Birmingham Research Unit of the Royal College of General Practitioners. Communicable and respiratory disease report for England and Wales. 2006. http://www.rcgp.org.uk/.

# Asthma 14

## DEFINITION AND BACKGROUND

Asthma is a chronic inflammatory disorder of the airways characterized by recurrent episodes of typical symptoms (wheeze, chest tightness, breathlessness and cough) with periods of no/minimal symptoms between episodes. The pathophysiology of asthma involves variable airflow obstruction, airway hyperresponsiveness and airway inflammation. There is no gold standard diagnostic test and therefore it is a clinical diagnosis.

## Prevalence

Asthma is the most common lung condition in the UK. Asthma + Lung UK data shows that in the UK, 5.4 million people have asthma. This is roughly equivalent to 1 in 12 adults and 1 in 11 children. Unfortunately, according to the National Review of Asthma Deaths 2024, every day four people die from an asthma attack with 2/3 of these deaths found to be preventable.

## CLASSIFICATION

Over recent years, asthma has been increasingly recognized as a heterogeneous clinical syndrome rather than a single disease entity. It may be classified phenotypically according to clinical and physiological characteristics or by endotype according to distinct pathophysiology. The phenotypic model classifies asthma as 'extrinsic' (atopic childhood asthma) or 'intrinsic' (adult onset, nonatopic; Table 14.1). Occupational asthma can be considered as a separate group.

## Extrinsic asthma

This is classical asthma with onset in childhood or young adolescence, commonly with a previous history of atopy (allergic rhinitis, food allergy or eczema). It is triggered by inhalation of allergens and typically responds to treatment.

## Intrinsic asthma

This subtype tends to be of adult onset, is more progressive and is less responsive to therapy. It is less likely to be related to a previous history of atopy.

**Table 14.1** Classification of asthma

|  | Extrinsic asthma | Intrinsic asthma |
|---|---|---|
| Underlying abnormality | Immune reaction (atopic) | Abnormal autonomic regulation of airways |
| Onset | Childhood | Adulthood |
| Distribution | 60% | 40% |
| Allergens | Recognized | None identified |
| Family history | Present | Absent |
| Predisposition to form IgE antibodies | Present | Absent |
| Association with chronic obstructive pulmonary disease | None | Chronic bronchitis |
| Natural progression | Improves | Worsens |
| Eosinophilia | Sputum and blood | Sputum |
| Drug hypersensitivity | Absent | Present |

## PRECIPITATING FACTORS

Recognized precipitating factors for asthma include:

- Allergens: house dust mite, flour, animal danders.
- Occupational factors: solder (colophony) fumes, flour, isocyanates.
- Viral infections: parainfluenza, respiratory syncytial virus, rhinovirus.
- Drugs: β-blockers, nonsteroidal anti-inflammatory drugs, aspirin.
- Other factors: cold air, exercise, emotion.

## OCCUPATIONAL ASTHMA

Occupational asthma is caused by specific sensitizers in the workplace and can occur in individuals without previously diagnosed asthma. Occupational asthma may be classified as:

- Allergic – immunologically mediated with a latent period between exposure and symptoms during which the worker becomes sensitized to the causal agent.

- Nonallergic – immediate response after exposure to an irritant, e.g., to high concentrations of a toxic gas.

Occupational asthma can be difficult to diagnose owing to the latency period between exposure and symptoms. It is important to ask questions in the history about worsening symptoms at work or improved symptoms when on holiday, as well as possible exposures at work. Currently, over 200 materials encountered at the workplace are implicated (Table 14.2). Diagnosis is based on confirming the diagnosis of asthma in the usual manner, confirming the relationship between asthma and work and identifying the specific cause. Bronchial provocation tests may be used in specialist centres to demonstrate bronchospasm to a particular agent.

## PATHOGENESIS

The pathogenesis of asthma is very complex; however, three main processes are responsible for the majority of symptoms. These are bronchospasm, smooth-muscle hypertrophy and mucus plugging (Fig. 14.1). Allergen-induced airway inflammation results in:

- Smooth-muscle constriction
- Thickening of the airway wall (smooth-muscle hypertrophy and oedema)
- Basement membrane thickening
- Mucus and exudate in the airway lumen.

Microscopically, the viscid mucus contains:

- Desquamated epithelial cells
- Whorls of shed epithelium (Curschmann whorls)
- Charcot–Leyden crystal (eosinophil cell membranes)
- Infiltration of inflammatory cells, particularly CD4$^+$ T lymphocytes.

**Table 14.2** Factors implicated in occupational asthma

| Agents | Workers at risk |
|---|---|
| **High-molecular-weight agents** | |
| Cereals | Bakers, millers |
| Animal-derived allergens | Animal handlers |
| Enzymes | Detergent users, pharmaceutical workers, bakers |
| Gums | Carpet makers, pharmaceutical workers |
| Latex | Health professionals |
| Seafoods | Seafood processors |
| **Low-molecular-weight agents** | |
| Isocyanates | Spray painters, insulation installers, etc. |
| Wood dusts | Forest workers, carpenters |
| Anhydrides | Users of plastics, epoxy resins |
| Fluxes | Electronic workers |
| Chloramine | Janitors, cleaners |
| Acrylate | Adhesive handlers |
| Drugs | Pharmaceutical workers, health professionals |
| Metals | Solderers, refiners |

## Inflammatory mediators

Inflammatory mediators play a vital role in the pathogenesis of asthma. Inflammatory stimuli activate mast cells, epithelial cells,

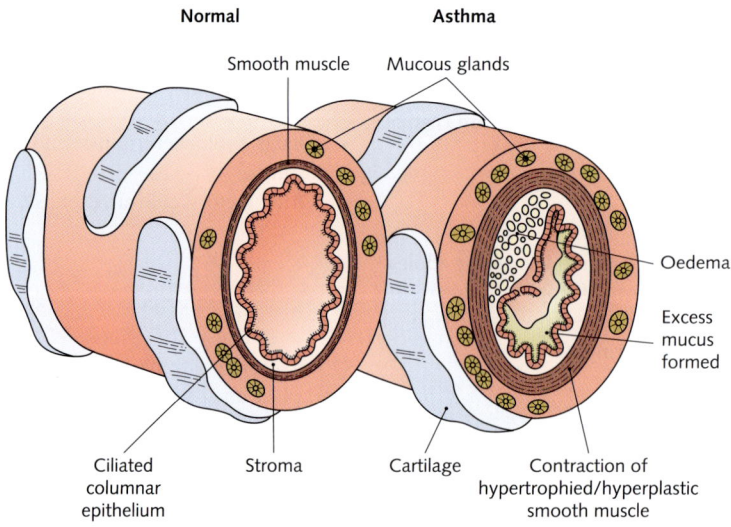

**Fig. 14.1** Mechanisms of airway narrowing in asthma.

alveolar macrophages and dendritic cells resident within the airways, causing the release of mediators that are chemotactic for cells derived from the circulation – secondary effector cells (eosinophils, neutrophils and platelets). Mediators that are thought to be involved in asthma include:

- Preformed mediators – present in cytoplasmic granules ready for release. They are associated with human lung mast cells and include histamine, neutral proteases and chemotactic factors for eosinophils. These are responsible for the early response.
- Newly generated mediators – manufactured secondary to the initial triggering stimulus after release of preformed mediators. Some of these mediators are derived from the membrane phospholipids and are associated with the metabolism of arachidonic acid (e.g., prostaglandins and leukotrienes). The production of inflammatory cytokines and chemokines is important in the activation and recruitment of inflammatory cells, ultimately leading to a so-called late response.

## Early and late responses

Two patterns of response can be considered; in practice, most asthmatics show evidence of both responses, although either may be absent.

### Immediate (early) reaction

The release of preformed mediators (predominantly from mast cells) causes vascular leakage and smooth-muscle contraction within 10–15 minutes of challenge, with a return to baseline within 1–2 hours. The mast cells are activated by allergens that cross-link with the immunoglobulin E (IgE) molecules that are bound to high-affinity receptors on the mast cell membrane.

### Late reaction

The influx of inflammatory cells (predominantly eosinophils) and the release of their inflammatory mediators cause airway narrowing after 3–4 hours, which is maximal after 6–12 hours. This is much more difficult to reverse than the immediate reaction and there is an increase in the level of airway hyperreactivity.

The biphasic nature of asthma attacks is the basis behind patients being admitted for observation for approximately 24 hours after a moderate or severe attack.

The asthmatic process is overviewed in Fig. 14.2: panel A shows the cellular and mediator response to allergen, whereas panel B shows the pathophysiological effects of this process.

## Airway remodelling

This is a term used to describe the specific structural changes that occur in long-standing asthma with severe airway inflammation. The characteristic features include:

- Increased vascular permeability.
- Loss of surface epithelial cells and hypertrophy of goblet cells.
- Hypertrophy of smooth muscle.
- Myofibroblast accumulation and increased collagen deposition, hence causing basement membrane thickening.

Airway remodelling may cause a fixed airway obstruction, which may not be reversible with antiinflammatory agents or bronchodilators.

## CLINICAL FEATURES

## Symptoms and clinical history

The typical symptoms of asthma are wheeze, breathlessness, chest tightness, cough and noisy breathing. Symptoms are episodic with a return to normal or near normal in between. Classically, symptoms show a diurnal variation, often being worse at night or in the early morning. Symptoms may also be seasonal. Nocturnal coughing is a common presenting symptom, especially in children. This in part may be due to reduced cortisol levels and thus steroid at night with levels increasing again during the day. Symptoms are intermittent and can be associated with specific triggers listed earlier in the chapter. It is important to try and discern the exact timing of symptoms, as this can be crucial not only in diagnosing asthma but also in identifying the underlying trigger. Asking about worsening of symptoms at work (with reduction when on holiday or at the weekend/between shifts) can be very useful in those with occupational asthma.

Other features to look out for in the history include a personal or family history of atopic illness, including eczema and hay fever, nasal symptoms, food allergies, pets and a history of gastrooesophageal reflux disease (which can worsen asthma).

## Examination

Owing to the variability of airflow obstruction in asthma, examination of a patient's respiratory system may be completely normal. During an exacerbation, a polyphonic expiratory wheeze is classically heard. In severe and life-threatening asthma, however, the chest may be silent as airflow in the small airways is almost completely obstructed.

## INVESTIGATIONS AND DIAGNOSIS

There is no single diagnostic test for asthma. An assessment of clinical probability of asthma based on symptoms and signs should take place initially. If the diagnosis is uncertain, further objective diagnostic tests looking for variable airflow obstruction or airway inflammation can then be used to help make the diagnosis. It is important to note that BTS, NICE and SIGN 2024 guidelines state to not confirm a diagnosis of asthma without a

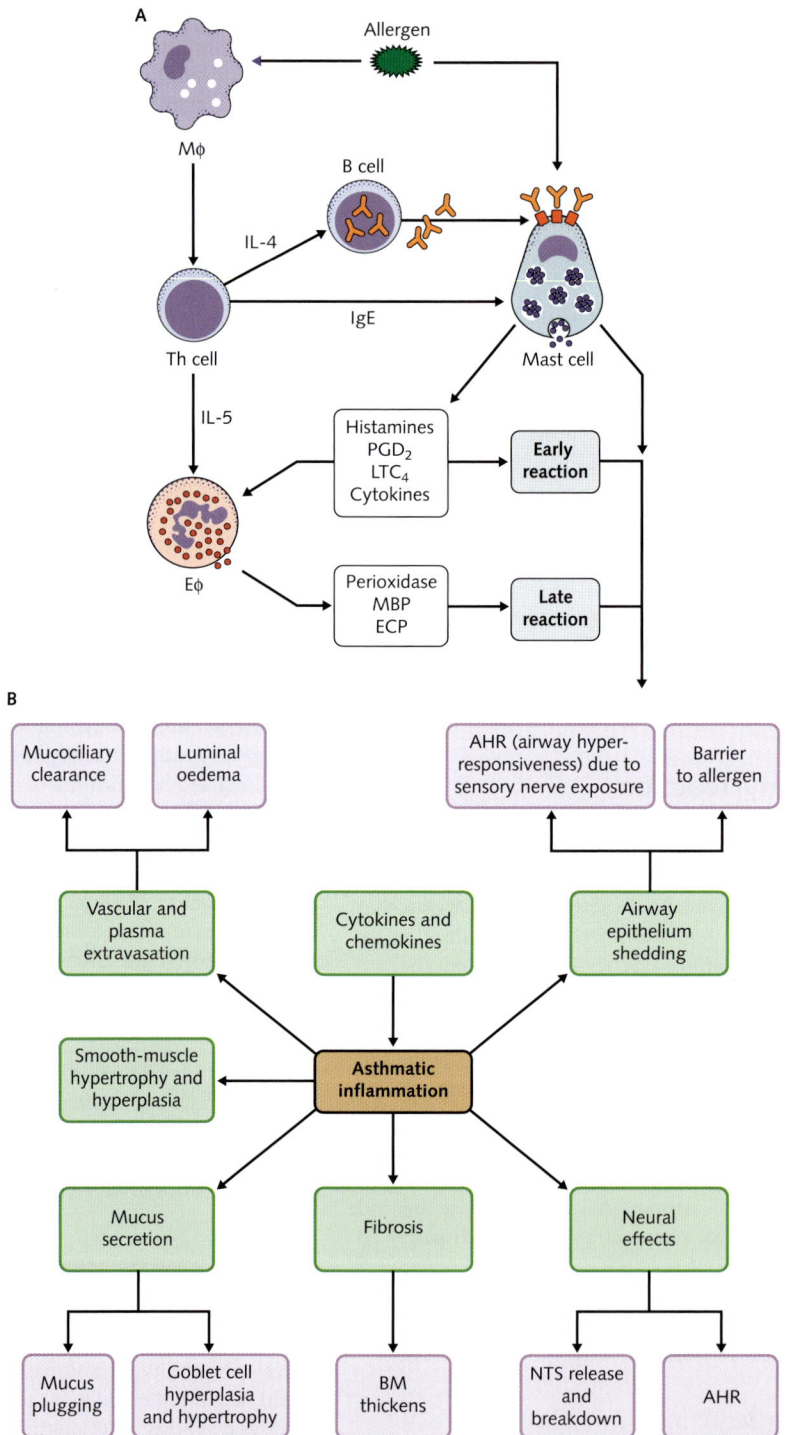

**Fig. 14.2** (A) Pathogenesis of asthma. (B) The pathophysiological effects of cellular processes in asthma. *AHR,* Airway hyperresponsiveness; *BM,* basement membrane; *ECP,* eosinophil cationic protein; *IgE,* immunoglobulin E; *IL-4,* interleukin 4; *IL-5,* interleukin 5; *MBP,* major basic protein; *LTC₄,* leukotriene C₄; *NTS,* neurotransmitter substance; *PGD₂,* prostaglandin D₂.

**Table 14.3** Comparison between asthma and chronic obstructive pulmonary disease

|  | Asthma | Chronic obstructive pulmonary disease |
|---|---|---|
| Genetic components | Polygenetic | Fewer genes involved, e.g., $\alpha_1$-antitrypsin |
| Age of onset | Can occur at any age but more common during childhood | Mainly affects the adult population |
| Inflammatory cells involved | Eosinophils and mast cells are the main culprits | Mainly neutrophils |
| Symptoms | Variable – wheeze, cough | Persistent – shortness of breath on exertion, cough |
| Investigations | Diurnal variation in $FEV_1$ | Progressive decline in $FEV_1$ over time |
| Reversibility | Marked | Sometimes |
| Most effective bronchodilator | $\beta_2$-adrenoceptor agonist, e.g., salbutamol | Anticholinergics, e.g., ipratropium bromide |
| Steroid treatment | Beneficial | Not very beneficial but useful in acute exacerbations |

$FEV_1$, Forced expiratory volume in 1 second.

suggestive clinical history and a supporting objective test. Initial objective tests for diagnosing asthma in adults are: blood eosinophil count – if the count is above the lab reference range then, alongside a supportive clinical history, asthma can be diagnosed; fractional exhaled nitric oxide (FeNO) level – this measures the amount of nitric oxide in a person's breath, with high levels indicating airway inflammation and so can be used to diagnose asthma. According to these guidelines, a FeNO level of 50 ppb or more with the clinical features of asthma is diagnostic. However, it is worth noting that steroids (oral or inhaled) and cigarette smoking can reduce the FeNO score.

If asthma is not confirmed by either the blood eosinophil count or FeNO levels, then the next objective test is to assess for bronchodilator reversibility with spirometry. Forced expiratory volume in 1 second ($FEV_1$) is reduced in airway obstruction caused by bronchospasm but may be normal between episodes. Reversibility tests look for variability of airflow obstruction with bronchodilators. An improvement in $FEV_1$ of $\geq$12% from baseline and an improvement of $\geq$200 mL (or $\geq$10% of predicted normal) after bronchodilator administration is diagnostic of asthma. If there is no improvement with bronchodilators and the patient has a smoking history, consider alternative diagnoses such as chronic obstructive pulmonary disease (COPD). The main differences between asthma and COPD are described in Table 14.3.

If spirometry is not immediately available then the next step is to measure the peak expiratory flow (PEF) twice a day for 2 weeks. Astham is diagnosed if PEF variability is $\geq$20%. If asthma is not confirmed by eosinophil count, FeNO levels, bronchodilator reversibility or PEF variability but is still clinically suspected, then the next test is to refer for a bronchial challenge test. Asthma is diagnosed if bronchial hyperresponsiveness is present.

A basic diagnostic algorithm is shown in Fig. 14.3. Where there is diagnostic uncertainty or symptoms persist despite treatment, referral to a specialist should be considered. Further diagnostic tests may include:

- Methacholine chloride challenge testing – this measures bronchial hyperresponsiveness by measuring $FEV_1$ before and after sequential inhaled dosing of methacholine chloride, an airway irritant. The recorded PC20 result is the provocative concentration of agent that caused a 20% fall in the $FEV_1$. The lower the PC20, the more likely the diagnosis of asthma.
- Skin prick tests to aeroallergens – allergen injections into the epidermis of the forearm, which are used to show atopy and identify potential triggers. Look for wheal development in sensitive patients.
- Laryngoscopy to investigate for upper airway obstruction or vocal cord dysfunction may be useful.

## Differential diagnosis of asthma

The differential diagnosis for asthma is wide and should include COPD, as already discussed, especially where there is a history of smoking. Other important differentials include:

- Disorders of the upper airway – obstruction, tracheal tumour, foreign body aspiration
- Congestive cardiac failure
- Chronic thromboembolic disease
- Vocal cord dysfunction
- Pulmonary hypertension
- Interstitial lung disease
- Gastroesophageal reflux disease
- Eosinophilic granulomatosis with polyangiitis – a vasculitis affecting the small- and medium-sized vessels of the respiratory tract and causing asthma, eosinophilia, sinusitis, neuropathy and pulmonary infiltrates on chest X-ray.

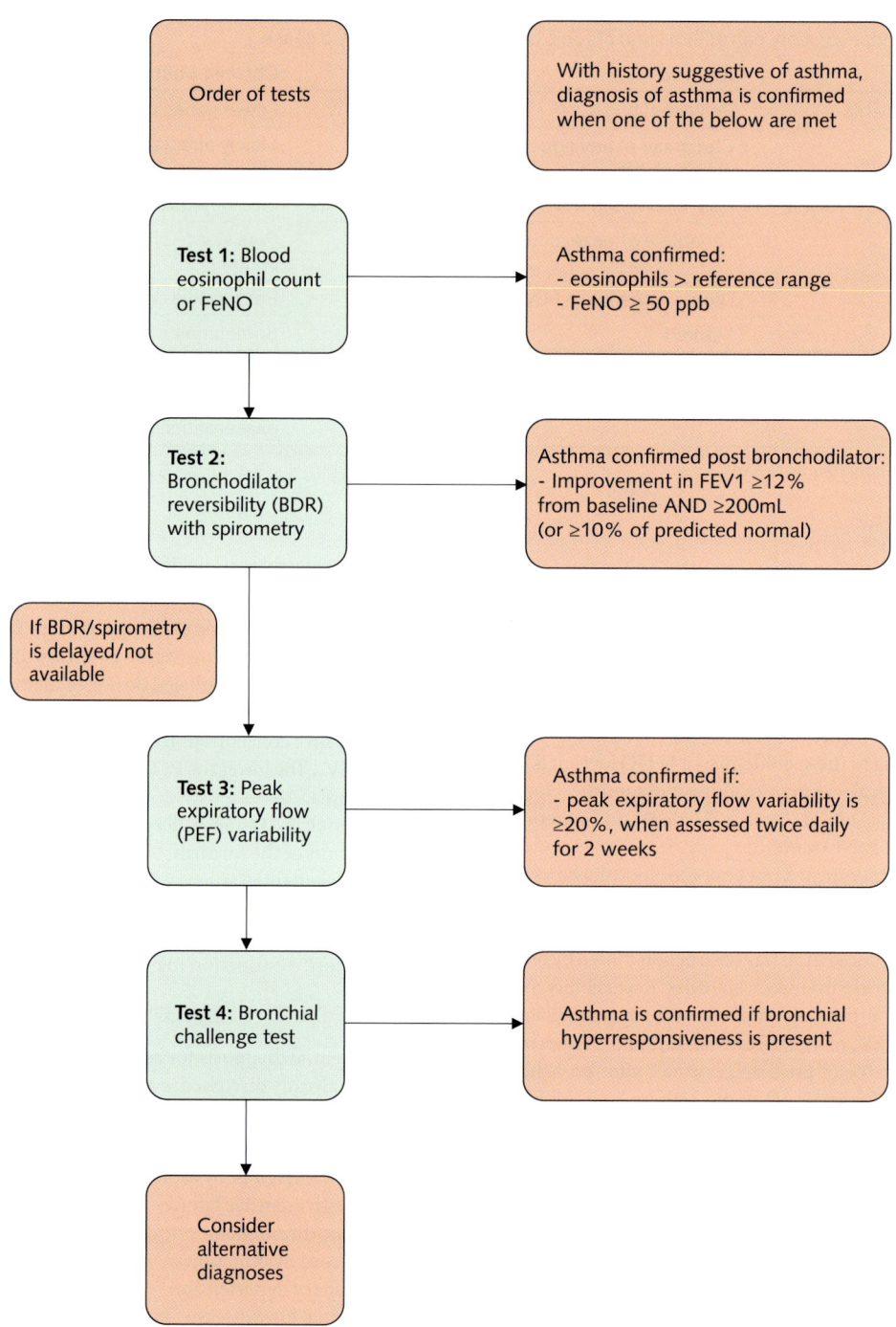

Order of tests

With history suggestive of asthma, diagnosis of asthma is confirmed when one of the below are met

**Test 1:** Blood eosinophil count or FeNO

Asthma confirmed:
- eosinophils > reference range
- FeNO ≥ 50 ppb

**Test 2:** Bronchodilator reversibility (BDR) with spirometry

Asthma confirmed post bronchodilator:
- Improvement in FEV1 ≥12% from baseline AND ≥200mL (or ≥10% of predicted normal)

If BDR/spirometry is delayed/not available

**Test 3:** Peak expiratory flow (PEF) variability

Asthma confirmed if:
- peak expiratory flow variability is ≥20%, when assessed twice daily for 2 weeks

**Test 4:** Bronchial challenge test

Asthma is confirmed if bronchial hyperresponsiveness is present

Consider alternative diagnoses

**Fig. 14.3** A useful approach to asthma diagnosis (from BTS, NICE and SIGN guidelines).

## TREATMENT OF STABLE ASTHMA

The aim of asthma treatment is to control the disease, with complete control of asthma defined as:

– The patient is not experiencing daytime symptoms
– Not waking up in the night due to asthma
– No asthma attacks
– No limitations on activity including exercise or time off work/school due to asthma
– Normal lung function
– No need for rescue medication (amount of reliever inhaler needed, number of courses of oral corticosteroids), all while minimizing drug side effects.

Patients should perform peak expiratory flow (PEF) monitoring in the morning and evening. The measurements should be entered into a PEFR diary. A characteristic morning dipping pattern is seen in poorly controlled asthma and once treatment starts the daily PEFR should improve (Fig. 14.4). In occupational asthma, a reduction in peak flow can be seen during working hours, with return to normal when the patient is off work. Note that regular PEF monitoring should not be used to assess asthma control unless there is a specific reason for this. BTS, NICE and SIGN guidelines suggest the use of a validated symptom questionnaire such as the Asthma Control Questionnaire in adults at any review. Also to consider FeNO monitoring at regular review and before and after changing asthma therapy.

## Nonpharmacological treatment

Smoking cessation and avoidance of passive smoking should be encouraged as smoking reduces the effect of inhaled corticosteroids. This also includes vaping using e-cigarettes. In obese patients, weight reduction may help. It is important to identify and avoid triggering factors such as air pollution or indoor mould exposure. However, this may be easier said than done. For

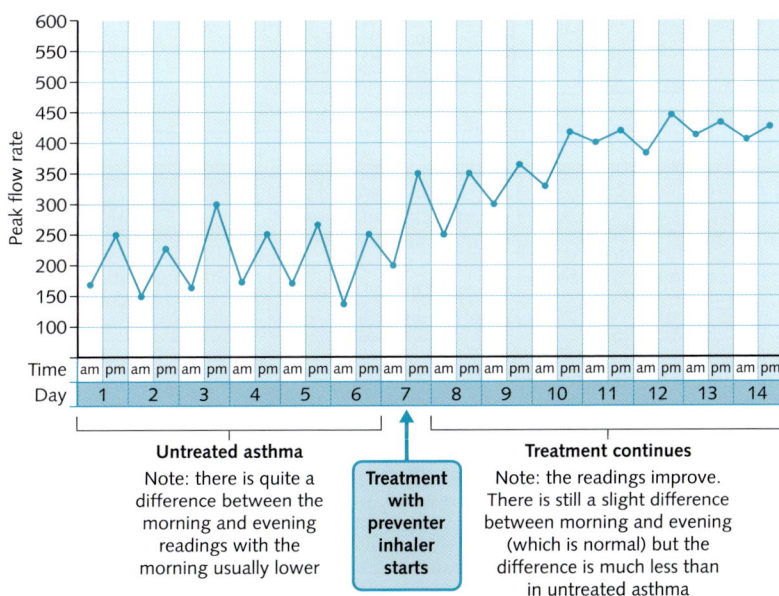

**Fig. 14.4** Example of a peak expiratory flow rate diary showing characteristic diurnal variation of peak flow and improvement following treatment initiation.

example, if the patient is suffering from occupational asthma, this may involve giving up their job. Similarly, it is difficult to avoid house dust mites as they are present on most soft furnishings in a house. Removal of a pet may be required if the clinical history is suggestive of a trigger.

## Pharmacological treatment

If a patient has uncontrolled asthma, before starting/adjusting medicines, clinicians should try to address possible reasons for this, such as those mentioned previously, lack of adherence or suboptimal inhaler technique.

BTS, NICE and SIGN guidelines 2024 for asthma management follows a stepwise approach (illustrated in Fig. 14.5):

- Step 1: Offer a low-dose ICS/formoterol combination inhaler to be used as needed for symptom relief.
- Step 2: If the patient still presents very symptomatic (such as waking up in the night due to asthma), start treatment with low-dose MART (Maintenance and Reliever Therapy). Note if their asthma becomes controlled then patients can be stepped down to step 1.
- Step 3: Offer moderate-dose MART if asthma not controlled on low-dose MART.

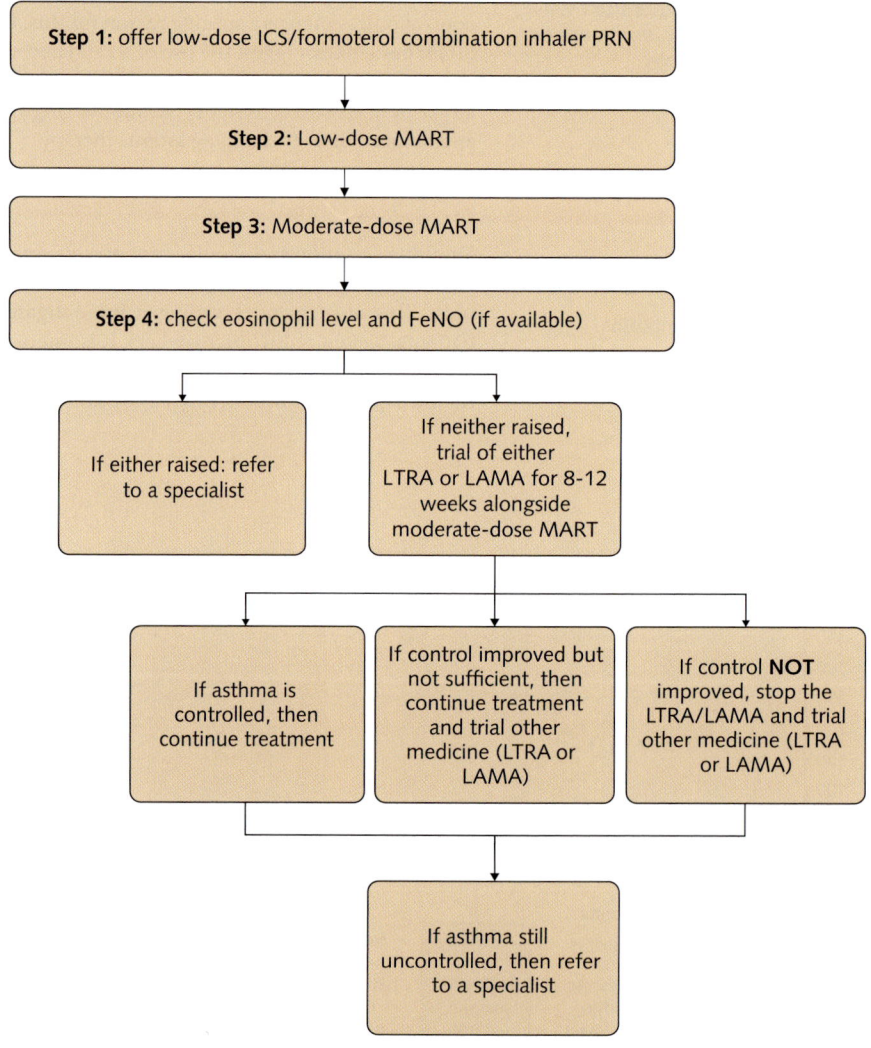

**Fig. 14.5** BTS, NICE and SIGN 2024 guidelines for treatment of asthma in adults. *ICS*, inhaled corticosteroid; *LAMA*, long-acting muscarinic receptor antagonist; *LTRA*, leukotriene receptor antagonist; *MART*, maintenance and reliever therapy; *FeNO*, Fractional Exhaled Nitric Oxide.

– Step 4: Consider adding a leukotriene receptor antagonist (LTRA) to the moderate-dose MART for 8-12 weeks; stop LTRA if it is ineffective.

– Step 5: Consider adding a long-acting muscarinic receptor antagonist (LAMA) to moderate-dose MART +/− LTRA for 8-12 weeks. Stop LAMA if it is ineffective.

– Step 6: If asthma is still uncontrolled, then referral to a specialist is required.

> ### CLINICAL NOTES
>
> Changes in the new BTS, NICE and SIGN 2024 guidelines: 2024 guidelines on asthma state to not prescribe a short-acting $\beta_2$-agonist to people of any age with asthma without a concomitant prescription of an inhaled corticosteroid.
>
> There is now a move towards MART for asthma control. This is because regular low-dose ICS/LABA was found to be better than regular low-dose ICS in improving lung function and reducing exacerbations.

The key point to remember about the stepwise management of asthma is to step down the treatment once the patient has good symptom control. A patient should be maintained on the lowest possible inhaled corticosteroid dose to adequately control their asthma symptoms. After starting or adjusting medicines for asthma, the response to this treatment should be reviewed in 8–12 weeks. Remember to always check inhaler technique at any consultation with a patient.

The pharmacology of inhaled therapy, corticosteroids and oral theophylline used in asthma is discussed in Chapter 7. Other medications used in asthma include:

1. Leukotriene receptor antagonists (e.g., montelukast) – may be useful in atopic or exercise-induced asthma as an add-on therapy. Patients should trial for 1 month and stop if there is no benefit. Of note, side effects of montelukast include neuropsychiatric reactions such as sleep disturbance, depression and agitation, so it is important to clearly explain the side effects to patients/families.

2. Monoclonal antibodies against IgE (omalizumab) or interleukin 5 (IL-5) (mepolizumab) are given as subcutaneous injections to patients with continued asthma symptoms despite maximal inhaled therapy. There are criteria for their use and, therefore, currently these medications can only be prescribed after review by a specialist asthma physician.

## Patient education

Education with inhaler technique and drug compliance can also contribute to the management of asthma. For those who find inhalers difficult to use, a wide variety of spacers are available, which are much simpler to use and allow good delivery of inhaled therapies.

> ### RED FLAG
>
> ## ASTHMA ACTION PLANS
>
> Patients should be provided with a personalized asthma action plan that tells them what to do if their symptoms worsen, for example, how to escalate their treatment and when to seek medical attention. The personalized asthma plan should be reviewed by an asthma specialist nurse during each hospital admission and at community asthma check-ups. Plans improve outcomes for patients, reducing hospital admissions and frequency of exacerbations. An example of an asthma action plan can be found on the Asthma + Lung UK website (https://shop.asthmaandlung.org.uk/collections/health-advice-resources/products/adult-asthma-action-plan-1). These plans should also include self-management programmes on contacting a healthcare professional if asthma control deteriorates.

## ACUTE ASTHMA

### Definition

An acute asthma attack occurs when a patient experiences worsened asthma symptoms over a period of hours to days that are not responsive to the patient's normal asthma medications. It requires either an increase in the patient's normal treatments or new, more complex treatment.

### Prevalence

According to NICE, asthma accounts for 60,000 hospital admissions each year in the UK.

### Clinical features

Severe asthma is a life-threatening medical emergency and critical care input should be sought early in patient management. Features of moderate, severe and life-threatening asthma are summarized in Table 14.4.

### Management

Acute asthma should be managed by following the British Thoracic Society guidelines, summarized in Fig. 14.6. Continuous monitoring by pulse oximetry, electrocardiography and blood

**Table 14.4** Symptoms and signs of acute asthma according to severity

| Features | Moderate | Severe (any one of below) | Life-threatening (any one of below) | Near-fatal |
|---|---|---|---|---|
| Talking | Able to complete sentences | Unable to complete sentences in one breath | Unable to speak | Raised $P_aCO_2$ and/or requiring mechanical ventilation with raised inflation pressures |
| Distress | Minimal | Marked | Very severe | |
| Accessory muscles | No | Yes | Yes | |
| Peak flow | >50%–75% predicted | 33%–50% predicted | <33% predicted | |
| Other | No features of severe asthma | RR ≥ 25 breaths/min HR ≥ 110 beats/min | $O_2$ saturation < 92% or $P_aO_2$ < 8 kPa Normal $PCO_2$ (4.6–6 kPa) Silent chest Cyanosis Arrhythmia Exhaustion Poor respiratory effort Hypotension Altered conscious level | |

*HR, Heart rate; RR, respiratory rate.*

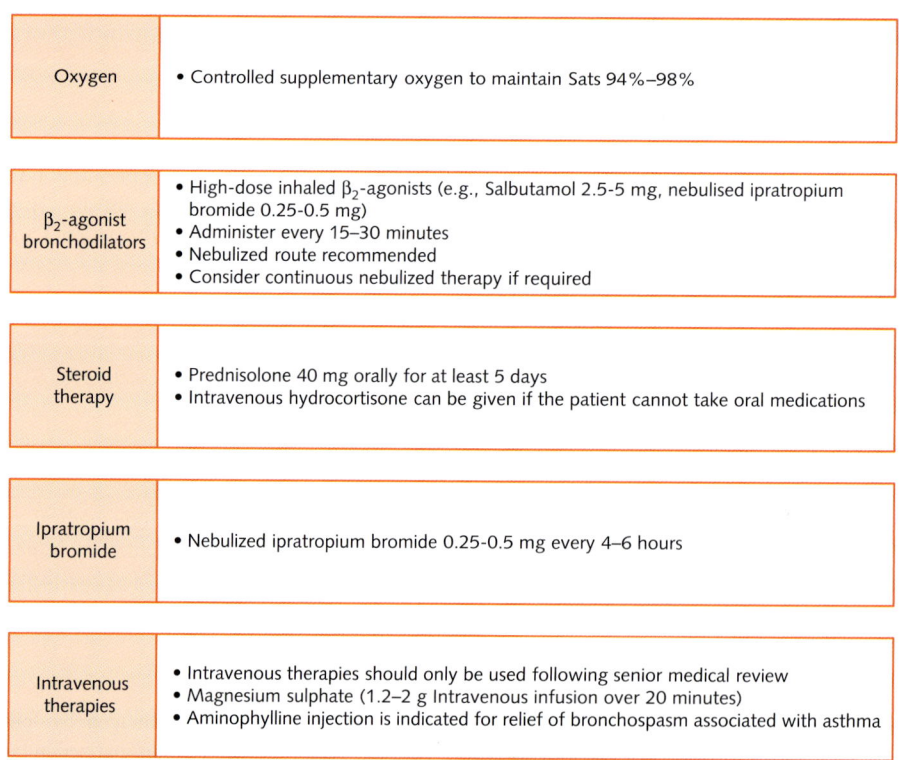

| Oxygen | • Controlled supplementary oxygen to maintain Sats 94%–98% |
|---|---|
| $β_2$-agonist bronchodilators | • High-dose inhaled $β_2$-agonists (e.g., Salbutamol 2.5-5 mg, nebulised ipratropium bromide 0.25-0.5 mg)<br>• Administer every 15–30 minutes<br>• Nebulized route recommended<br>• Consider continuous nebulized therapy if required |
| Steroid therapy | • Prednisolone 40 mg orally for at least 5 days<br>• Intravenous hydrocortisone can be given if the patient cannot take oral medications |
| Ipratropium bromide | • Nebulized ipratropium bromide 0.25-0.5 mg every 4–6 hours |
| Intravenous therapies | • Intravenous therapies should only be used following senior medical review<br>• Magnesium sulphate (1.2–2 g Intravenous infusion over 20 minutes)<br>• Aminophylline injection is indicated for relief of bronchospasm associated with asthma |

**Fig. 14.6** Management of acute asthma.

pressure measurement is necessary. PEFR monitoring is a useful measure of airway calibre and should be compared with a patient's previous best or predicted value. Arterial blood gas measurements should be obtained if there are features of life-threatening asthma or if oxygen saturations are <92%. Chest X-ray is not routinely required unless pneumothorax or consolidation are suspected or features of life-threatening asthma persist. If the patient is unresponsive to treatment and features of severe asthma persist, refer to the intensive therapy unit for consideration of possible noninvasive or invasive ventilation. As per BTS guidelines, it is essential that the patient's GP is informed within 24 hours of discharge from A&E or the hospital following an asthma attack. The British Thoracic Society has also launched an asthma attack care bundle which set out four actions – 'The Asthma 4' – to help improve patient outcomes following an asthma attack. They are:

– Action 1: Medication review
– Action 2: A personalized Asthma Action plan
– Action 3: Tobacco dependence advice and support for current smokers
– Action 4: Clinical review within 4 weeks.

## ● Chapter Summary

- Asthma is a heterogeneous clinical syndrome that is diagnosed following assessment of the clinical probability of disease based on symptoms, signs and investigation results.
- Asthma can be classified phenotypically as intrinsic or extrinsic asthma.
- Investigations used to diagnose asthma focus on finding evidence of variable airflow obstruction, airway hyperresponsiveness and airway inflammation.
- Asthma should be managed via the stepwise approach detailed in the Combined BTS, NICE and SIGN guidelines.
- A severe acute asthma attack is a life-threatening medical emergency requiring urgent medical attention.

### MLA Conditions
Asthma
Bronchiectasis
Chronic obstructive pulmonary disease
Gastrooesophageal reflux disease
Occupational lung disease

### MLA Presentations
Breathlessness
Cough
Wheeze

## Further reading

Asthma + Lung, UK. www.asthmaandlung.org.uk/.
British Thoracic Society/Scottish Intercollegiate Guidelines Network. British guideline on the management of asthma. 2019. Quick Reference Guide.

McCracken JL, Veeranki SP, Ameredes BT, Calhoun WJ. Diagnosis and management of asthma in adults. *JAMA*. 2017;318(3):279–290. doi:101001/jama.20178372.

# Chronic obstructive pulmonary disease 15

## INTRODUCTION

Chronic obstructive pulmonary disease (COPD) is a progressive lung disease, characterized by airflow obstruction with little or no reversibility. The Global Initiative for Obstructive Lung Disease (GOLD) defines COPD as 'a common, preventable and treatable disease that is characterized by persistent respiratory symptoms and air flow limitation that is due to airway and/or alveolar abnormalities usually caused by a significant exposure to noxious particles or gases'.

Patients with smoking-related lung disease were previously thought of as developing either chronic bronchitis or emphysema. However, we now realize that most patients actually develop varying combinations of these two processes (Table 15.1). Thus the term COPD represents a spectrum of disease in which several pathological processes occur.

## EPIDEMIOLOGY

COPD is a common lung condition and its prevalence is estimated to be 2%–15% in industrialized countries. COPD is a major cause of mortality and morbidity. COPD is currently the third most common cause of death worldwide.

Currently, COPD is more common in men, tends to present in those over the age of 40 years and becomes more common with age. However, prevalence is increasing in women and by the next decade, it is estimated that COPD will affect both men and women equally.

## AETIOLOGY

Worldwide, the most commonly encountered risk factor for developing COPD is tobacco smoke (including cigarettes, pipes, cigars, shisha, other types of tobacco and environmental exposure, i.e., passive smoking). The relationship between smoking and COPD is well proven; it is estimated that 80% of patients with COPD have a significant smoking history.

Other environmental risk factors include:

- Indoor air pollution, i.e., biomass fuels used for indoor cooking and heating—a significant risk factor for women in developing countries.
- Occupational dusts and chemicals.
- Outdoor air pollution (minimal effect in COPD).
- Marijuana smoking.

A person's risk of developing COPD is related to the total burden of inhaled particles he or she encounters over a lifetime.

## GENETIC RISK FACTORS

Despite a strong relationship between smoking and COPD, not all smokers go on to develop COPD. In fact, studies have demonstrated that only 15%–20% of smokers develop COPD. This implies that there must be a genetic susceptibility that predisposes some individuals to developing COPD when exposed to environmental risk factors such as tobacco smoke.

The best-described genetic risk factor is $\alpha_1$-antitrypsin deficiency, which affects 2% of COPD patients. $\alpha_1$-Antitrypsin is a serum acute-phase protein produced in the liver; it acts as an antiprotease in the lung and inhibits neutrophil elastase. Deficiency creates a protease–antiprotease imbalance, resulting in unopposed neutrophil elastase action and, consequently, alveolar destruction and early-onset emphysema. $\alpha_1$-Antitrypsin deficiency should be suspected in individuals who develop COPD under 40 years of age. Genetic inheritance of this deficiency is autosomal dominant with equal distribution between sexes.

## PATHOPHYSIOLOGY

Cigarette smoke and exposure to other noxious environmental particles trigger the pathological processes that occur within the lungs of COPD patients. Tobacco smoke has been shown to damage the lungs via three main mechanisms (Fig. 15.1):

- Inflammatory cell activation: cigarette smoke stimulates epithelial cells, macrophages and neutrophils to release inflammatory mediators and proteases (neutrophil elastase).

| Table 15.1 Definitions of chronic bronchitis/emphysema | |
|---|---|
| | **Definition** |
| Chronic bronchitis | Clinically defined: presence of cough and sputum production for most days for 3 months of 2 consecutive years |
| Emphysema | Histologically defined: dilatation of the air spaces distal to the terminal bronchioles with destruction of the alveoli |

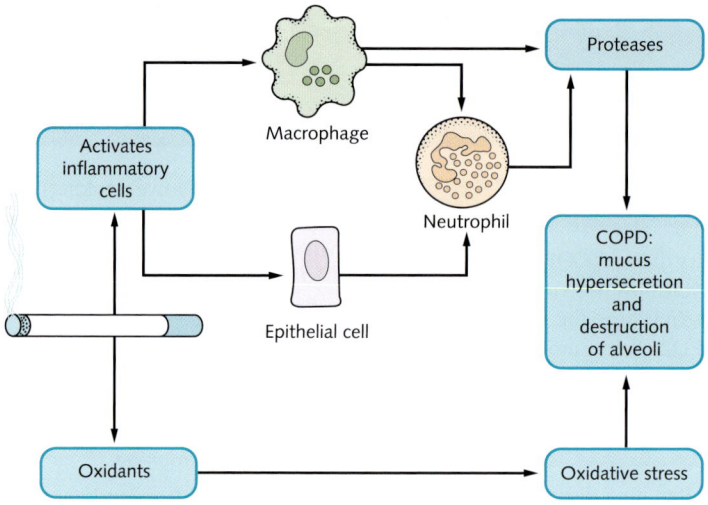

**Fig. 15.1** Overall pathogenesis of chronic obstructive pulmonary disease (COPD).

- Oxidative stress: oxidants in cigarette smoke act directly on epithelial and goblet cells, causing inflammation.
- Impaired mucociliary clearance, thus leading to retained mucus secretions.

The two main pathological processes in COPD are alveolar destruction (emphysema) and mucus hypersecretion (chronic bronchitis). As previously discussed, there are many different phenotypes of COPD. Whereas some patients may have a more emphysematous or bronchitic phenotype, the majority of patients develop a combination of these two pathological processes and have a mixed phenotype.

## Alveolar destruction (emphysema)

Cigarette smoke and other inhaled noxious particles cause inflammatory cell activation within the lung, inducing cells to release inflammatory mediators and proteases. Importantly, in COPD, cigarette smoke induces the release of neutrophil elastase from neutrophils. In healthy lung tissue, antiproteases neutralize these proteases; however, in COPD the volume of proteases produced overwhelms antiproteases (protease–antiprotease imbalance). Consequently, there is unopposed action of neutrophil elastase within the lung, which destroys alveolar attachments. As the distal airways are held open by the alveolar septa, destruction of alveoli causes the airways to collapse, resulting in airway obstruction and gas trapping (Fig. 15.2).

Destruction of the parenchyma increases compliance of the lung and causes a mismatch in ventilation:perfusion. Increased compliance, that is, reduced elastic recoil of the lungs, means the lungs do not deflate as easily, contributing to air trapping. As more alveolar walls are destroyed, compliance of the lungs increases and bullae (dilated air space > 10 mm) form, which may rupture, causing pneumothoraces.

Classification of emphysema is based on anatomical distribution (Fig. 15.3). The two main types are centriacinar and panacinar.

## Centriacinar (centrilobular) emphysema

Septal destruction and dilatation are limited to the centre of the acinus and around the terminal bronchiole, and predominantly affect the upper lobes (Fig. 15.3B). This pattern of emphysema is associated with smoking.

## Panacinar (panlobular) emphysema

The whole of the acinus is involved distal to the terminal bronchioles, and lower lobes are predominantly affected. This is characteristic of $\alpha_1$-antitrypsin deficiency (Fig. 15.3C).

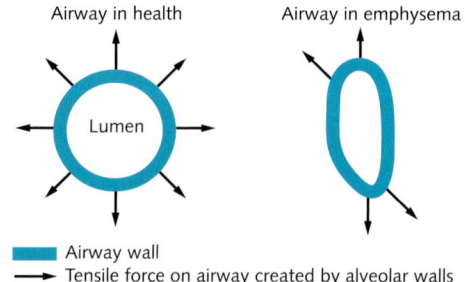

**Fig. 15.2** The mechanism of underlying airway obstruction in emphysema.

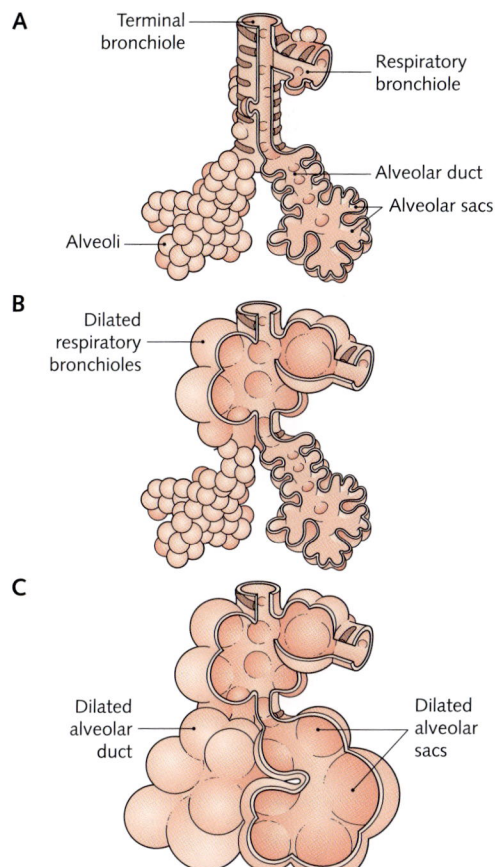

**Fig. 15.3** Main patterns of alveolar destruction. (A) Normal distal lung acinus; (B) centriacinar emphysema; (C) panacinar emphysema.

# MUCUS HYPERSECRETION

Cigarette smoke causes hyperplasia and hypertrophy of mucus-secreting glands found in the submucosa of the large cartilaginous airways. Mucous gland hypertrophy is expressed as gland:wall ratio, known as the Reid index (normally <0.4; >0.5 indicates chronic bronchitis). Hyperplasia of the intraepithelial goblet cells occurs at the expense of ciliated cells in the lining epithelium. Regions of epithelium may undergo squamous metaplasia.

Small airways become obstructed by intraluminal mucus plugs, mucosal oedema, smooth-muscle hypertrophy and peribronchial fibrosis. Secondary bacterial colonization of retained products occurs (Fig. 15.4).

The effect of these changes is to cause obstruction, increasing resistance to airflow. A mismatch in ventilation:perfusion occurs, impairing gas exchange.

# CLINICAL FEATURES

The clinical presentation of COPD is variable, but patients predominantly complain of:

- Progressive shortness of breath
- Reduced exercise tolerance
- Persistent cough
- Chronic sputum production.

Weight loss and peripheral muscle weakness or wasting may also occur.

Breathlessness is one of the primary symptoms of COPD and it is useful to assess this objectively using a modified version of the Medical Research Council (MRC) Dyspnoea Scale (see Chapter 8 for more discussion; Table 15.2). Other COPD-specific severity scores exist and may be used instead.

Typical signs found on examination are shown in Table 15.3.

---

**HINTS AND TIPS**

**DIFFERENTIAL DIAGNOSIS**

There is a significant crossover in the presentation of chronic obstructive pulmonary disease and other respiratory diagnoses, particularly asthma, which can make a single diagnosis difficult. Other important differential diagnoses include bronchiectasis, congestive cardiac failure, tuberculosis, obliterative bronchiolitis and diffuse panbronchiolitis.

---

**CASE STUDY**

Bob, a 71-year-old man, presented to his general practitioner with a 12-month history of shortness of breath and reduced exercise tolerance. He was noted to have smoked 30 cigarettes a day for the last 25 years. Examination revealed him to be cachectic and breathing through pursed lips. A diagnosis of chronic obstructive pulmonary disease was made on spirometry.

---

# COMPLICATIONS

## Exacerbations

A COPD exacerbation can be defined as an acute episode where patients experience worsening of their usual symptoms necessitating additional therapy. They are usually caused by an infection, which can be viral (e.g., influenza) or bacterial (commonly *Haemophilus influenzae*). A mild exacerbation may only require

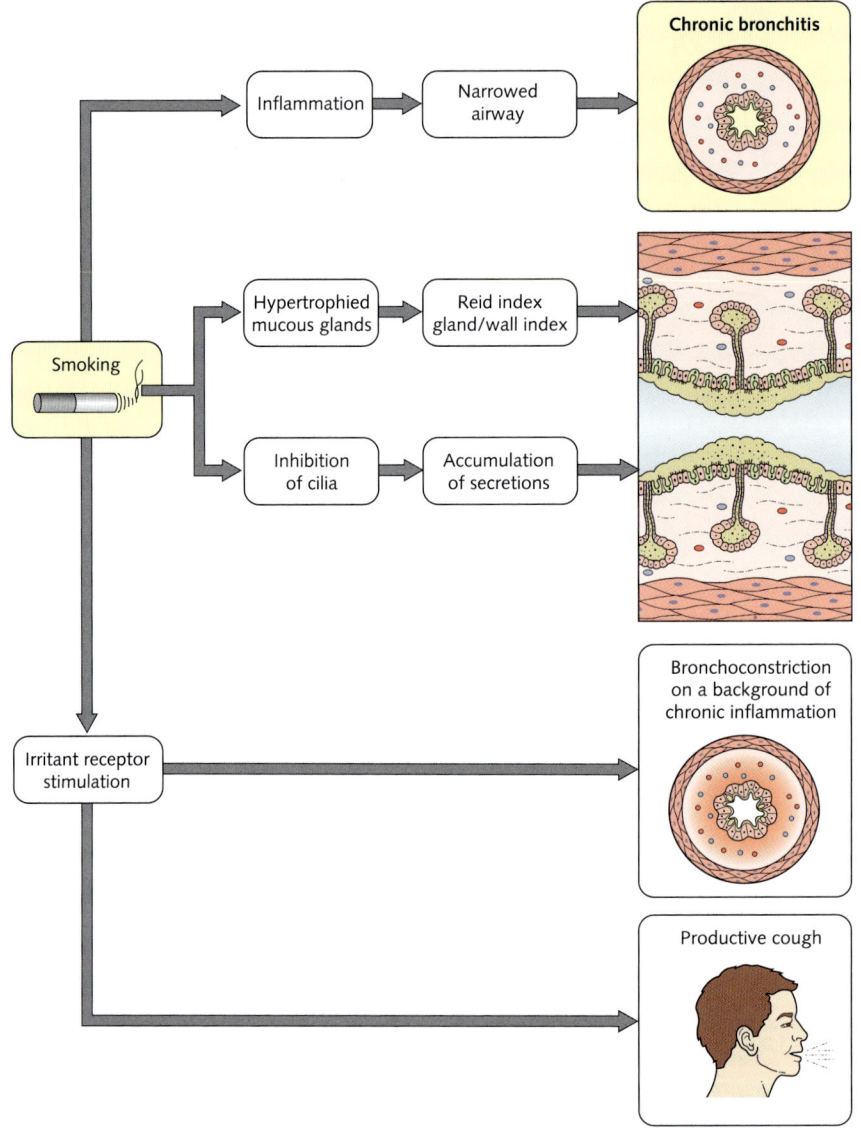

**Fig. 15.4** Pathogenesis of mucus hypersecretion.

an increase in usual inhaled therapy at home, whereas a moderate exacerbation needs antibiotics +/− steroids, and a severe exacerbation is one which needs hospital attendance.

## Respiratory failure

In severe exacerbations the patient may be unable to maintain adequate oxygenation. This state is known as acute respiratory failure and is discussed in more detail in Chapter 12. As COPD progresses, the lungs are unable to perform adequate gas exchange and a chronic respiratory failure develops. Respiratory failure is the leading cause of death in patients with COPD and is often hypercapnic (type 2 respiratory failure).

## Cor pulmonale

Mortality increases in those patients with COPD who develop cor pulmonale, or right ventricular failure secondary to disorders affecting the lungs. In COPD, it is pulmonary hypertension that causes the right ventricle to hypertrophy and eventually fail. This is clinically manifested as peripheral oedema, raised JVP, right ventricular heave, tricuspid regurgitation and palpable liver edge.

**Table 15.2** Modified Medical Research Council (mMRC) Dyspnoea Scale: A useful tool for objectively assessing breathlessness

| mMRC Grade | Degree of breathlessness related to activities |
|---|---|
| 0 | Breathlessness with strenuous exercise |
| 1 | Short of breath when hurrying on the flat or walking up a slight hill |
| 2 | Walks slower than contemporaries on level ground because of breathlessness, or has to stop for breath when walking at own pace |
| 3 | Stops for breath after walking about 100 metres or after a few minutes on level ground |
| 4 | Too breathless to leave the house, or breathless when dressing or undressing |

**Table 15.3** Signs of chronic obstructive pulmonary disease

| On inspection | Central cyanosis<br>Barrel chest<br>Use of accessory muscles<br>Intercostal indrawing<br>Pursed-lip breathing<br>Flapping tremor<br>Tachypnoea |
|---|---|
| On palpation | Tachycardia<br>Tracheal tug<br>Reduced expansion |
| On percussion | Hyperresonant lung fields |
| On auscultation | Wheeze<br>Prolongation of expiration<br>Silent chest |

## Lung cancer

Smoking and smoke inhalation, as well as potentially causing COPD, are significant risk factors for the development of bronchial carcinomas and other forms of lung cancer. As a result, lung cancers are a major cause of death in the COPD population and doctors need to be vigilant to assess for symptoms or signs suggesting underlying malignancy. See Chapter 17 for more information.

---

**RED FLAG**

**CLUBBING**

Note that chronic obstructive pulmonary disease (COPD) alone is not a cause of clubbing of the nail beds. In a COPD patient with clubbed nails, suspect underlying malignancy until proven otherwise. Other causes of clubbing with crossover for COPD symptoms include bronchiectasis and pulmonary fibrosis.

---

## INVESTIGATION

The gold standard for diagnosis of COPD is spirometry. A post-bronchodilator forced expiratory volume in 1 second ($FEV_1$)/forced vital capacity (FVC) ratio of <0.7 confirms the presence of persistent airflow limitation and thus of COPD.

The severity of COPD can also be classified in terms of its effect on lung function (Table 15.4).

Other tests include:

- Pulse oximetry.
- Chest X-ray (classically, hyperinflated lung fields with flattened hemidiaphragms; however, may be normal).
- Full blood count (polycythaemia secondary to chronic hypoxaemia is a late complication).
- Sputum culture (identify persistent organisms).
- $\alpha_1$-Antitrypsin level (all COPD patients should be tested once; especially consider in younger patients).
- Electrocardiograph/echocardiogram may be useful in end-stage COPD with features of cor pulmonale.

These tests are helpful but not essential in making a diagnosis of COPD.

## Chronic obstructive pulmonary disease assessment

Once the diagnosis is confirmed and classification of airflow severity limitation made, the impact of symptoms on the individual must be considered. This combined information is then used to stratify patient groups and guide future management. The GOLD classification system takes into account the spirometry findings, number of exacerbations and the mMRC Dyspnoea Scale score to stratify patients using the refined ABE assessment tool (Fig. 15.5).

## MANAGEMENT

Management of COPD is holistic and incorporates both pharmacological and conservative treatments. There is no cure for

**Table 15.4** Classification of chronic obstructive pulmonary disease

| Classification of COPD | $FEV_1$ % compared with predicted value |
|---|---|
| Mild/GOLD 1 | $FEV_1 > 80$ |
| Moderate/GOLD 2 | $FEV_1$ 50–80 |
| Severe/GOLD 3 | $FEV_1$ 30–49 |
| Very severe/GOLD 4 | $FEV_1 < 30$ |

*COPD, Chronic obstructive pulmonary disease; $FEV_1$, forced expiratory volume in 1 second; GOLD, Global Initiative for Obstructive Lung Disease.*

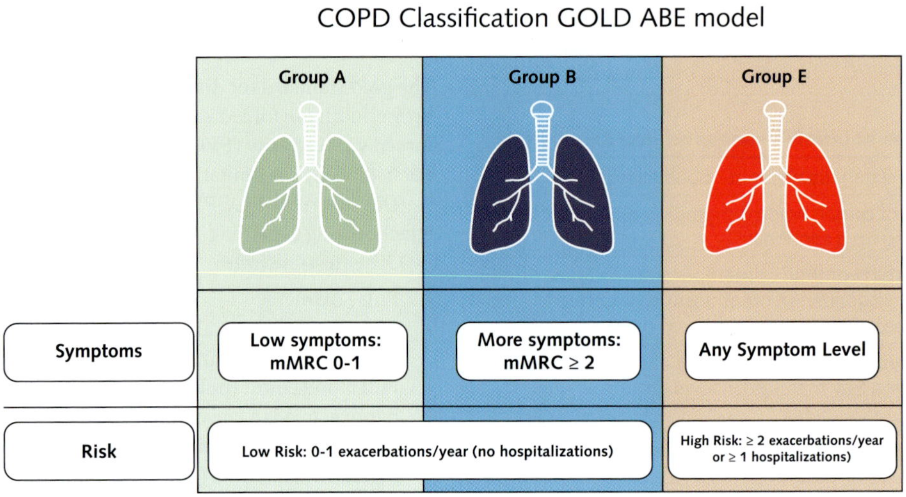

## COPD Classification GOLD ABE model

Fig. 15.5 ABE assessment tool from the 2023 Global Initiative for Obstructive Lung Disease (GOLD) guide. The mildest form of COPD would be GOLD 1 group A, with the most severe being GOLD 4 group E.

COPD and no treatment available that can reverse the damage caused to the lungs by exposure to tobacco smoke or other noxious particles. The aim of treatment in COPD is to control symptoms and reduce exacerbations of disease.

## Conservative measures

The single most important intervention in COPD is smoking cessation. Numerous studies have demonstrated that this has the single greatest impact on the natural history of COPD. Counselling and support should always be provided when discussing COPD management. Smoking cessation has been shown to be aided by a variety of pharmacological and nicotine replacement agents, discussed in Chapter 7. At present, the effectiveness of e-cigarettes to aid smoking cessation is unclear.

Other important conservative measures include:

- Physical activity
- Improved nutrition
- Regular vaccination—yearly influenza and 5-yearly pneumococcus have been shown to reduce the number of COPD exacerbations
- Counselling and education.

### Pulmonary rehabilitation

A pulmonary rehabilitation programme is increasingly essential in the management of COPD. It is one of the few interventions in COPD (along with smoking cessation) proven to reduce symptoms and improve both quality of life and survival.

Pulmonary rehabilitation normally occurs in an outpatient setting with a multidisciplinary team aiming to coordinate optimum management. Courses usually last 6–12 weeks and aim to improve patients' exercise tolerance and provide management strategies enabling patients to cope with symptoms of breathlessness.

## Pharmacological treatments

The use of pharmacological treatment should be guided by the severity of disease, symptoms and frequency of exacerbations, as outlined by the ABE assessment tool. Patients are divided into three distinct groups and therapy escalation is divided up to provide tailored improvement in symptom control. See Fig. 15.6 for a breakdown of treatments.

### Inhaled bronchodilators

The mainstay of pharmacological treatment in patients with COPD is inhaled bronchodilator therapy, used to control symptoms of breathlessness. More details on the classes of drugs described are given in Chapter 7. Initially, patients start with a short-acting $\beta_2$-agonist (SABA, i.e., salbutamol) and/or a short-acting muscarinic antagonist (SAMA, i.e., ipratropium) inhaler, using only when symptomatic.

While guidelines differ, they all have the same underlying principles of management. Patients who have minimal symptoms and minimal exacerbation history (GOLD group A) can be started on a single bronchodilator agent regularly. If patients are symptomatic but have infrequent exacerbations (GOLD group B), then they should be offered a long-acting $\beta$2-agonist (LABA)

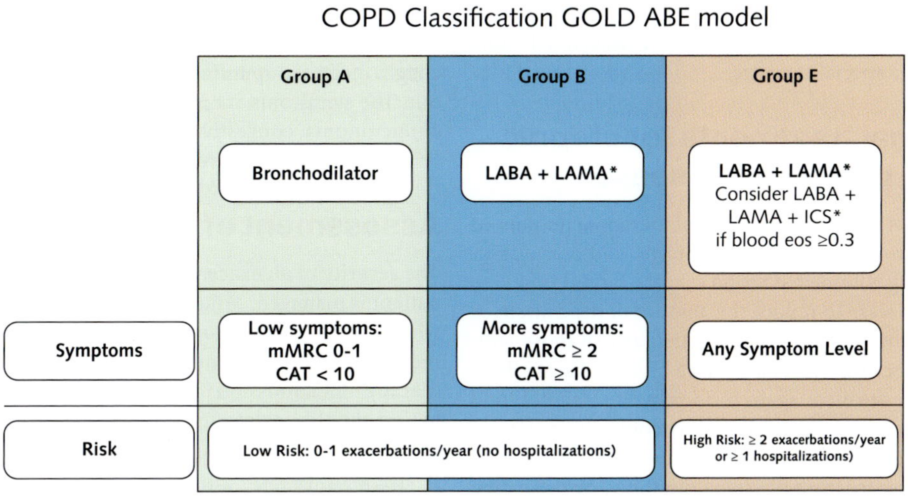

## COPD Classification GOLD ABE model

| Group A | Group B | Group E |
|---|---|---|
| Bronchodilator | LABA + LAMA* | LABA + LAMA*<br>Consider LABA +<br>LAMA + ICS*<br>if blood eos ≥0.3 |

| | Group A | Group B | Group E |
|---|---|---|---|
| Symptoms | Low symptoms:<br>mMRC 0-1<br>CAT < 10 | More symptoms:<br>mMRC ≥ 2<br>CAT ≥ 10 | Any Symptom Level |
| Risk | Low Risk: 0-1 exacerbations/year (no hospitalizations) | | High Risk: ≥ 2 exacerbations/year<br>or ≥ 1 hospitalizations) |

**Fig. 15.6** Global Initiative for Chronic Obstructive Lung Disease guide to the ABE management of chronic obstructive pulmonary disease. *ICS*, inhaled corticosteroids; *LABA*, long-acting β₂-agonist; *LAMA*, long-acting muscarinic antagonist; *blood eos*, blood eosinophils.

and long-acting muscarinic antagonist (LAMA) combination inhaler. If, despite this, they continue to have ongoing symptoms, an inhaled corticosteroid (ICS) inhaler can be added. However, if there is no improvement in their symptoms in 3 months, then patients should be de-escalated back to LAMA + LABA.

In patients who frequently exacerbate (GOLD group E), they should be started on LABA + LAMA combination inhaler in the first instance with ICS added if the exacerbations continue. However, in patients who are deemed to have asthmatic type features such as a blood eosinophil level of ≥0.3, atopy history or substantial variation in their FEV$_1$ over time of at least 400 mL or substantial diurnal variation in their peak expiratory flow rate of 20%, they should get ICS therapy earlier in their management trajectory. This can either be with LABA + ICS or LABA + LAMA + ICS.

It is important to remember that ICS has an increased risk of pneumonia in this patient population and therefore their use should be judicious. Furthermore, combination inhalers, which are once-daily preparations, are likely to be preferred by patients and improve patient use and compliance. Patients with COPD should never be prescribed isolated ICS inhalers.

### Oral therapy

Oral medications tend to be reserved for refractory disease not responding to other treatments. Oral agents used include:

- PDE4 inhibitors (e.g., roflumilast).
- Long-term macrolide antibiotics (can reduce exacerbations, must be balanced against risk of antibiotic resistance).
- Theophylline (requires level monitoring, may be used as an adjunct to treatment).

- Carbocisteine (mucolytic, particularly in patients with chronic productive cough).
- Rescue pack antibiotics (enable patients to treat exacerbations preemptively).

Note that long-term oral corticosteroid use is not recommended in routine COPD management.

### Long-term oxygen therapy

Management with home oxygen is an indicator of severe end-stage COPD. In patients with evidence of hypoxaemia (peripheral oxygen saturation < 92%) in stable COPD, arterial blood gas measurement should be performed for consideration of long-term oxygen therapy (LTOT). National Institute for Health and Care Excellence guidance indicates that patients with the following features should be considered to receive oxygen:

- Patients who have a $P_aO_2$ less than 7.3 kPa when stable.
- Patients with a $P_aO_2$ between 7.3 and 8 kPa, with evidence of one or more of the following:
  - Polycythaemia
  - Peripheral oedema
  - Pulmonary hypertension.

To benefit from LTOT, patients should breathe supplemental oxygen for at least 15 hours per day. If patients can adhere to this, an MRC study has demonstrated that LTOT is associated with a 50% reduction in mortality at 3 years. Note that smoking is a relative rather than absolute contraindication to home oxygen therapy. Smoking should be strongly discouraged and carries significant risk of fire injury.

In patients who become hypercapnic or acidotic on LTOT, regular noninvasive ventilation (NIV) must be considered—this requires referral to a specialist centre.

## Interventional treatments for chronic obstructive pulmonary disease

In severe COPD not responsive to medical therapy, a number of treatments exist to improve both symptoms and survival in selected cases. Lung volume reduction surgery is used in severe emphysematous disease to reduce the amount of dead airspace trapping and improve gas exchange, particularly in those with localized upper lobe emphysema. In large bullous disease, bullectomy may be performed, again to improve functional lung area performing gas exchange. Bronchoscopic intervention, either by endobronchial valve or lung coil insertion, also aims to reduce the dead airspace in emphysematous lungs, by collapsing targeted lung segments. Finally, lung transplantation has been shown to improve quality of life and functional capacity.

As the COPD population often has multiple comorbidities, strict selection criteria are in place for the use of any interventional therapies, which each carry significant risks on implementation.

## Palliative care and chronic obstructive pulmonary disease

COPD is a progressive disease that can be highly symptomatic. While some patients have stable disease for many years, for others the disease progression and failure of treatment options mean that they will eventually die of the condition. Early recognition of when the patient is in the terminal phase or last 6 months of life is a key part of good COPD management. Discussions with the patient and relatives, including resuscitation orders, advanced directives and preferences for the place of death, should be performed where possible. Hospice and hospice-at-home services can be utilized for ongoing community palliative support.

Symptomatic treatments for breathlessness can include a combination of using a fan to blow air onto the face, oxygen therapy and opiates. Nutritional support, education and talking therapies can also improve fatigue and symptom management.

## MANAGEMENT OF ACUTE EXACERBATIONS OF CHRONIC OBSTRUCTIVE PULMONARY DISEASE

An exacerbation is a sustained worsening of the patient's symptoms from his or her usual stable state that is beyond normal day-to-day variations, and is acute in onset. Exacerbations are triggered by an event, most commonly by respiratory tract infection with either viral or bacterial culprits. Commonly reported symptoms are worsening breathlessness, wheeze, cough, increased sputum production and change in sputum colour. The symptoms are nonspecific, and differential diagnoses of pneumonia, congestive cardiac failure, pulmonary embolism or acute coronary syndrome (ACS) must also be considered.

## Assessment of severity

The severity of an exacerbation determines how and where the patient is managed. Mild exacerbations can be treated at home, while severe exacerbations require hospital attendance and can require ventilator support and high-dependency unit/intensive therapy unit admission if appropriate. The severity of an exacerbation should be determined by the clinical assessment made, including:

- Respiratory rate (>30 breaths per minute suggests a moderate to severe exacerbation)
- Use of accessory muscles
- Altered mental status (confusion or drowsiness)
- Evidence of hypoxaemia and response to oxygen therapy if required (this should trigger arterial blood gas assessment)
- Evidence of hypercarbia or respiratory acidosis (confirmed with arterial blood gas analysis)
- Failure of community or initial medical management of acute exacerbation.

If there is no evidence of concerning features or respiratory failure, the exacerbation can be managed at home if enough support is in place for this. Any evidence of concern or respiratory failure should prompt further assessment or hospitalization.

## Investigation

- Observations and clinical assessment—ABCDE assessment of any critically unwell patient to assess for evidence of end organ dysfunction. Wheeze or silent chest may be present and clues for alternative pathology can be found. Oxygen saturations and respiratory rate are key.
- Biochemical—evidence of a raised white cell count and C-reactive protein indicates the presence of infection (isolated neutrophilia can also be seen in recent glucocorticoid use). Assessing urea and electrolytes, liver function and clotting for evidence of end organ dysfunction or electrolyte imbalances may also be appropriate.
- Arterial blood gas assessment—perform if there are any indicators of respiratory failure, and is mandatory if the patient requires supplemental oxygen. It provides indicators of severity, i.e., hypoxia, hypercapnia and acidosis, as well as guiding treatment options for either type 1 or type 2 respiratory failure. Serial measurements are often required for monitoring purposes and to assess response to treatment.

- Sputum culture—enables targeted antibiotic use. Recommended in moderate or severe exacerbations but should not routinely be performed in community management. Common bacterial pathogens include *H. influenzae*, *Streptococcus pneumoniae* and *Moraxella catarrhalis*.
- Chest radiograph—assess for evidence of pneumonia or other infective process, or alternative cause for acute exacerbation. Always consider the ruptured bullae causing a spontaneous pneumothorax in any sudden deterioration of a COPD patient.
- Electrocardiogram—may be required if ACS is suspected or to assess for evidence of arrhythmia.

## Management of acute exacerbations

Management is dictated by severity. If deemed to be mild/moderate and otherwise safe, the patient may be managed in the community with a combination of steroids, antibiotics and increased inhaler use. If severe with respiratory failure, then ventilation may be required. The following treatment options are described and often used in combination:

- Controlled oxygen to maintain oxygen saturations between 88% and 92%; this is normally achieved with a Venturi mask. Over oxygenation can result in hypercapnoea and iatrogenic type 2 respiratory failure, hence the importance of controlled oxygen delivery.
- Nebulized short-acting bronchodilators (salbutamol and ipratropium) may be used in combination in those requiring hospitalization.

- A short course of oral steroids (usually 30 mg prednisolone for 5–7 days) is given to reduce airway inflammation. If patients have received multiple courses of steroids, they will require a reducing-dose regimen to avoid rebound exacerbations when the steroids are stopped.
- Antibiotics, if exacerbation is thought to be infective (e.g., 5–7 days of oral doxycycline).
- NIV should be the first mode of ventilation in patients with acute respiratory failure in the absence of contraindications. Indications for NIV include type 2 respiratory failure with accompanying respiratory acidosis ($P_aCO_2 > 6$ kPa and arterial pH < 7.35). Bilevel positive airway pressure is used to treat type 2 respiratory failure.
- Invasive ventilation—used if patients are unable to tolerate or fail the trial of NIV or have severe hypoxia or signs of fatigue or have other severe pathology such as post respiratory or cardiac arrest. Full discussion of the management of respiratory failure is in Chapter 12.

Patients may stay in hospital for several days, depending on their response to treatment. Once stabilized, treatments should be stepped down gradually (such as reducing oxygen and reducing the frequency of nebulizers) and, if they remain stable, the patient can be deemed suitable for discharge. Follow-up within 1 month of the event is recommended following any acute exacerbation and has been shown to reduce further exacerbations and hospital admission. This may require alteration and increase of stable COPD treatment and is often performed by respiratory specialist nurses.

## Chapter Summary

- Chronic obstructive pulmonary disease (COPD) is a disease process causing persistent respiratory symptoms and airflow limitation owing to airway and/or alveolar abnormalities, usually caused by a significant exposure to noxious particles or gases.
- The majority of COPD is caused by cigarette smoking, although other pollutant exposure can cause the condition. There are genetic risk factors, the most important being $\alpha_1$-antitrypsin deficiency.
- COPD symptoms include persistent cough, shortness of breath and reduced exercise tolerance. Diagnosis is made using spirometry and excluding other underlying pathology.
- Management of COPD can be divided into conservative, medical and surgical therapies, with management stratified depending on degree of airflow limitation, number of exacerbations and impact on daily life. The most important management step is smoking cessation.
- Acute exacerbations of COPD are managed depending on severity, with steroid therapy, bronchodilators, antibiotics, oxygen or ventilator support used.

**MLA Conditions**
Asthma COPD overlap syndrome
Chronic obstructive pulmonary disease

**MLA Presentations**
Breathlessness
Cough
Weight loss
Wheeze

### Further reading

British Medical Journal Learning Module. COPD: diagnosis and management of exacerbations. www.learning.bmj.com.

British Thoracic Society. Guidelines for COPD. www.brit-thoracic.org.uk.

GOLD. Guideline for COPD. www.goldcopd.org.

Lopez AD, Murray CC. The global burden of disease, 1990–2020. *Nat Med*. 1998;4:1241–1243.

Medical Research Council Working Party. Long-term domiciliary oxygen therapy in chronic hypoxic cor pulmonale complicating chronic bronchitis and emphysema. *Lancet*. 1981;1:681–686.

NICE. Guideline for COPD. www.nice.org.uk.

## INTERSTITIAL LUNG DISEASE

The interstitial lung diseases (ILDs) are a diverse group of over 300 different lung diseases (see Table 16.1 for an overall classification of the different types of ILD) that all affect the lung interstitium, that is, the space between the alveolar epithelium and capillary endothelium (see Chapter 3). Terminology in ILD is continually evolving and the term 'diffuse parenchymal lung disease' may be used interchangeably with ILD. An integrated clinical, radiological and pathologic approach allows a formal classification. Key radiological patterns include usual interstitial pneumonia (UIP) which describes a peripheral distribution of disease predominantly at the bases consisting of a reticular pattern with honeycombing, and this is often seen in idiopathic pulmonary fibrosis (IPF), a nonspecific interstitial pneumonia (NSIP) radiological pattern is often associated with an underlying connective tissue lung disease, drug-induced ILD or chronic hypersensitivity pneumonitis. NSIP is often associated with improved morbidity. Although separately each disease is rare, collectively they affect 1/2000 of the population. Outcome varies according to the individual phenotype of disease.

## Aetiology

ILDs are a heterogeneous group of disorders with many known causes. However, only approximately one-third of cases of ILD currently have a known cause—see Fig. 16.1.

Firstly, we will go through the common clinical features of a patient with ILD and their diagnostic work-up. Secondly, we will look at some common specific diseases associated with ILD in more detail—idiopathic interstitial pneumonias (IIPs), HP and occupational lung disorders. Further information on systemic diseases associated with ILD, including sarcoidosis, connective tissue disorders and vasculitis, can be found in Chapter 23.

## Clinical features of interstitial lung disease

Patients typically present with breathlessness on exertion, with or without an associated dry cough. The symptoms are usually of progressive and gradual onset; however, some ILDs can present acutely or subacutely over days to weeks. In addition to taking a detailed history of the complaint and previous medical history, it is important to ask about:

- Myalgia, joint pains, sicca symptoms, Raynaud disease—is there an underlying connective tissue disorder?
- Dry eyes, dry mouth, dry skin—these are common in Sjögren syndrome.
- Dysphagia and weight loss—dysphagia is common in systemic sclerosis.
- Skin changes on the fingers and face particularly—rashes such as erythema nodosum may be found in sarcoidosis while mechanic's hands and Gottron papules can be found in myositis.
- Medications, especially the use of nitrofurantoin for urinary tract infections, prior or current use of amiodarone, chemotherapy, methotrexate or other drugs that affect the lungs—check for all prescribed and over-the-counter medications.
- Check for prior or current radiation treatment to the chest.
- Occupational history—any history of occupational dust or asbestos, coal or silica exposure?
- Environmental exposures—mould, animals, antigens from birds, hay, water humidifiers and hot tubs can all cause an HP.

**Table 16.1** Classification of types of interstitial lung disease

| Types of interstitial lung disease | |
|---|---|
| Idiopathic interstitial pneumonias | Idiopathic pulmonary fibrosis<br>Idiopathic nonspecific interstitial pneumonia<br>Cryptogenic organizing pneumonia<br>Desquamative interstitial pneumonia<br>Cryptogenic organizing pneumonia<br>Acute interstitial pneumonia<br>Idiopathic lymphoid interstitial pneumonia<br>Idiopathic pleuroparenchymal fibroelastosis |
| Autoimmune interstitial lung disease | Mixed connective tissue disease<br>Sjögren syndrome<br>Systemic lupus erythematous<br>Polymyositis and dermatomyositis<br>Systemic sclerosis<br>Other connective tissue disease ILDs |
| Granulomatous interstitial lung disease | Sarcoidosis |
| Other ILDs | Hypersensitivity pneumonitis<br>Drug associated ILD<br>ILD related to other occupational exposures<br>Vasculitis<br>Langerhans' cell histiocytosis<br>Lymphangioleiomyomatosis |

155

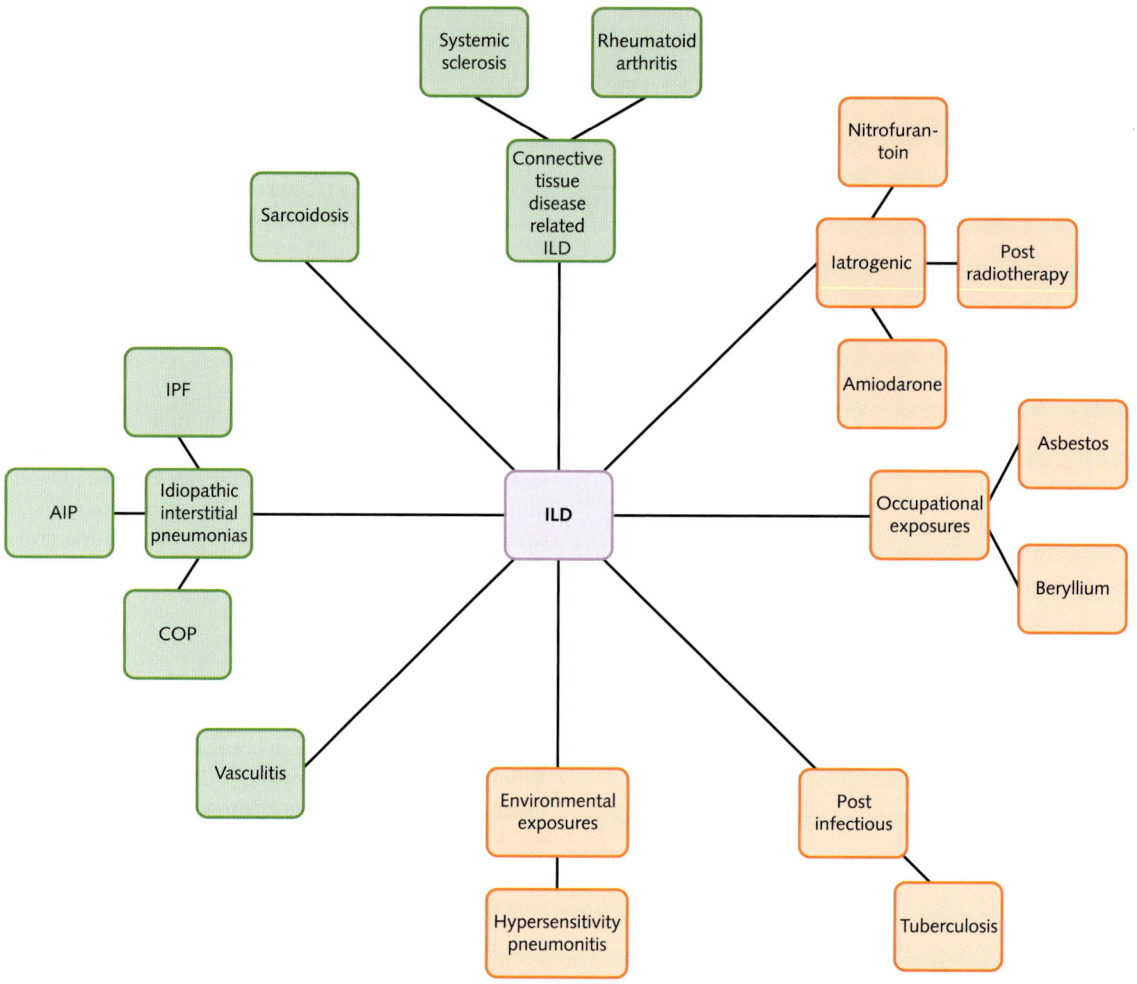

**Fig. 16.1** Disorders related to interstitial lung disease. *Green boxes* represent disorders of unknown cause and *orange boxes* represent those with known cause. *AIP,* Acute interstitial pneumonia; *COP,* cryptogenic organizing pneumonia; *ILD,* interstitial lung disease; *IPF,* idiopathic pulmonary fibrosis.

- Smoking history—chronic obstructive pulmonary disease is a key differential diagnosis.

Examination may reveal a patient who is hypoxic at rest or, in earlier stages, only on exertion. Typically, fine end-inspiratory crackles are heard on chest auscultation—these may be bilateral and are often basal or in the apices of the lungs, depending on the underlying condition. Examination should include careful inspection of the patient for signs of systemic illnesses related to ILD, as mentioned previously.

## Investigations of interstitial lung disease

Lung function tests demonstrate a restrictive pattern along with a decreased transfer factor. Repeated testing aids in monitoring the progression of the disease, which is important to target eligibility for antifibrotic or immunosuppressive treatment where indicated. Specialist blood tests may be requested to seek out underlying causes in addition to routine blood tests. Table 16.2 summarizes the pertinent investigations needed.

The British Thoracic Society (BTS) recommends after seeing a respiratory physician, patients with suspected ILD should be discussed with an ILD multidisciplinary team (MDT), with whom a diagnosis and treatment plan can be made.

If there is diagnostic uncertainty, the MDT may recommend a lung biopsy to aid diagnosis. Transbronchial biopsy at bronchoscopy is possible if the disease has a central distribution. If the disease is well localized and peripheral, percutaneous image-guided biopsy may be possible. Otherwise, patients require surgical biopsy using a video-assisted thoracoscopic surgery method (VATS

**Table 16.2** Autoantibody blood tests useful to aid diagnosis of differential ILDs

| Autoantibody | Disease associations |
|---|---|
| ANA | SLE, Sjögren syndrome, SS, PM, DM, mixed connective tissue disease |
| ENA | SLE, Sjögren syndrome |
| Scl70 | SS |
| dsDNA | SLE |
| Rheumatoid factor | RA, Sjögren syndrome |
| Anti-CCP antibody | RA, Sjögren syndrome |
| Myositis-specific antibodies (Jo-1, PL-7, PL-12, EJ, OJ KS, SRP, Mi2, NXP2, TIF1γ) | PM, DM, antisynthetase syndromes |
| Myositis-associated antibodies (Ku, PMScl75, PMScl00) | PM, DM, SS, SLE |
| ANCA including MPO and PR3 | ANCA-associated vasculitis |
| Serum calcium and angiotensin-converting enzyme levels | Sarcoidosis |

DM, Dermatomyositis; PM, polymyositis; RA, rheumatoid arthritis; SLE, systemic lupus erythematous; SS, systemic sclerosis.

biopsy) or open lung biopsy (the latter requires a general anaesthetic and is therefore not without risk). Full discussion of biopsy risks versus possible benefits should be had prior to the procedure.

## Treatment of interstitial lung disease

Treatment for ILD depends on the underlying cause. If the cause is known, underlying triggers or stimuli should be removed or avoided where possible. Current therapy for ILD of unknown cause includes antifibrotic and antiinflammatory or immunosuppressant drugs, which will be discussed in later sections.

When patients develop advanced ILD, home oxygen therapy may be required. A multidisciplinary approach is recommended by the BTS, and subjective and objective benefits may be achieved through pulmonary rehabilitation. Lung transplantation should be considered in appropriate patients where there is a potential postoperative survival of more than 5 years with a quality of life acceptable to the recipient.

Specific criteria for transplantation for IPF include:

– A 10% or greater decrement in forced vital capacity (FVC) during 6 months of follow-up
– A DLCO of less than 40% with clinical deterioration and/or a greater than 15% decline in DLCO over 6 months of follow-up
– A rapid decrease in pulse oximetry below <88% during a 6-minute walk test

Towards the end of life, palliative care involvement is important for patients and their family.

## Complications of interstitial lung disease

An acute deterioration in ILD symptoms often requires admission to hospital for investigation and treatment. An acute deterioration may be caused by:

• Infection—bacterial or viral pneumonia
• Cardiac failure
• Pulmonary embolism.

## IDIOPATHIC INTERSTITIAL PNEUMONIAS

This is a group of diffuse parenchymal lung disorders that involve the pulmonary interstitium. The most common disorder in the group is IPF, which is discussed in more detail later. Rare IIPs include:

• Cryptogenic organizing pneumonia (COP)—previously bronchiolitis obliterans organizing pneumonia
• Nonspecific interstitial pneumonia
• Acute interstitial pneumonia
• Respiratory bronchiolitis associated ILD
• Desquamative interstitial pneumonia
• Lymphoid interstitial pneumonia.

Each disorder is distinct with different patterns of involvement seen on high-resolution computed tomography (HRCT), different histology and different prognoses. The underlying aetiology for this group is as yet unknown; however, genetic predisposing factors and multiple environmental factors have been linked as triggers for disease.

## Idiopathic pulmonary fibrosis

### Definition
Previously known as cryptogenic fibrosing alveolitis, IPF is a progressive chronic pulmonary fibrosis of unknown aetiology. It is the most common IIP. Predicted incidence rates vary but are estimated in the United Kingdom at 5 per 100,000 people per year and appear to be increasing. There is a male predominance and the median age of onset is mid-60s. The familial form of IPF is rare and has an identical clinical picture.

### Pathology
IPF is characterized by scar tissue in the lungs that decreases lung compliance, that is, the lungs become stiffer. The pathogenesis is complex and not completely understood. The main features are:

• A lesion affecting the alveolar–capillary basement membrane.
• Cellular infiltration and thickening with collagen of the interstitium of the alveolar wall.
• Fibroblasts proliferate, leading to further collagen deposition.

## Clinical features

IPF typically presents with progressive, gradual-onset (e.g., 9 months) exertional breathlessness and a dry cough. Examination reveals fine bilateral basal late inspiratory crackles on auscultation. Clubbing is present in 50% of cases. As the disease progresses, the patient may develop cyanosis, respiratory failure and signs of cor pulmonale.

## Investigations

The patient is often hypoxic with reduced oxygen saturations, especially on exertion. Arterial blood gas sampling may demonstrate type I respiratory failure. Lung function tests show a restrictive pattern with reduced gas transfer.

HRCT in IPF has a classical 'usual interstitial pneumonia' (UIP) pattern. This is classified as:

- Fibrosis and reticulation with a subpleural, peripheral and basal predominance
- 'Honeycombing'
- Architectural distortion with traction change
- Minimal ground glass change.

Diagnosis of IPF can usually be made on clinical and radiological grounds without the need for a biopsy. If biopsy does take place, histology shows a UIP pattern with areas of fibrosis at different stages within the biopsy sample. Normal lung will be interspersed with areas of acute fibroblastic infiltrates, mature fibrosis and honeycombing, leading to distortion of the lung architecture (established fibrosis).

---

### HINTS AND TIPS

#### TERMINOLOGY—USUAL INTERSTITIAL PNEUMONIA

Usual interstitial pneumonia (UIP) is a radiological and histological pattern, not a separate disease entity. Idiopathic pulmonary fibrosis is the clinical syndrome most associated with UIP, however, the UIP pattern is also found in interstitial lung disease secondary to connective tissue disease (particularly rheumatoid arthritis), asbestos exposure and chronic hypersensitivity pneumonitis. UIP is associated with a worse prognosis than other histological patterns.

---

## Treatment

Treatment options for IPF are supportive, medical or lung transplant. Supportive treatments include:

- Oxygen therapy—if the patient is breathless and $pO_2 < 7.3$ kPa or $< 8$ kPa with evidence of pulmonary hypertension.
- Pulmonary rehabilitation.
- Palliative care support—opioids may be required for symptomatic severe breathlessness.

Treatment with antifibrotic medications such as pirfenidone and nintedanib are licensed in the United Kingdom by the National Institute for Health and Care Excellence (NICE) for patients whose FVC is between 50% and 80% predicted, for a 12-month trial period. The drugs have significant gastrointestinal side effects and are not always well tolerated.

Lung transplantation is the only surgical option for IPF currently and patients should be referred where appropriate; however, this option is still rare in the United Kingdom. Prognosis of patients with IPF remains poor, with an average life expectancy of 3 years following diagnosis.

## Cryptogenic organizing pneumonia

In contrast to IPF, COP is an IIP with a much better prognosis. It is characterized by plugging of the alveolar spaces with fibrin-containing granulation tissue. The aetiology can be unknown ('cryptogenic'), but COP can occur secondary to infection, medication, connective tissue disorders or malignancy.

It presents with a subacute (e.g., 3-month) history of cough and exertional breathlessness, often associated with systemic features of fever, malaise or myalgia. It is not associated with clubbing and chest auscultation may be normal or reveal crackles. Inflammatory markers are raised. Imaging of the chest shows patchy consolidation with a basal, subpleural and peribronchial predominance that may spontaneously migrate to other areas of the lung. As the consolidation is often next to the bronchi (peribronchial), transbronchial biopsy at bronchoscopy can provide histological diagnosis.

Treatment is with high-dose steroids for 3 months prior to slowly weaning, for a total course of 6–12 months. Prognosis is generally good; however, relapse is common during steroid weaning.

## HYPERSENSITIVITY PNEUMONITIS

### Definition

HP (previously known as extrinsic allergic alveolitis) is an immunological reaction within the lung parenchyma caused by the inhalation of an organic antigen to which the patient has previously been sensitized.

### Pathogenesis

The pathogenesis is not completely understood but is thought to be driven by either T cell–mediated immunity and granuloma formation (type IV hypersensitivity reaction), immune complex formation (type III hypersensitivity reaction) or a combination of the two processes. Histological specimens show an inflammatory infiltrate within the interstitium, poorly differentiated noncaseating granuloma formation and, in later disease stages,

**Table 16.3** Common Investigations used to diagnose ILDs

| Investigation | |
|---|---|
| Blood tests | Erythrocyte sedimentation rate, C-reactive protein and full blood count including eosinophil count Autoantibody screen—may suggest underlying connective tissue disease (see Table 16.3 for a list of these tests) |
| Chest X-ray (CXR) | May initially show fine reticular (linear), nodular or reticulonodular infiltration (Fig. 16.2) As the disease progresses, fibrotic changes can be seen on the CXR |
| Electrocardiogram and echocardiogram | To exclude left ventricular failure as an underlying cause of dyspnoea and to assess for signs of right heart failure and pulmonary hypertension secondary to ILD |
| High-resolution computed tomography (HRCT) | HRCT is the gold standard imaging in ILD. Changes such as a 'ground glass' appearance and fine reticulation may be seen earlier in the process, while fibrotic distortion and a 'honeycomb' appearance may be evident later (Fig. 16.3). The pattern of changes on HRCT depends on the underlying cause and it is important that the images are reviewed by a specialist chest radiologist |
| Six-minute walk test | Measuring oxygen desaturation on exercise testing can be useful for functional assessment and to assess whether oxygen is needed either as ambulatory oxygen therapy or long-term oxygen therapy |
| Bronchoscopy and bronchial lavage (BAL) | BAL differential cell counts can provide useful diagnostic clues |

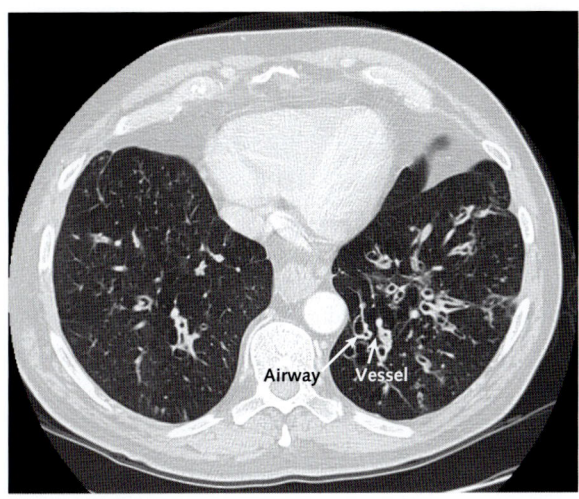

**Fig. 16.2** Chest X-ray of a patient with an idiopathic pulmonary fibrosis. Note the 'meshwork' reticulation appearance in the lung fields. Here it is predominantly basal and peripheral. (From Corne J, Pointon K. *Chest X-Ray Made Easy*. 3rd ed. Churchill Livingstone, Elsevier; 2009.)

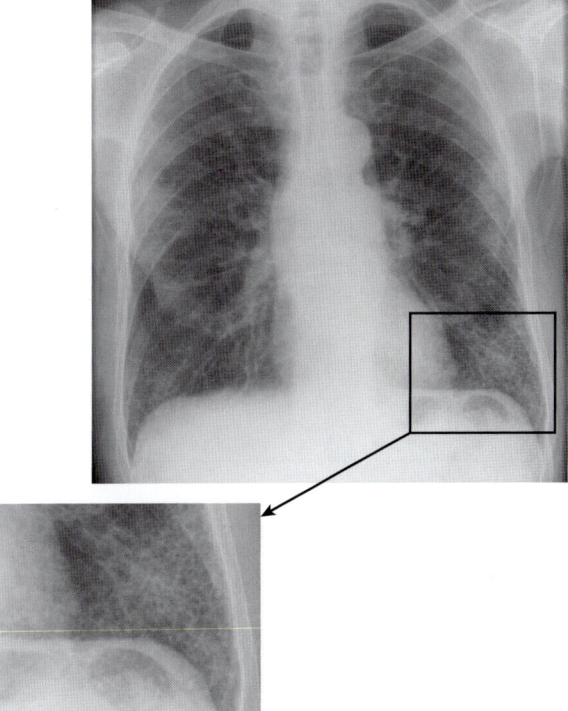

**Fig. 16.3** A section of a high-resolution computed tomography scan showing typical bilateral basal 'honeycombing'. This is typically seen in idiopathic pulmonary fibrosis. (From Corne J, Pointon K. *Chest X-Ray Made Easy*. 3rd ed. Churchill Livingstone, Elsevier; 2009.)

established fibrosis. More than 200 antigens have been identified, ranging from plant and animal proteins, chemicals and microbes that cause a range of diseases. Table 16.4 shows examples of diseases, their antigens and the source.

## Clinical features

HP presents in three recognized patterns:

1. Acute—following a short exposure to an antigen at a high concentration.
2. Chronic—following a long exposure to an antigen at a lower concentration.
3. Subacute—between acute and chronic.

Acute HP presents within 4–6 hours of heavy exposure to the causative antigen. Patients have symptoms of cough and

**Table 16.4** Antigens causing hypersensitivity pneumonitis and their sources

| Disease | Source | Causative antigens |
|---|---|---|
| Farmer's lung | Mouldy hay, grain | Thermophilic actinomycetes *Aspergillus* species |
| Malt worker's lung | Mouldy barley | *Aspergillus fumigatus* |
| Bird fancier's lung | Bird feathers, droppings | Bird proteins |
| Bat lung | Bat droppings | Bat serum protein |
| Hot tub lung | Hot tub mist | *Mycobacterium avium* complex |
| Mushroom worker's lung | Mushrooms | Mushroom spores |
| Cheese washer's lung | Mouldy cheese | *Aspergillus clavatus Penicillium casei* |

**Table 16.5** Imaging finding in hypersensitivity pneumonitis

| | Chest X-ray | High-resolution computed tomography |
|---|---|---|
| Acute | May be normal Bilateral small nodules or infiltrates | Homogenous ground glass and alveolar opacities bilaterally |
| Subacute HP | May be normal Bilateral small nodules or infiltrates | Ground glass and nodular opacities in a centrilobular distribution Mosaic attenuation |
| Chronic HP | Predominantly upper and midzone reticulation/fibrosis | Ground glass and nodular opacities in a centrilobular distribution Mosaic attenuation Pulmonary fibrosis and honeycombing— typically upper lobe predominance |

*HP, Hypersensitivity pneumonitis.*

breathlessness, and systemic symptoms such as fever. Chronic HP presents as an insidious onset of cough, breathlessness and weight loss over months to years. The subacute disease may present over weeks to months, with infrequent acute attacks.

## Investigations

In acute HP, blood tests may show a neutrophilia but, importantly, the eosinophil count is normal. Serum antibody (IgG) precipitin may be tested against suspected antigens—for example, avian precipitins in a patient owning pigeons presenting with HP. The imaging findings in acute and chronic HP are summarized in Table 16.5.

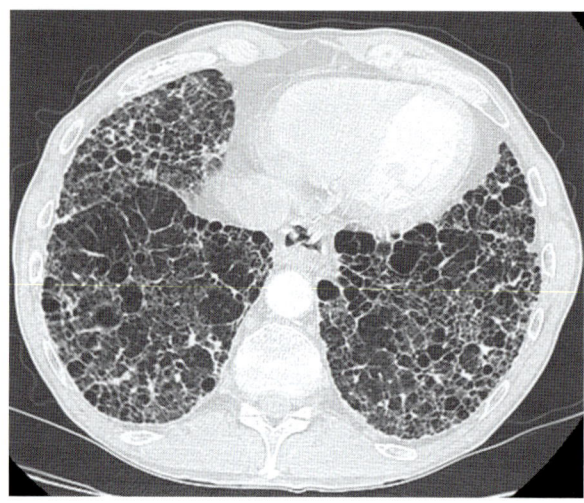

**Fig. 16.4** Ground glass opacity on high-resolution computed tomography shown by *arrows* 1 and 2. (From Corne J, Pointon K. *Chest X-Ray Made Easy*. 3rd ed. Churchill Livingstone, Elsevier; 2009.)

An example of ground glass opacity on HRCT can be seen in Fig. 16.4; this is a common sign in HP but not specific, as it can also be found in many other conditions including IIPs, infections (pneumocystis pneumonia [PCP]; cytomegalovirus [CMV]) and pulmonary oedema. Lung function tests typically show a restrictive pattern with reduced gas transfer.

## Treatment

Treatment of HP includes removal of the causative antigen. With acute HP, symptoms may resolve spontaneously within a few days following removal from the exposure. Patients with chronic HP may also improve; however, underlying fibrosis is irreversible.

Steroids are used in all forms of HP to speed recovery to normal pulmonary function; however, evidence for their long-term benefit is lacking. Prognosis of HP is variable—acute HP may not progress to chronic disease with antigen avoidance, if possible.

## OCCUPATIONAL LUNG DISEASES

## Pneumoconioses

### Definition

The pneumoconioses are a group of nonmalignant disorders caused by inhalation of mineral or biological dusts. The incidence in the United Kingdom is decreasing as working conditions improve.

**Table 16.6** Causative mineral dusts and their associated pneumoconioses

| Disease | Mineral dust | Exposure |
|---|---|---|
| Silicosis | Silica | Sandblasting and stone cutting Hard rock mining |
| Acute berylliosis Chronic berylliosis | Beryllium | Mining Electrical equipment manufacture |
| Siderosis | Iron oxide | Welding |

## Pathogenesis

Small dust particles (<5 microns in diameter) are inhaled and settle on the epithelial lining of the alveoli where they cause an inflammatory reaction. Diseases caused by coal dust and asbestos exposure are discussed below and further examples of pneumoconioses caused by mineral dusts are shown in Table 16.6.

## Coal worker's pneumoconiosis

There are two conditions caused by exposure to coal dust:

1. Simple pneumoconiosis
2. Progressive massive fibrosis

The incidence of coal worker's pneumoconiosis is related to total dust exposure with the highest risk in those with the largest exposure.

In recent years, thousands of patients have lodged claims for compensation for work-related exposure to coal dust. The Coal Workers Pneumoconiosis Scheme has been set up specifically for this purpose. Although not all claims are successful, many patients are able to get some compensation for the disease that they have subsequently developed.

---

### HINTS AND TIPS

#### DEATH RELATED TO OCCUPATIONAL LUNG DISEASES

When writing a death certificate, it is important to note if the cause of death is related to the patient's employment history. In the United Kingdom, the coroner must be notified if the death may have been caused by an industrial disease or poisoning.

---

### Simple pneumoconiosis

Simple pneumoconiosis is the commonest type of pneumoconiosis, reflecting coal dust deposition within the lung. It is asymptomatic, and diagnosis is made on the basis of small round opacities in the upper zone on CXR. Those with severe disease may go on to develop progressive massive fibrosis.

### Progressive massive fibrosis

In progressive massive fibrosis, large, round fibrotic nodules measuring more than 10 mm in diameter are seen, usually in the upper lobes. Scarring is present. Nodules may show central liquefaction and become infected by tuberculosis. The associated emphysema is always severe.

Symptoms include dyspnoea, cough and sputum production (which may be black as cavitating lesions rupture). Lung function tests show a mixed restrictive and obstructive pattern.

The disease may progress once exposure has ceased (unlike simple coal worker's pneumoconiosis) and there is no specific treatment.

### Caplan syndrome

Caplan syndrome is the association of coal worker's pneumoconiosis and seropositive rheumatoid arthritis. Rounded lesions, measuring 0.5–5.0 cm in diameter, are seen on CXR and may cavitate, but are normally asymptomatic.

## Asbestos-related lung diseases

Asbestos is a group of naturally occurring compounds composed of a mixture of silicates of iron, nickel, magnesium, aluminium and cadmium mined from the ground. In the United Kingdom, asbestos was used in multiple industries up until the 1970s and many people were exposed through their occupation or at home through remodelling of contaminated buildings. Occupations at risk of exposure include:

- Asbestos mining and transport
- Construction and demolition industry
- Friction materials such as brake lining
- Insulation, e.g., boiler fitting and lagging.

Several types of asbestos exist: serpentine fibres (white) and amphibole fibres. The serpentine fibres are considered less toxic than amphibole fibres. The most important type of amphibole asbestos is crocidolite (blue asbestos), a straight fibre 50 μm long and 1–2 μm wide that cannot be cleared by the immune system. Fibres remain in the lung indefinitely and become coated in iron (haemosiderin) to form the classic drumstick-shaped asbestos bodies.

In the United Kingdom, peak exposure to asbestos was in the early 1970s; however, there is a long latency period of 20–40 years between exposure and disease development. The use of asbestos in the United Kingdom and the United States has been restricted since the 1970s; however, use continues to increase in developing countries.

Asbestos causes four distinct patterns of lung disease:

1. Benign asbestos-related pleural disease—pleural plaques, effusion and thickening
2. Asbestosis—discussed later
3. Mesothelioma (see Chapter 20)
4. Lung cancer.

## Asbestosis

Asbestosis is a chronic interstitial fibrosis resulting from asbestos inhalation. The risk of developing asbestosis is increased with higher exposure to asbestos, and with concurrent smoking. Clinical symptoms are a gradual onset of dyspnoea and a dry cough; signs include clubbing and bibasal late inspiratory crackles on auscultation. HRCT appearances show parenchymal bands, traction change and honeycombing. Associated asbestos-related pleural disease including plaques and thickening may also be seen on imaging. Biopsy is rarely required for diagnosis; however, if histology is performed, it classically shows asbestos bodies (Fig. 16.5).

There is no specific treatment for asbestosis; it is usually supportive, with oxygen therapy as required and treatment of complications including cor pulmonale.

## Compensation

Compensation for asbestos-related diseases is available both through the Diffuse Mesothelioma Payment Scheme and from the civil courts directly from the previous employer. There must be a clear history of asbestos exposure, and time restrictions exist from the time of

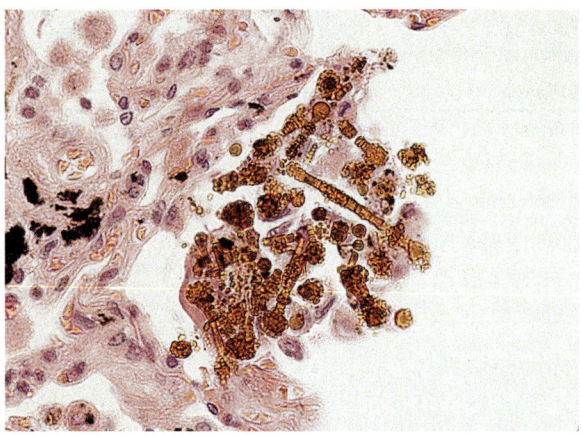

**Fig. 16.5** Asbestos body. (From Stevens A, Lowe J, Scott I. Respiratory system. In: *Core Pathology*. 3rd ed. Elsevier; 2009.)

diagnosis to making a claim. It is therefore important that patients see a specialist respiratory nurse at diagnosis who can provide them with the information and contacts required to make a claim.

---

### ● Chapter Summary

- Interstitial lung diseases (ILDs) are a heterogeneous group of over 300 lung diseases that all affect the lung interstitium. Their pathology can be broadly classed as granulomatous, inflammatory or fibrotic.
- Lung function tests in ILD typically demonstrate a restrictive pattern with a decreased transfer factor.
- Idiopathic pulmonary fibrosis (IPF) is a progressive chronic pulmonary fibrosis of unknown aetiology. It presents with progressive, gradual-onset exertional breathlessness and a dry cough. Examination reveals fine bilateral basal late inspiratory crackles on auscultation and clubbing may be present.
- The appearance of IPF on high-resolution computed tomography is of a 'usual interstitial pneumonia' pattern. This appears as reticulation with a subpleural, peripheral and basal predominance, honeycombing, architectural distortion with traction change and minimal or absent ground glass change.
- Hypersensitivity pneumonitis is an immunological reaction within the lung parenchyma caused by the inhalation of an organic antigen. It can present as an acute, subacute or chronic disease.
- The pneumoconioses are a group of nonmalignant disorders caused by inhalation of mineral or biological dusts. Asbestosis and coal worker's lung are two important examples.

**MLA Conditions**
Asbestos-related lung disease
Fibrotic lung disease
Occupational lung disease
Sarcoidosis

---

### USEFUL LINKS

European Respiratory Society. European Lung White Book – Interstitial Lung Disease.

National Institute for Health and Care Excellence. Idiopathic pulmonary fibrosis in adults: diagnosis and management. 2013. http://www.decc.gov.uk/en/content/cms/funding/coal_health/coal_health.aspx.

# Lung cancer 17

## BRONCHIAL CARCINOMA

Bronchial carcinoma accounts for 95% of all primary tumours of the lung and is one of the commonest malignant tumour in the developed world. It is one of the leading causes of cancer deaths worldwide. Bronchogenic carcinoma was traditionally seen to affect men more than women, but its incidence is rising in females and it is now the second commonest cancer in both sexes (behind prostate cancer in men and breast cancer in women). This trend is thought to be partly linked to the increased proportion of female smokers, despite an overall reduction in smoking as a habit in developed countries, with a current male to female ratio for new lung cancer diagnoses being 11:10 in the United Kingdom. The incidence of bronchial carcinoma is strongly linked to age, with the highest rates in the over-75 years population; less than 1% occur in people under 35 years old in the United Kingdom.

## Aetiology

Cigarette smoking is by far the largest independent risk factor for lung cancer, accounting for over 85% of cases.

- It is related to the amount smoked, duration of habit and cigarette tar content.
- Lung cancer death risk is 15 times higher in smokers compared with nonsmokers.
- The rise in incidence of lung cancer correlates closely with the increase in smoking over the 20th century.
- The risk in those who give up smoking decreases with time.
- Smoking cessation improves life expectancy compared with continuing smokers. This includes long-term smokers and smokers who quit after lung cancer diagnosis.
- Passive smoking also increases lung cancer risk.
- Other forms of smoking including shisha use and cigars are also linked to increased cancer risk. There is not enough current evidence to assess a link between e-cigarettes and lung cancer.

Environmental and occupational factors also play a significant role. Independent of smoking, there is a higher incidence of lung cancer in urban as opposed to rural areas.

Risk factors include:

- Radon released from granite rock.
- Asbestos exposure (increases risk of bronchial carcinoma as well as mesothelioma).
- Air pollution (e.g., beryllium emissions).
- Occupational exposure to nickel, arsenic, chromium, aromatic hydrocarbons and many others.

Host factors also play a role, with a positive family history and underlying lung disease showing association with increased lung cancer rates.

## Histological types

Bronchial carcinomas have traditionally been subdivided into small-cell (20%) and non–small-cell (80%) carcinomas, based on histological appearance. This distinction predicts tumour behaviour and provides information on prognosis and treatment options. 'Non–small cell' is a broad term, and can be subdivided further into squamous cell carcinoma (SCC) (30%), adenocarcinoma (40%) and large-cell anaplastic carcinoma (10%–15%).

The different types of tumour are summarized in Table 17.1. Tumours may occur as discrete, but up to 20% show mixed histological patterns. Owing to significant advances in immunohistochemistry and genetic testing, these broad categories of bronchogenic carcinoma can be further subcategorized based on specific gene mutations. This allows for more personalized treatment and targeted therapy in even advanced disease, and has revolutionized lung cancer management in the last decade.

### Small-cell carcinoma

Small-cell carcinomas arise from neuroendocrine cells and are the most aggressive form of bronchogenic tumour. Their incidence is directly related to cigarette consumption. Most originate in the proximal large bronchi, and tend to invade locally with blood-borne and lymphatic metastases.

Histologically, these tumours have hyperdense nuclei. Occasionally, almost no cytoplasm is present and the cells are compressed into an ovoid form giving rise to the alternative name of oat-cell carcinoma. On radiography, the small-cell carcinoma tends to lie close to the hilum and does not cavitate – it may present with lobar collapse.

As small-cell carcinoma is a neuroendocrine tumour, neurosecretory granules are often present within the cell. A variety of polypeptide hormones can be released from these granules, such as adrenocorticotrophic hormone, antidiuretic hormone and calcitonin, which can lead to paraneoplastic syndromes. However, the most common presenting complaint is coughing. As spread is rapid, metastatic lesions may be the presenting sign.

Owing to the aggressive nature of small-cell carcinoma up to 70% of patients have disseminated or extensive disease at presentation. As a result, prognosis is often very poor, with a

**Table 17.1** Summary of tumour types

| | Non–small-cell tumours | | | Small-cell tumours |
|---|---|---|---|---|
| | Squamous cell | Adenocarcinoma | Large-cell | |
| Incidence (%) | 30 | 40 | 10%–15% | 20 |
| Male/female incidence | M > F | F > M | M > F | M > F |
| Location | Hilar | Peripheral | Peripheral/central | Hilar |
| Histological features | Keratin | Mucin | Mixed | Oat cell |
| Relationship to smoking | High | Low | High | High |
| Growth rate | Slow | Medium | Rapid | Very rapid |
| Metastasis | Late | Intermediate | Early | Very early |
| Treatment Stage 1 | Surgery ± adjuvant chemotherapy, radiotherapy | | | Rarely surgery, often radiochemotherapy |
| Treatment Stage 4 | Chemotherapy, biological agents, palliation | | | Palliative chemotherapy |
| Prognosis stage 1 | 5-year survival 45% mean survival time 50 months | | | 5-year survival 10% mean survival time 15 months |
| Prognosis stage 4 | 5-year survival 2% mean survival time 6 months | | | 5-year survival 1% mean survival time 10 months |

mean survival time for untreated patients with stage 4 small-cell carcinoma of 7 weeks after diagnosis. Death is generally caused by metastatic disease. Overall 5-year survival rates are around 7%.

## Non–small-cell lung carcinoma

### Squamous cell carcinoma

SCC arises from squamous epithelium in the large bronchi, characterized by keratinization. It is the second commonest form of non–small-cell lung cancer. There is a strong association between cigarette smoking and SCC.

Most SCCs arise proximally in large bronchi (although they can occur peripherally). The major mass of the tumour may occur outside the bronchial cartilage and encircle the bronchial lumen, producing obstructive phenomena. Presentation may be through postobstructive infection.

These tumours are almost always hilar and are prone to massive necrosis and cavitation, with upper-lobe lesions more likely to cavitate. Of SCCs, 13% show cavitation on chest radiographs. If squamous carcinoma occurs in the apical portion of the lung, it may produce Pancoast syndrome (see Pancoast syndrome section).

SCCs are associated with paraneoplastic syndromes: the cancer commonly produces a substance similar to parathyroid hormone (parathyroid hormone–related peptide), which leads to hypercalcaemia and bone destruction (Table 17.2).

SCC is the least likely type to metastasize and, untreated, it has the longest patient survival of any of the bronchogenic carcinomas.

### Adenocarcinoma

Bronchial adenocarcinomas are neoplastic tumours derived from glandular epithelium such as mucus goblet cells, type II pneumocytes and Clara cells. They are less clearly linked with smoking (the most common cell type in nonsmokers) and are more common in women than in men. Adenocarcinoma is the most common cancer subtype in patients under 45 years. Incidence is rising in the United Kingdom and it is now the single most common lung cancer subtype as smoking decreases as a habit.

Adenocarcinomas can arise from lung scar tissue and are associated with fibrotic lung disease. Bronchogenic tumours associated with occupational factors are mainly adenocarcinomas.

As the tumour is commonly at the lung periphery (visible on chest radiograph or computed tomography [CT] imaging), obstructive symptoms are rare, so the tumour may be clinically silent. Symptoms include coughing, haemoptysis, chest pain and weight loss.

Diagnosis is usually via imaging, demonstrating a solitary peripheral nodule confirmed with external biopsy, although sputum cytology may detect malignant cells. Adenocarcinomas tend to metastasize relatively late and in certain cases, resection is possible. However, owing to the silent nature of adenocarcinomas, metastases may be seen by the time of diagnosis – typically occurring in the pleura, lymph nodes, bone, brain and adrenal glands.

Further subdivisions of bronchial adenocarcinoma have been made based on genetic subtyping. This reflects great advancement in the multidisciplinary management of adenocarcinoma. For example, the epidermal growth factor receptor (EGFR) mutation has been shown to be a predictive marker for response

**Table 17.2** Paraneoplastic disorders associated with lung cancer

| | Mechanism | Clinical features | Lung cancer association |
|---|---|---|---|
| SIADH | Excess secretion of ADH | Headache, nausea, muscle weakness, drowsiness, confusion, eventually coma | Small-cell |
| Ectopic ACTH | Adrenal hyperplasia and secretion of large amounts of cortisol | Cushing: polyuria, oedema, hypokalaemia, hypertension, increased pigmentation | Small-cell or carcinoid |
| Hypercalcaemia | Ectopic PTH secretion | Lethargy, nausea, polyuria, eventually coma | Squamous cell (but may be caused by bone metastases) |
| Hypertrophic pulmonary osteoarthropathy | Unknown | Digital clubbing and periosteal inflammation | Adenocarcinoma, squamous cell |
| Lambert–Eaton myasthenic syndrome | Autoimmune attack on presynaptic motor voltage-gated calcium channels | Proximal muscle weakness, reduced tendon reflexes and autonomic dysfunction. Can initially be confused with myasthenia gravis | Small-cell most commonly (can present in others) |
| Gonadotrophins | Ectopic secretion | Gynaecomastia, testicular atrophy | Large-cell |

ACTH, Adrenocorticotrophic hormone; ADH, antidiuretic hormone (vasopressin); PTH, parathyroid hormone; SIADH, syndrome of inappropriate antidiuretic hormone.

to targeted therapy (EGFR tyrosine kinase inhibitors) in advanced adenocarcinomas, and so testing for the EGFR mutation is now routine.

### Large-cell anaplastic tumour

Large-cell anaplastic tumours are often poorly differentiated and are diagnosed by a process of elimination, officially only by resected specimen, the appearance of which does not fit with other carcinoma subtypes. No clear-cut pattern of clinical or radiological presentation distinguishes them from other malignant lung tumours. These tumours are variable in location, but are usually centrally located. The point of origin of the carcinoma influences the symptomatic presentation of the disease: central lesions present earlier than peripheral lesions as they cause obstruction.

As with most poorly differentiated tumours, large-cell carcinomas tend to demonstrate more aggressive behaviour and metastasize relatively early.

The tumour causes coughing, sputum production and haemoptysis. When a tumour occurs in a major airway, obstructive pneumonia can occur.

On electron microscopy, these tumours turn out to be poorly differentiated variants of SCC and adenocarcinoma; they are extremely destructive lesions that metastasize early.

### Other bronchial tumours

Other bronchial tumours exist which are often considered benign or were not previously considered clinically relevant to the management of bronchial carcinoma. The 2015 World Health Organization guidance on lung tumours creates different subcategories to encompass tumour subtypes outside of the four categories described previously, as well as intensively subcategorizing existing tumours – for example, both small-cell carcinoma and carcinoid tumours are subdivided into a 'neuroendocrine tumour' category. These subcategories better incorporate the mixed histological patterns currently seen.

Carcinoid tumours are rare, slow-growing and often benign neuroendocrine tumours which can occur in any tissue derived from the embryonic gut. While the majority arise in the gastrointestinal system, they may also grow in a multitude of organs, including the lung, and make up a small subset (<5%) of bronchial tumours. They are often asymptomatic although can become metabolically active owing to hormone secretion or eventual mass effect and, rarely, metastatic spread. Carcinoid syndrome is a result of the release of active mediators, including prostaglandins, somatostatin and other neuropeptide hormones, and typically presents as facial flushing, as well as diarrhoea, palpitations, wheezing and altered mental state. Management of carcinoid tumours is typically surgical unless widespread metastases are present. Octreotide, a form of somatostatin analogue, is often used to manage symptoms of carcinoid syndrome by decreasing the release of serotonin by the tumour. Targeted therapy via octreotide hormonal manipulation has been proposed to provide a new form of cancer treatment, and is another current area of research.

## Clinical features

While there are no specific signs of bronchogenic carcinoma, a variety of different features can point you towards the diagnosis. Details specific to the histological types have already been introduced above. A good clinician will always look for red flag symptoms and have a high index of suspicion in high-risk groups (Box 17.1). Diagnosis always needs to be excluded in cigarette smokers who present with recurrent respiratory symptoms:

- Persistent cough – commonest presentation; may be productive if obstruction leads to recurrent infection.
- Haemoptysis – occurs at some stage in disease in 50%, owing to tumour bleeding into an airway or bronchial ulceration.
- Dyspnoea – rarely at presentation but occurs as disease progresses, as central tumours obstruct large airways.
- Chest pain – often sharp pleuritic pain caused by peripheral tumours invading the pleura (which is well innervated). May be a dull central ache as a result of large-volume mediastinal node disease.
- Wheezing – monophonic, owing to partial airway obstruction.
- Hoarse voice – owing to either mediastinal node compression or direct tumour invasion of the left recurrent laryngeal nerve.
- Unexplained weight loss.
- Night sweats.
- Finger clubbing – in 10%–30% of patients, finger clubbing is present on examination.
- Signs of metastatic disease – patients may present for the first time late in their disease. Classic signs of metastatic disease are described below.

# Complications

## Local complications

Symptoms of local complications may be caused by:

- Bronchial obstruction: the lumen of the bronchus becomes occluded; distal collapse and retention of secretions subsequently occur. This clinically causes dyspnoea, secondary infection and lung abscesses.
- Central necrosis: carcinomas can outgrow their blood supply, leading to central necrosis. The main complication is then the development of a lung abscess.
- Pleural effusion: as a result of tumour spread to the pleural space. Can lead to progressive breathlessness and pleuritic pains, and may require symptomatic drainage.

- Paralysis of the hemidiaphragm: caused by direct invasion of the phrenic nerve. Can produce sudden onset of breathlessness and gives a classic chest radiograph appearance.

## Pancoast syndrome

Pancoast syndrome can be caused by all types of bronchogenic carcinoma, although two-thirds originate from squamous cells. As the tumour grows outward from the pulmonary parenchymal apex, it encroaches on anatomical structures, including:

- Chest wall
- Subpleural lymphatics
- Sympathetic chain
- Brachial plexus.

Pancoast tumours can affect the sympathetic chain, resulting in loss of sympathetic tone and an ipsilateral Horner syndrome (ptosis, meiosis, enophthalmos, conjunctival injection and reduced sweating on ipsilateral side of the head and neck). Intractable shoulder pain occurs when the upper rib is involved. The subclavian artery and vein may become compressed. Destruction of the inferior trunk of the brachial plexus leads to pain in ulnar nerve distribution and may lead to small-muscle wasting of the hand.

## Superior vena cava obstruction

The obstruction of the superior vena cava by external pressure, direct tumour invasion or blood clot is considered an oncological emergency. While it can occur through any upper mediastinal mass, bronchial carcinoma is the most common cause (with lymphoma being the next most common). The onset may be gradual or acute, depending on the speed of vessel occlusion, resulting in worsening venous congestion. Symptoms include headaches, breathlessness, dysphagia, stridor and swollen oedematous face and upper limbs, as well as venous congestion of the neck. Symptoms may be aggravated with postures that increase venous pressure such as bending over or lying down. Complete airway obstruction may occur if untreated, owing to oedema. While the diagnosis may be made clinically, investigation via chest X-ray (CXR) (widened mediastinum) and CT chest (more detail) is usually required. The treatment aim is to shrink the mass and resolve the obstruction. This is achieved with immediate high-dose steroids, and consideration for emergency mediastinal radiotherapy. In tumours highly responsive to chemotherapy (such as small-cell lung cancer), this may be the preferred initial treatment. Surgical resection or vascular stents may also be considered in certain cases.

## Metastatic complications

Bronchial carcinoma typically spreads to mediastinal, cervical or even axillary lymph nodes, which may become palpable. Distant metastases occur in the liver, bone, brain, adrenal glands and skin:

- Liver – may present with nausea, weight loss or right upper quadrant pains (tumour growth resulting in liver capsular pains). Can be palpated as an enlarged irregular liver edge.

- Bone – most commonly presenting as a gnawing bone pain, bony metastases can also present with pathological fractures. Rarely, these may present as spinal cord compression, an oncological emergency resulting in neurological symptoms and eventual paralysis below the level of compression. Any clinical suspicion requires urgent investigation with magnetic resonance imaging of the spine and treatment with high-dose steroids and either radiotherapy or decompressive surgery.
- Brain – metastases may present in a variety of different ways, from headache and confusion to focal neurological lesions to seizures to raised intracranial pressure and mass effect. While rarely operable, symptoms of brain metastases may be treated with steroid therapy to reduce cerebral oedema and mass effect.
- Adrenal – these are usually asymptomatic and rarely produce adrenal insufficiency.
- Skin – although uncommon, may present as cutaneous or subcutaneous nodules. Usually solitary and fast growing, they tend to be mobile, painless and firm. Can be investigated with punch biopsy.

## Paraneoplastic syndromes

Paraneoplastic syndromes are clinical presentations of malignancy that cannot be explained by direct invasion of the tumour. They are caused by production of polypeptides that mimic various hormones by the tumour cells. Although possible with all bronchial carcinomas, paraneoplastic syndromes are most commonly associated with small-cell lung cancer. They may result in electrolyte abnormalities, physical deformity or other symptoms seemingly unexplained by the initial presentation. The commonest of the paraneoplastic syndromes is the syndrome of inappropriate antidiuretic hormone secretion, a syndrome produced by a variety of conditions, including neurological, infective and iatrogenic as well as malignant disease. Excessive antidiuretic hormone results in increased water resorption in the collecting ducts of the kidney, leading to low total body sodium (dilutional hyponatraemia), low serum osmolality and a high urine osmolality in an otherwise euvolaemic patient. This creates symptoms of headache and nausea, eventually leading to confusion, drowsiness and even coma, caused by cerebral oedema. Treatment is through fluid restriction and, occasionally, cautious salt replacement.

Other paraneoplastic syndromes are outlined in Table 17.2.

## Investigations

The key to any tumour investigation is to find where the primary tumour is and the extent of the disease (imaging), and to find out the underlying tissue diagnosis (usually performed through biopsy, histology and cytological analysis). This allows for prediction of tumour progression and establishes parameters for treatment.

## Chest radiography

An initial erect chest radiograph (posteroanterior image) is a vital initial screening tool in anyone presenting with symptoms suggestive of lung cancer. Seventy percent of bronchial carcinomas arise centrally, and chest radiography demonstrates over ninety percent of carcinomas. The mass needs to be 1–2 cm in size to be recognized reliably. Lobar collapse, raised hemidiaphragm and pleural effusions may be present. A routine lateral image is not required, and further assessment of any mass is performed by more detailed imaging such as CT to confirm the diagnosis.

## Computed tomography scan

This is the diagnostic method of choice for suspected lung cancer, as well as giving information on tumour staging and spread. It gives good visualization of the mediastinum and is good for identifying small lung lesions. While imaging of the chest is essential for lung cancer diagnosis, inclusion of the neck, upper abdomen and adrenals are essential for staging (via the tumour – node – metastasis (TNM) system, see Table 17.3), and may include the head if cerebral metastases are clinically suspected. The CT scan also acts as a mode of triage that defines the next appropriate investigative step: a central mass may be accessible via bronchoscopy for biopsy, while a peripheral lesion may be more amenable to radiologically guided percutaneous biopsy.

**Table 17.3** Staging in non–small-cell lung cancer (based on the TNM 8th edition)

| T1 | ≤3 cm | | |
|---|---|---|---|
| T2 | >3 cm but ≤5 cm or tumour of any size involving visceral pleura, main bronchus (not carina) or atelectasis to hilum. | | |
| T3 | >5 cm but ≤7 cm or extending into the chest wall, pericardium, phrenic nerve; or separate tumour nodule(s) in the same lobe. | | |
| T4 | Tumour >7 cm or tumour invading mediastinum, diaphragm, heart, great vessels, recurrent laryngeal nerve, carina, trachea, oesophagus, spine; or tumour nodule(s) in a different ipsilateral lobe. | | |
| | **Regional lymph nodes** | | **Distant metastases** |
| N0 | No nodal involvement | M0 | No metastases |
| N1 | Ipsilateral pulmonary and/or ipsilateral hilar nodes | M1a | Malignant pleural or pericardial effusion/ nodules or separate nodule in a contralateral lobe |
| N2 | Ipsilateral mediastinal and/or subcarinal lymph nodes | M1b | Single extrathoracic metastasis |
| N3 | Contralateral mediastinal, hilar node involvement or supraclavicular | M1c | Multiple extrathoracic metastases (1 or >1 organ) |

## Positron emission computed tomography

While not an initial diagnostic test, the positron emission computed tomography (PET-CT) scan is a useful complementary scan for assessing lymph node spread and metastatic disease, and is useful in the accurate staging and treatment planning for bronchogenic carcinoma. It works by using a radiolucent tracer marker as a measure for glucose uptake, indicating areas of high cell turnover. These metabolically active areas light up on the scan as hotspot areas suggesting metastatic spread if positive, and are particularly useful in assessing mediastinal disease and nodes suitable for biopsy, as well as assessing distant metastatic disease. PET-CT scanning should now be available for all those being considered for radical (curative) treatment.

## Bronchoscopy

Bronchoscopy is a safe and effective diagnostic and staging investigation. It confirms central lesions, assesses operability and allows accurate cell type to be determined through biopsy. Mediastinal lymph nodes can be sampled by a technique called transbronchial needle aspiration. This is increasingly performed using endobronchial ultrasound (EBUS) to guide mediastinal lymph node biopsy. Mucus secretions plus sputum can be examined for the presence of malignant cells, either endoscopically through a process called bronchoalveolar lavage (see Chapter 10) or directly via sputum sampling, although these techniques are far less sensitive and are not routinely relied upon unless no other techniques are possible.

## Mediastinoscopy

Mediastinoscopy is the current gold standard for preoperative nodal assessment in mediastinal disease and involves direct visualization. However, with advances in PET and EBUS techniques, the role of mediastinoscopy is diminishing.

## Transthoracic fine-needle aspiration biopsy

While bronchoscopy is useful in assessing central lesions, peripheral lesions are approached externally through radiological guidance. In transthoracic fine-needle aspiration biopsy, the needle is guided by ultrasound or CT. Direct aspiration of peripheral lung lesions takes place through the chest wall; 25% of patients suffer pneumothorax caused by the procedure, which may require admission for monitoring or drainage (see Chapter 20). Implantation metastases do not occur.

## Assessing fitness for treatment

It is vital to assess whether a patient is suitable to undergo radical treatment. This includes assessment of their existing comorbidities and current level of baseline fitness. Grading systems are available to aid in this assessment such as the American Society of Anesthesiologists performance status classification and the Medical Research Council Dyspnoea Scale. These are discussed in more detail in Chapter 8.

Any patient considered a candidate for treatment should undergo full lung function testing with transfer capacity assessment. Other underlying diseases may also warrant further investigation – for example, significant cardiovascular disease may require echocardiography or further cardiologist review.

## Lung cancer staging

Staging of lung cancer using the methods described previously is a vital part of assessment, as it affects both prognosis and treatment options. Small-cell and non–small-cell cancers are both staged using the tumour–node–metastasis (TNM) system (Table 17.3), as recommended by the International Association for the Study of Lung Cancer.

However, small-cell cancers are often additionally staged as either limited or extensive using the Veterans Administration Lung Cancer Study Group system, owing to the aggressive nature of the disease. Limited-stage disease is confined to an area that can feasibly be treated by one radiation area – meaning the cancer is confined to one lung with the inclusion of nearby lymph nodes. It automatically excludes cancers with pleural and pericardial effusions. All other small-cell lung cancers not confined to the hemithorax are extensive-stage in this scheme.

## Multidisciplinary team assessment

All patients thought to have lung cancer should be referred to a member of a lung cancer multidisciplinary team (MDT). Often the initial referral is through a rapid access lung clinic to aid faster diagnosis and reduce patient anxiety (these are part of the 2-week wait pathway in the United Kingdom). Individual cases are then discussed by a group of experts from different fields at an MDT meeting. These meetings include a respiratory physician, an oncologist, a thoracic surgeon, a histologist, a radiologist, a clinical nurse specialist and a palliative care specialist. The team reviews the type of cancer, the staging and underlying comorbidities to decide on the best course of action available. Each team member provides a different area of expertise to the patient's care, and multidisciplinary care is the gold standard in all cancer management.

## Treatment

Treatment of lung cancer is complex and ever evolving. While there are a variety of treatment options available, the majority of patients are diagnosed at an advanced stage, meaning curative treatment is often not possible. We aim to outline broad treatment principles, with recommendations for further reading outlined later.

## Communication and lifestyle advice

Treatment begins with informing the patient of the diagnosis. How this is done will affect the patient for the rest of their life and should not be taken lightly. As patient-centred care is key to good medical practice, honest and open discussions on available treatment options, prognosis and MDT recommendations can be had with the patient. Anyone undergoing treatment should be aware of the risks involved and the likely outcomes – some treatment is for curative intent while others are to prolong life expectancy or improve quality of life.

Lifestyle factors should be taken into account. Patients should be advised to stop smoking and should be aware of why this is important. Smoking cessation therapies and counselling should be made available to all patients who require it.

### COMMUNICATION

### BREAKING BAD NEWS

Having a structured approach will help you to present bad news in a manner that is both factual and considerate. This framework may help you when breaking bad news.

S–P–I–K–E–S

S – Setting

Prepare and rehearse what you will say, pick an appropriate and quiet setting, involve relatives, and manage time constraints to avoid interruption.

P – Perception

Ask the patient what they already know and understand about what is happening. You can then correct misinformation and tailor your input to what the patient already knows. This will also reveal any denial or unrealistic expectations of treatment.

I – Invitation

Establish whether the patient wants the full information available. Some patients would rather not know their full prognosis, as part of their coping mechanism.

K – Knowledge

Give a warning shot before giving full information. Use simple and understandable language. Give information in small chunks and check the patient's understanding.

E – Empathy

Take time to pause and understand the patient's emotional response to the bad news. An empathic response can provide support.

S – Strategy and summary

Giving a clear treatment plan or next steps will avoid patient uncertainty and reduce anxiety. Summarizing key information will help with retention of information. Always allow time for questions and prompt the patient, who may not feel comfortable enough to ask.

For more information, see Baile et al.: SPIKES – A Six-Step Protocol for Delivering Bad News: Application to the Patient with Cancer, *The Oncologist* 2000, Society for Translational Oncology.

## Surgery

Surgery is used in early-stage disease in non–small-cell lung cancer (NSCLC) and is considered the best option for curative intent. Likewise, surgery is now also offered for very early-stage small-cell lung cancer in otherwise healthy patients, although these cases are even rarer than in NSCLC. The goal of surgery is complete tumour resection. Surgical procedures include lobectomy (either open or thoracoscopic) as the treatment of choice, with extensive surgeries such as pneumonectomy reserved for more extensive disease. The patient needs to be fit enough for the surgery and be prepared for postoperative reduction in lung function depending on the extent of the surgery planned. Patient fitness is assessed via patient performance status (see Chapter 8).

Where nodal disease is associated with NSCLC, surgery is offered with postoperative chemotherapy if the patient's performance status is good enough to tolerate treatment.

## Radiation therapy

This is the treatment of choice if the tumour is inoperable or the patient is not fit for surgery, and radiotherapy can be administered with curative intent in NSCLC. Again, baseline assessment and adequate lung function need to be considered. In early-stage NSCLC, high-dose radiotherapy or continuous hyperfractionated accelerated regimens can provide outcomes almost comparable to surgery. Even if the patient's lung function is poor, radiation therapy can still be of benefit as long as the area irradiated is small. While radiotherapy has less of a role in small-cell lung cancer, it can be useful in certain instances to prolong life rather than to cure disease. Again, treatment can be combined with chemotherapy to produce better response rates and extend median survival in NSCLC in certain instances.

Radiotherapy can also be used in the palliation of symptoms of lung cancer. This includes management of bone pain from metastatic disease and the management of local invasion of the thoracic wall, bronchial occlusion or invasion with subsequent haemoptysis, superior vena cava obstruction or spinal cord compression.

Radiotherapy is not without its risks. Radiation pneumonitis occurs in up to 15% of cases, resulting in acute infiltration within 3 months of radiotherapy. Radiation fibrosis occurs later and is much more common, although is rarely clinically significant.

## Chemotherapy and immunotherapy

Medical therapies can be offered as an adjuvant to other treatment modalities for curative intent or to prolong survival and improve quality of life. Agents used depend on the underlying histological type, with newer biologic agents providing survival benefits compared with traditional chemotherapy in responsive patients.

Small-cell lung cancer in limited-stage disease responds well to combination chemoradiotherapy, although this is not with curative intent. Platinum-based agents such as cisplatin or carboplatin plus a combination agent often show significant response. Even in extensive disease, median survival can be increased from 6 to 12 months with combination chemotherapy. If first-line chemotherapy fails, second-line chemotherapy can provide further palliation in patients with a good performance status.

SCC rarely demonstrates active mutations for targeted agents and so chemotherapy is often used as first line. A third-generation agent such as gemcitabine plus cisplatin is the standard first-line treatment, although a variety of agents may be used.

In adenocarcinoma, targeted biological agents are used on the EGFR if the mutation is present, with the EGFR tyrosine kinase inhibitor afatinib providing survival and quality of life benefits compared with first-line chemotherapy. Immunotherapy using immune checkpoint inhibitors such as with PD-L1 inhibitors has also shown to be highly successful in NSCLC treatment. These act to upregulate the host immune system to destroy cancer cells. Other genetic mutations are tested for and other biological agents, with significant advances to treatment being made. Chemotherapy options include a third-generation drug in combination with a platinum agent, with maintenance chemotherapy prolonging survival rates significantly.

Side effects and intolerances of chemotherapy should not be underestimated. Nausea and vomiting are the commonest effects but can be debilitating, inducing life-threatening renal impairment, and requiring hospital admission. Other effects include immunosuppression, and patients can be susceptible to neutropenic sepsis following treatment. Specific chemotherapy agents will have specific side effect profiles and should be considered in all treatment plans and reviews.

## Palliative care

As most disease is diagnosed at an advanced stage and multiple comorbidities are associated with the smoking population, much lung cancer treatment is with palliative intent. This encompasses both anticancer treatment and symptom management. The role of palliative radiotherapy and chemotherapy treatments are discussed previously. Endoscopic therapy and transbronchial stenting are used to provide symptomatic relief in patients with terminal disease. Daily corticosteroids may improve appetite. Opioid analgesia is given to control pain and laxatives should be prescribed to counteract the opioid side effects. Candidiasis is a common, treatable problem. Specific problems of breathlessness may also occur and can be treated with opiates and oxygen therapy. Both patients and relatives require counselling. Involvement

of Macmillan nurses and palliative care and community teams is paramount for effective management of end-stage disease.

## Prognosis

Overall prognosis for lung cancer is poor. Survival rates are very variable and depend on tumour type and stage at diagnosis. For all lung cancer types in the United Kingdom, the 5-year survival rate is 20%. Small-cell lung cancer carries the worst prognosis, with the median survival time for those with extensive disease being around 12 months if treated.

## METASTATIC MALIGNANCY TO THE LUNG

Metastases to the lung are a common clinical and radiological finding. They are often found on CXR in patients with known malignancy, but can be the first presentation. Metastases are more likely to be multiple than solitary. Most haematogenous metastases are sharply circumscribed with smooth edges, and the appearance of multiple smoothly circumscribed nodules is highly suggestive of metastatic disease. Cavitation is unusual in metastatic lesions.

Solitary pulmonary metastases do occur as sarcomas of soft tissue or bone, and carcinoma of the breast, colon and kidney. Multinodular lung metastases may be of varying sizes (Table 17.4):

- Very large dimensions – cannonball pattern.
- Many small nodules – snowstorm pattern.

Carcinoma of the breast, stomach, pancreas and prostate can involve mediastinal lymph nodes. This can lead to spread along the lymphatics of both lungs and lymphatic congestion, resulting in a condition known as lymphangitis carcinomatosis, which causes severe breathlessness. On CXR, bilateral lymphadenopathy is seen with associated widespread basal shadowing spreading across both lung fields owing to the lymphatic congestion. Management is to treat the underlying malignancy.

**Table 17.4** Metastatic malignancy of lung and the resulting radiological appearance

| Multinodular | | Solitary nodule |
|---|---|---|
| **Cannonball** | **Snowstorm** | |
| Salivary gland | Breast | Breast |
| Kidney | Kidney | Kidney |
| Bowel | Bladder | Bowel |
| Uterus/ovarian | Thyroid | |
| Testis | Prostate | |

## LUNG NODULES

As CT scans are increasingly used for a variety of medical assessments, the incidental detection of asymptomatic small lung nodules has been increasing. The majority of these nodules are benign, but some may be early signs of malignant disease. Recent guidance has been developed on the monitoring of such nodules based on their original size and appearance as well as patient risk factors, and should be performed with interval CT scanning. For example, a new solitary 7-mm nodule seen on chest CT scan should be followed up with a further CT scan in 3 months to assess for evidence of growth.

## MESOTHELIOMA

See Chapter 20.

## ● Chapter Summary

- Bronchial carcinoma is a common malignancy, linked to smoking and age. It is divided into small-cell lung cancer (20%) and non–small-cell lung cancer (80%).
- Typical presenting symptoms include persistent cough, haemoptysis, weight loss or shortness of breath. The key initial investigation in anyone with high risk features is chest radiography.
- Paraneoplastic syndromes are rare manifestations or complications of malignancy caused by ectopic hormone secretion. Management includes correcting the underlying disturbance and, ultimately, treating the malignancy.
- Diagnosis of lung cancer is performed with a mixture of computed tomography (CT) imaging and histological sampling, usually from endobronchial biopsy or radiologically guided lung biopsy.
- Management of lung cancer is with a multidisciplinary team approach. Communication, education, surgery, radiotherapy, chemotherapy, immunotherapy and targeted therapy may all play a role in active management. Palliative treatment is often key to managing patients with bronchial carcinoma with advanced-stage disease.

**MLA Conditions**
Lung cancer
Lymphadenopathy
Metastatic disease

**MLA Presentations**
Breathlessness
Chest pain
Cough
Haemoptysis
Hoarseness and voice change
Weight loss

## PNEUMONIA

Pneumonia is an infection within the lung parenchyma. It is a common condition, with an annual incidence in the community of 5–10 per 1000 adult population. Mortality of those admitted to hospital with pneumonia is between 5% and 14%, and increases to 30% in those who require admission to intensive care.

## Useful definitions

**Lower respiratory tract infection (LRTI)** – an acute illness (<21 days duration) with cough as the main symptom, and with at least one other lower respiratory tract symptom (e.g., fever, sputum production, breathlessness, wheeze or chest pain) and no alternative explanation for the symptoms. This definition encompasses pneumonia, acute bronchitis and infective exacerbation of airways disease.

**Community-acquired pneumonia (CAP)** – pneumonia acquired outside hospital. Patients present with symptoms and signs of LRTI and have a chest X-ray (CXR) demonstrating new parenchymal infiltrates.

**Hospital-acquired pneumonia (HAP)** – pneumonia that develops >48 hours after hospital admission.

**Ventilator-associated pneumonia** – pneumonia in a mechanically ventilated patient that develops >48 hours postintubation.

**Aspiration pneumonia** – pneumonia following aspiration of bacteria normally present in the upper airways or gastrointestinal tract. Note this differs from aspiration of substances that are toxic to the lower respiratory tract (e.g., vomit) that cause a chemical pneumonitis in the absence of bacterial infection. This is common in patients with swallowing difficulties, and causes include stroke or dementia.

## Pathophysiology

The infecting pathogen reaches the alveolar epithelium via inhalation, direct spread or microaspiration. It triggers both the lung's innate and adaptive immune defences and an acute exudate is formed within the alveoli. Recognition of the pathogen through toll-like receptors leads to release of proinflammatory cytokines that attract neutrophils. Alveolar macrophages phagocytose the bacteria and remove acute inflammatory cells, eventually leading to resolution of the host response.

Pneumonia can be classified by site. Lobar pneumonia refers to involvement of a pulmonary lobe while bronchopneumonia is more diffuse, involving lung lobules and their associated bronchi and bronchioles.

## Aetiology

The aetiology and risk factors for CAP and HAP are summarized in Table 18.1. *Streptococcus pneumoniae* is the commonest organism identified in CAP, found in 50% of cases with a microbiological diagnosis. It is most common in the winter months. Pathogens causing pneumonia are described as typical or 'atypical'. Atypical pathogens do not respond to penicillin and include bacteria such as Legionella, *Mycoplasma pneumoniae*, *Chlamydophila psittaci* and *Coxiella burnetii*. Immunocompromised patients are at risk of infection with organisms usually not pathogenic in immunocompetent individuals, including viruses such as cytomegalovirus (CMV) and varicella-zoster virus (VZV), fungi, including Aspergillus, and Mycobacteria.

## Clinical features

Patients with pneumonia commonly present with:

- Cough
- Sputum production (typically yellow or green in colour)
- Shortness of breath

**Table 18.1** Risk factors and common causative organisms in community-acquired and hospital-acquired pneumonia

| | Risk factors | Common causative organisms |
|---|---|---|
| CAP | Extremes of age<br>Aspiration<br>Alcoholism<br>Diabetes<br>Cigarette smoking<br>COPD<br>Nursing home residents | Bacterial:<br>*Streptococcus pneumoniae*<br>*Haemophilus influenza*<br>*Legionella pneumophilia*<br>*Staphylococcus aureus*<br>Viral:<br>Influenza A |
| HAP | Age > 70 years<br>Chronic lung disease<br>Diabetes<br>Reduced conscious level<br>Chest/abdominal surgery<br>Poor dental hygiene<br>Immunosuppressant medications | Bacterial:<br>Gram-negative enteric bacilli<br>*Pseudomonas aeruginosa*<br>Anaerobic bacteria<br>*Staphylococcus aureus*<br>MRSA |

*CAP, Community-acquired pneumonia; COPD, chronic obstructive pulmonary disease; HAP, hospital-acquired pneumonia; MRSA, methicillin-resistant Staphylococcus aureus.*

**Table 18.2** Clinical features associated with causative organism

| Organism | Type | Clinical features |
|---|---|---|
| *Legionella* spp. | Small gram-negative bacillus | Severe infection<br>Younger patients<br>Multisystem disease (abnormal liver enzymes, raised creatinine kinase (CK), diarrhoea, vomiting, hyponatraemia)<br>Travel related, typically Mediterranean<br>Epidemics occur in water-containing systems |
| *Mycoplasma pneumonia* | Obligate intracellular organism | Epidemics 4-yearly in the UK<br>Associated autoimmune phenomena – erythema multiforme, haemolysis, hepatitis, cold agglutinins |
| *Staphylococcus aureus* | Gram-positive cocci | Common with influenza |
| *Chlamydophila psittaci* | Gram-negative bacterium | Zoonotic infection from birds/animals, commonly parrots<br>Severe pneumonia<br>Associated fevers, joint pain and nose bleeds |
| *Coxiella burnetii* | Gram-negative obligate intracellular | Zoonosis – exposure to sheep and goats<br>'Q fever' – fever, myalgia, headache, hepatitis |

- Chest pain
- Fever
- Confusion
- Nonspecific features – especially in elderly patients.

On examination the patient may be pyrexial, tachycardic and tachypnoeic. Focal signs of chest examination include reduced lung expansion, a dull percussion note and increased tactile fremitus over the affected area, with bronchial breathing and coarse crackles on auscultation.

Although the causative organism cannot be accurately predicted from clinical features alone, some features are particularly associated with certain bacteria. These are summarized in Table 18.2.

## Investigations

Patients admitted to hospital with suspected pneumonia should have:

- CXR – within 4 hours to confirm diagnosis and guide antimicrobial treatment.
- Tests of full blood count and C-reactive protein – markers of infection.
- Renal function assessment, including testing of urea – allows severity scoring and assessment for renal dysfunction in severe pneumonia.
- Liver function tests – these can be deranged in severe pneumonia or associated with Legionella.
- Measurement of arterial blood gas levels if hypoxic, to assess for respiratory failure.
- Electrocardiogram if chest pain present or tachycardic to assess for arrhythmias.
- Blood cultures – for all moderate to severe pneumonia or if there is clinical evidence of sepsis.
- Sputum microscopy, culture and sensitivity.

- Pleural fluid sampling if effusion present.
- Pneumococcal urinary antigen testing – if moderate or severe pneumonia.
- Legionella urinary antigen testing – if moderate or severe pneumonia or where clinically suspected (e.g., recent Mediterranean travel).
- Mycoplasma, Coxiella or *C. psittaci* serology if clinically suspected.

## Management

Each patient should have a CURB 65 severity score assessment. One point is scored for each of the following criteria that apply:

- *C*onfusion – new mental confusion (Abbreviated mental test score [AMTS] < 8)
- *U*rea > 7 mmol/L
- *R*espiratory rate $\geq$ 30 breaths per minute
- *B*lood pressure – systolic < 90 mmHg and/or diastolic $\leq$ 60 mmHg
- 65: Age $\geq$ 65 years.

Antibiotic treatment should be guided by clinical features, severity score and local treatment guidelines. Treatment includes:

- Supplementary oxygen – aim for oxygen saturation levels of $\geq$94% (unless known chronic obstructive pulmonary disease and confirmed to be a carbon dioxide retainer, where controlled oxygen therapy targeting oxygen saturations at 88%–92% may be appropriate)
- Fluids – assess fluid status and encourage per os or supplement with intravenous fluids
- Analgesia
- Nutrition – consider supplements
- Physiotherapy – airway clearance techniques.

**Table 18.3** Community-acquired pneumonia antibiotic treatment by severity

| CURB 65 Score | Antibiotic treatment | Mortality (%) |
|---|---|---|
| 0–1 = Low severity | Amoxicillin 500 mg TDS PO for 5 days<br>Consider home treatment<br>If penicillin allergic: Clarithromycin 500 mg BD PO for 5 days OR if pregnant, erythromycin 500 mg QDS PO for 5 days | 3 |
| 2 = Moderate severity | Amoxicillin 500 mg TDS PO plus clarithromycin 500 mg BD PO for 5 days<br>If penicillin allergic: same as for low severity | 3–5 |
| 3–5 = High severity | Co-amoxiclav 1.2 g TDS IV plus clarithromycin 500 mg BD IV<br>If penicillin allergic: levofloxacin 500 mg BD IV or PO | >15 |

*BD, Twice daily; IV, intravenously; PO, per os; TDS, three times daily.*

Poor prognostic factors include coexisting disease, acute respiratory failure, hypoalbuminaemia, bilateral or multilobar involvement on CXR and positive blood cultures (i.e., bacteraemic patients). Usual antibiotic treatment and prognosis are summarized in Table 18.3.

## Complications

Immediate complications of CAP include sepsis, respiratory failure and multiorgan dysfunction. Critical care should be considered in patients with severe pneumonia and admission to intensive care may be required. Later complications can include parapneumonic effusion, empyema and lung abscess formation.

## Follow-up

Patients with CXR infiltrates suggestive of pneumonia should have follow-up imaging 6 weeks after the initial CXR to ensure resolution of the change. Ongoing infiltrate on CXR may prompt further investigation such as computed tomography scan to assess for underlying cancer.

# TUBERCULOSIS

## Definition and epidemiology

Tuberculosis (TB) arises as a result of infection with *Mycobacterium tuberculosis* (MTB). In 2022, TB was the second leading cause of death from a single infectious agent worldwide (after COVID-19). Globally in 2022, an estimated 10.6 million people developed TB causing an estimated 1.3 million deaths. From this total, 410,000 people developed multidrug-resistant or rifampicin-resistant TB (MDR/RR-TB) in 2022.

In the United Kingdom, the incidence of TB has declined since a peak in 2011, until 2019 when there was a slight increase (this decreased in 2020, coinciding with the COVID-19 pandemic). In 2021, the annual incidence of TB in England was 7.8 per 100,000 people, of which 76% were from the non-UK-born population. TB infections are strongly correlated with deprivation; there is an incidence of 13 per 100,000 in the most deprived areas compared to 2 per 100,000 in the least deprived areas.

Risk factors for developing TB include:

- Close contact (relative) with TB
- HIV
- Social factors – drug and alcohol abuse, homelessness, imprisonment, mental health needs
- Medical factors – immunosuppression, end-stage renal failure, drugs including tumour necrosis factor α antagonists (e.g., infliximab).

## Pathology

### Transmission and dissemination

Transmission of the disease occurs via airborne droplets containing the bacterium being released through coughing or sneezing by an infected individual. The droplet nuclei are then inhaled by an uninfected person and can lodge in the distal airways. Fig. 18.1 shows the pathogenesis of TB and the different outcomes following initial exposure.

### Primary tuberculosis

The process of primary infection following inhalation is:

1. Initial inflammatory reaction – the innate immune system is triggered by the activation of alveolar macrophages by MTB.
2. Lymphatic spread of MTB to the hilar lymph nodes.
3. Caseating granulomas form at site of infection through the activated T-lymphocytes and macrophages and stop further MTB replication.

The focus of primary infection is termed the Ghon complex. The combination of tuberculous lymphadenitis and the Ghon complex is termed the primary complex. In 90% of cases, MTB

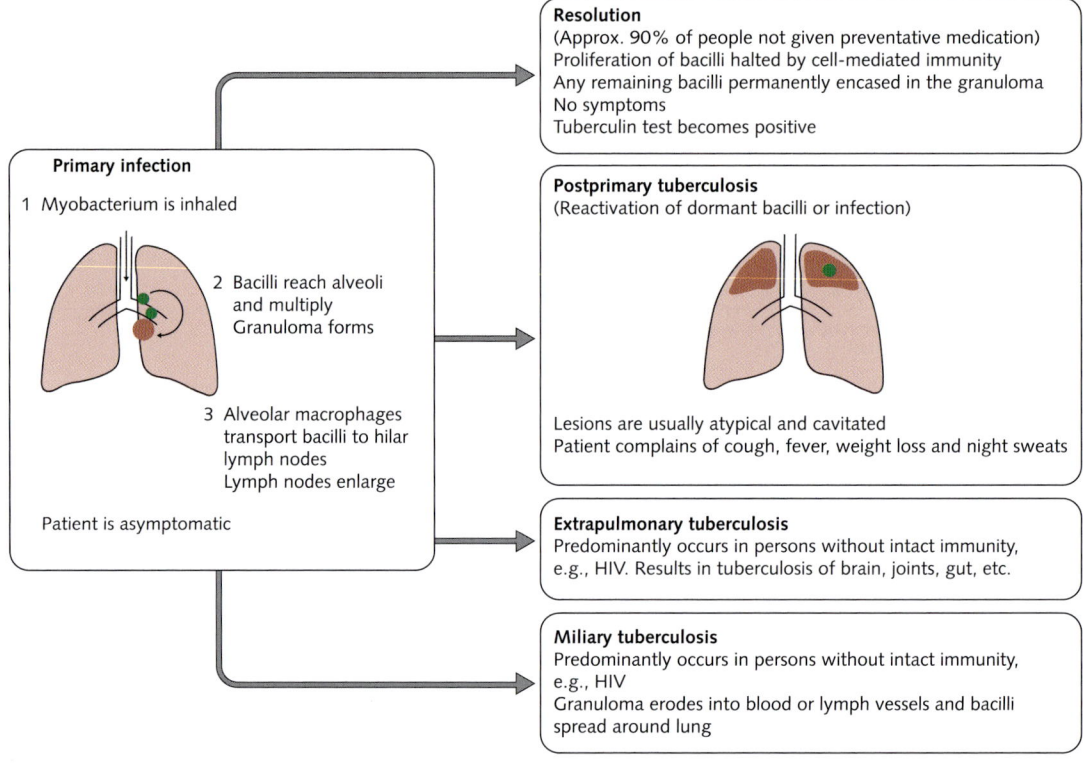

**Fig. 18.1** The pathogenesis of tuberculosis following primary infection.

replication is contained and the primary foci will organize and form a fibrocalcific nodule in the lung with no clinical symptoms. Active disease develops if the immune response of the host is unable to contain MTB replication. Approximately 10% of patients progress to primary progressive TB at this point.

### 'Postprimary' tuberculosis

Postprimary TB occurs following reactivation of a primary infection. In adults, this occurs if MTB lying dormant in the Ghon focus reactivates. The estimated lifetime risk of clinical disease in a child newly infected with MTB is 10%. Any form of immuno-compromise may allow reactivation.

### Miliary tuberculosis

In miliary TB, an acute diffuse dissemination of tubercle bacilli occurs through the bloodstream. Numerous small granulomas form in many organs, with the highest numbers found in the lungs. These form a characteristic pattern on CXR (Fig. 18.3). An important differential for this CXR is metastatic lung cancer, which may have similar appearances.

Miliary TB may be a consequence of either primary or secondary TB and is fatal without treatment.

## Clinical features

Primary TB is usually asymptomatic. Patients with secondary or progressive TB classically present with:

- Productive cough
- Haemoptysis
- Breathlessness
- Systemic features – fever, night sweats, weight loss.

## Extrapulmonary tuberculosis

TB can affect any organ via haematogenous spread, including gut, skin, kidney, genital tract and bone. Extrapulmonary TB is seen in roughly 20% of patients with TB. The most common manifestations include:

- Skin – erythema nodosum (Fig. 18.2A)
- Spine – tuberculoma causing vertebral collapse (Pott disease) (Fig. 18.2B)
- Brain – TB can cause chronic meningitis or a space-occupying lesion (Fig. 18.2C)
- Adrenal glands – adrenal TB is now rare in the United Kingdom but remains an important worldwide cause of adrenal failure.

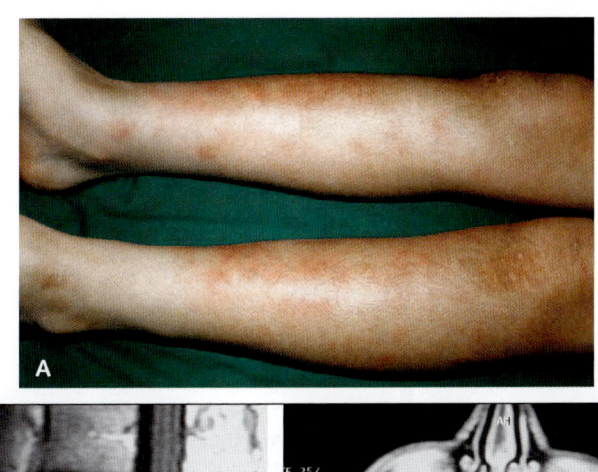
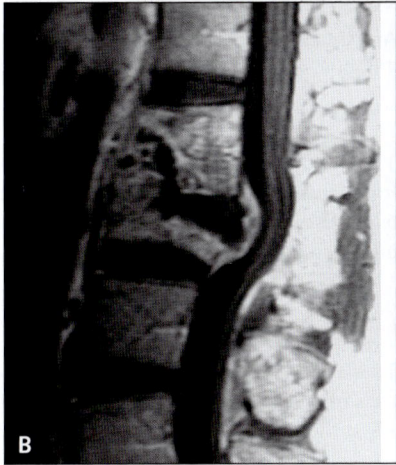
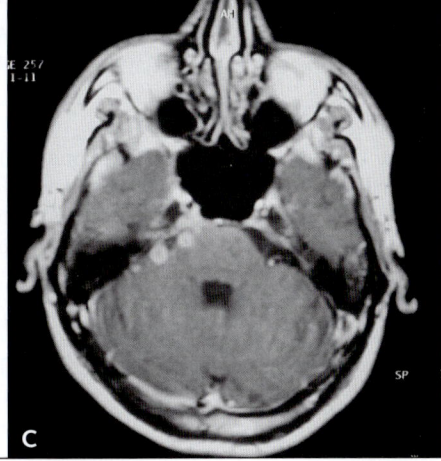

**Fig. 18.2** Extrapulmonary features of tuberculosis. (A) Erythema nodosum. (B) Magnetic resonance imaging of the spine demonstrating Pott disease. (C) Magnetic resonance imaging of the brain showing a tuberculoma. (From Mana J, Marcoval J. Erythema nodosum. *Clin Dermatol*. 2007;25:288–294.)

## Investigations

CXR features of TB include:

- Upper lobe infiltrates with cavitation.
- Hilar lymphadenopathy (Fig. 18.3A).
- Pleural effusion.
- Fibrous scar tissue and calcification – old TB infection, predominantly upper lobes (Fig. 18.3B).
- Miliary TB (disseminated small nodules throughout the lung field) (Fig. 18.3C).

Three deep sputum samples, one preferably an early morning sample, should be sent to the microbiology laboratory before starting treatment. If sputum cannot be produced spontaneously, the use of induced sputum or bronchoalveolar lavage specimens via bronchoscopy may be required.

Sputum is initially stained with a Ziehl–Neelsen stain, examined under microscopy to look for acid-fast bacilli and then sent for culture.

**HINTS AND TIPS**

- 'Smear-positive' tuberculosis (TB) = acid-fast bacilli (AFB) seen on sputum smear (Ziehl–Neelsen stain). These patients are very infectious and account for a high proportion of transmission (approximately 80%). They require isolation precautions in a negative pressure side room if a hospital inpatient.
- 'Culture positive' TB = AFB not seen on smear but TB grown on culture. Patients are much less infectious.

Sputum culture is the gold standard for TB diagnosis; however, this takes 6 weeks or more. Nucleic acid amplification techniques such as the Xpert MTB/RIF assay can detect MTB serotype and identify rifampicin resistance within hours. They are recommended by the World Health Organization (WHO) for use in regions with high TB incidence or coinfection with HIV.

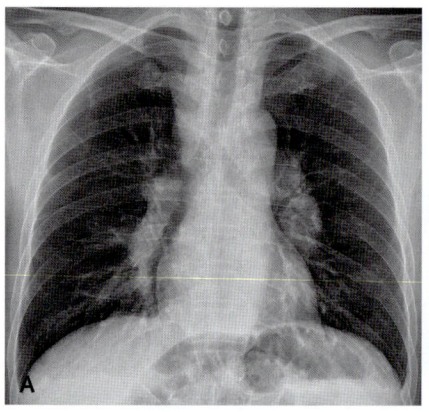
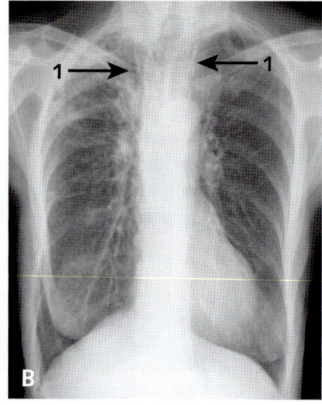
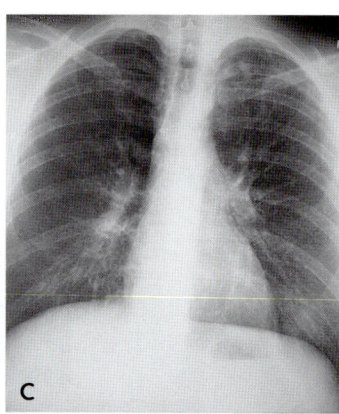

**Fig. 18.3** Chest X-ray (CXR) features suggestive of tuberculosis (TB). (A) CXR showing hilar lymphadenopathy. (B) Chronic bilateral upper lobe scarring from previous TB. (C) CXR showing miliary TB. (From Corne J, Pointon K. *Chest X-ray made easy*. 3rd ed. Churchill Livingstone, Elsevier; London; 2009.)

Diagnosis of extrapulmonary TB requires biopsy for tissue diagnosis, for example, lymph node or pleural biopsy. Patients diagnosed with TB should be tested for HIV and, where appropriate, the HIV specialist team should be involved in diagnosis and further treatment.

## Management

If a patient is smear-positive, treatment is usually started immediately. If smear-negative but with a high clinical suspicion of TB, treatment is usually started. Patients are treated for 6 months:

- Initial phase – 2 months of quadruple therapy, frequently *r*ifampicin, *i*soniazid, *p*yrazinamide plus *e*thambutol (mnemonic: RIPE)
- Continuation phase – 4 months of dual therapy, frequently rifampicin and isoniazid.

As therapeutic noncompliance is a major reason for treatment failure, patients should be followed up regularly by a TB team including a TB nurse specialist. Directly observed short-course therapy can be used to improve compliance by offering an incentive, for example, a free meal, for attending a daily clinic where medications are taken under supervision.

Side effects of TB medications (RIPE):

- Rifampicin: hepatitis, flu-like symptoms, orange secretions (tears, urine)
- Isoniazid: hepatitis, peripheral neuropathy (prevent with pyridoxine – a form of B6)
- Pyrazinamide: hepatitis, hyperuricaemia causing gout, arthralgia, myalgia
- Ethambutol: optic neuritis.

## Latent tuberculosis

Latent TB is defined by the presence of a small number of MTBs that are controlled by the patient's immune system. A person with latent TB is asymptomatic and not infectious. It is diagnosed differently from active TB as it follows a positive tuberculin skin test (Mantoux) or positive interferon-gamma release assay. Both of these tests examine a person's immune response to proteins within MTB (Table 18.4).

## Contact tracing

TB is a notifiable disease in the United Kingdom and any close contacts of the patient with pulmonary TB will be traced in order to assess their risk of having contracted TB. Persons in close contact are defined as those living within the same household or sharing kitchen facilities. If the index patient is smear-positive at diagnosis, casual contacts such as work colleagues may be screened too.

## Prevention

The Bacillus Calmette–Guérin (BCG) vaccine is a live attenuated vaccine made from modified live *Mycobacterium bovis*. From the 1950s to 2005, it was offered to all 10–14 year olds in UK schools. Since 2005, it has been offered only to children <16 years considered to be in high-risk groups or adults within certain settings. BCG is offered to:

- All 0–12 month olds where annual incidence is ≥40/100,000.
- Infants with a parent or grandparent born in a country with an annual incidence of ≥40/100,000.
- Adult healthcare workers and prison officers.

## INFLUENZA

## Definition and epidemiology

Influenza is an acute viral infection that usually affects the respiratory tract. Influenza occurs in annual seasonal epidemics

**Table 18.4** Diagnostic tests in latent tuberculosis

|  | Test type | Immunology | Pitfalls |
|---|---|---|---|
| Tuberculin skin test (Mantoux) | Skin test – intradermal injection | Tests cell-mediated immunity to intradermal tuberculin purified protein derivative | Low sensitivity in immunocompromised patients<br>Requires the patient to return 48 hours later to read result |
| IGRA (T-SPOT.TB; QuantiFERON-TB Gold) | Blood test | Detection of IFNγ released by T cells in response to MTB-specific antigens | Cannot be used to differentiate active and latent TB infection |

*IFNγ, Interferon γ; IGRA, interferon-gamma release assay; MTB, Mycobacterium tuberculosis; TB, tuberculosis.*

during the winter months in the temperate climates of the Northern and Southern hemispheres. The WHO predicts that in developed countries, seasonal influenza affects 10%–20% of the population annually. Worldwide, seasonal flu epidemics are estimated to result in between 250,000 and 500,000 deaths.

### HINTS AND TIPS

In 1918–1919, a new H1N1 influenza emerged – termed 'Spanish flu'. In 2 years, over 40 million people died in the Spanish flu pandemic.

In 2009, a new H1N1 emerged in Mexico – termed 'swine flu'. It caused mild or asymptomatic disease in the majority of cases but severe illness and death in a small proportion.

### HINTS AND TIPS: DEFINITIONS

**Epidemic**
An epidemic is the occurrence of more cases of a disease than would be expected in a community or region during a given time period.

**Pandemic**
A pandemic is the worldwide spread of a new disease. This occurs when a new influenza virus emerges to which most people do not have immunity.

## Pathology

Influenza viruses belong to the Orthomyxoviridae family and are single-stranded RNA viruses. There are three types of influenza virus:

1. Influenza A – common, potentially the most severe
2. Influenza B – common, less severe
3. Influenza C – uncommon, mild illness.

Type A influenza viruses are further subtyped according to the haemagglutinin (HA) and neuraminidase (NA) activity of their viral envelope glycoproteins (Fig. 18.4). Currently, influenza A (H1N1) and A (H3N2) subtypes are circulating in the human population.

Influenza viruses are antigenically unstable, that is, they are constantly changing and are therefore able to cause seasonal epidemics and, potentially, pandemics. Antigenic drift occurs owing to small genetic changes in the virus over time as it replicates. Once enough changes accumulate, the virus can infect an individual who has previously been infected, as the antibodies created against the old virus no longer recognize the new virus.

Antigenic shift occurs following a major change in the influenza A virus, leading to the formation of a new HA antigen. As with many other organisms, there is a large animal reservoir of influenza virus (mainly in domestic animals such as birds, cattle and pigs). Different strains of influenza affect animals compared to those that affect humans. If an animal subtype of influenza A

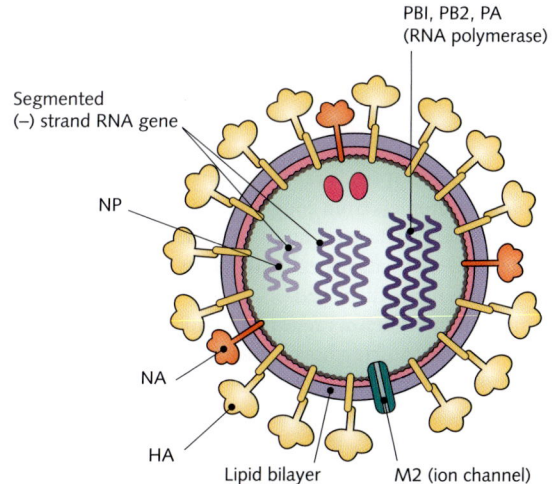

**Fig. 18.4** Structure of the influenza A virus. *HA*, Haemagglutinin; *NA*, neuraminidase; *NP*, nucleocapsid protein; *PBI, PB2, PA*.

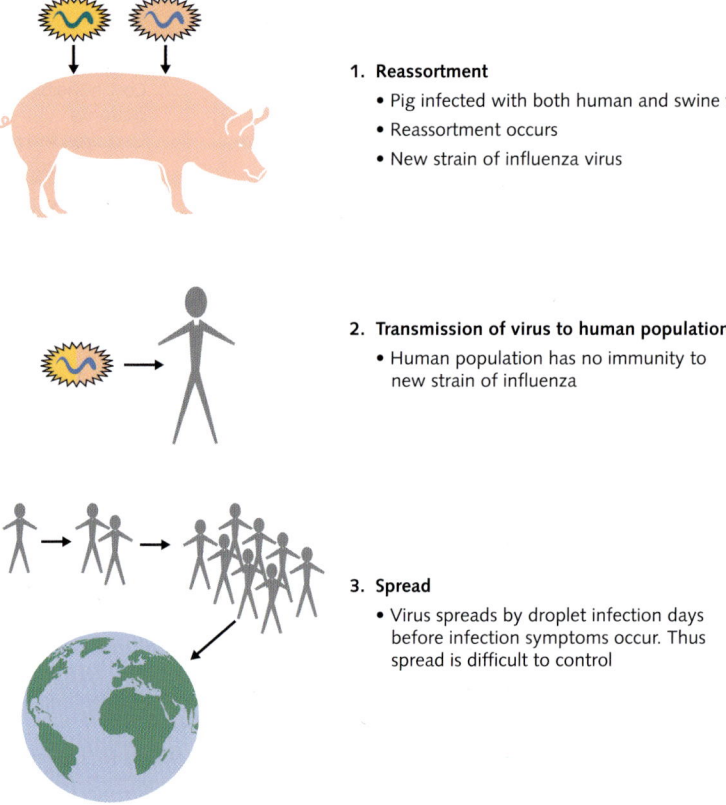

1. **Reassortment**
   - Pig infected with both human and swine virus
   - Reassortment occurs
   - New strain of influenza virus

2. **Transmission of virus to human population**
   - Human population has no immunity to new strain of influenza

3. **Spread**
   - Virus spreads by droplet infection days before infection symptoms occur. Thus spread is difficult to control

**Fig. 18.5** Stages of a pandemic.

combines with a human subtype of influenza A, a process called reassortment, then a new hybrid strain is formed (Fig. 18.5). Most people will not have immunity to this novel virus and therefore, in rare cases, a pandemic can occur if the virus is able to transmit easily between humans.

## Clinical features

Seasonal influenza spreads rapidly. Transmission of the virus is by respiratory droplets from coughing or sneezing. The virus can survive on a hard surface for up to 24 hours. Once an individual is infected, the incubation period in adults is typically 2–3 days before symptoms are displayed.

Symptoms of influenza range from a mild self-limiting illness to severe illness requiring hospitalization and in some cases are fatal. Symptoms include:

- High fever
- Dry cough
- Upper respiratory tract symptoms, e.g., coryza
- Myalgia and arthralgia
- Headache.

Patients at high risk of complicated infection include children under 5 years, the elderly, pregnant women and those with chronic medical conditions.

Common complications include primary viral pneumonia, secondary bacterial pneumonia (*S. pneumoniae* and *Staphylococcus aureus* are common pathogens), otitis media, sinusitis, neurological complications, including encephalitis and cardiovascular complications, including myocarditis.

## Investigation and management

Influenza is often a clinical diagnosis, not requiring formal investigation. In severe cases or during outbreaks, virology may be performed via nose and throat swabs in addition to the normal septic screen tests.

Management is usually symptomatic, with paracetamol and bed rest. In severe cases, supportive care and treatment of complications (such as secondary bacterial pneumonia) require hospital inpatient admission. Antiviral treatment may be indicated in immunocompromised patients, elderly patients or during a known pandemic. It is important to consult local microbiology guidelines at the time for treatment recommendations. Common antiviral medications available are:

1. Neuraminidase inhibitors (oseltamivir and zanamivir)
2. Adamantanes (amantadine and rimantadine).

## Prevention

Vaccination is the most effective way to prevent influenza and severe illness. It is especially important for people at higher risk of serious influenza complications, and for people who live with or care for high-risk individuals. An influenza vaccine is produced annually. The most common type for adults is a trivalent inactivated vaccine protecting against two subtypes of influenza A (H1N1 and H3N2) and one subtype of influenza B. A live attenuated vaccine in the form of a nasal spray is used in babies and children. Vaccine effectiveness varies annually but in the UK 2023/24 season, it was predicted between 30% and 60% by the UK Health Security Agency.

The WHO recommends annual vaccination for:

- Nursing home residents
- Individuals over 65 years of age
- Patients with chronic medical conditions
- Other groups, i.e., pregnant women, healthcare workers, children aged 6 months to 2 years.

## CORONAVIRUS DISEASE (COVID-19)

## Definition and epidemiology

COVID-19 is an infectious respiratory disease caused by the novel SARS-CoV-2 virus. Typically, presentation is that of a respiratory illness with symptoms ranging from mild/moderate flu-like illness to severe viral pneumonia that can cause fatal acute respiratory distress syndrome. The WHO declared COVID-19 a pandemic on 11 March 2020 and WHO data as of March 2024 demonstrated that globally there was a cumulative total of 775 million cases of COVID-19, with 7 million cumulative deaths.

## Pathology

The SARS-CoV-2 virus is part of the coronavirus family, a large family of enveloped RNA viruses, which have also caused other infections such as severe acute respiratory syndrome (SARS) and Middle Eastern respiratory syndrome (MERS). Currently, the origin of the virus is unknown, and zoonotic transmission (transmission of an infectious disease from a non-human animal to a human) has not been confirmed.

The exact pathophysiology of COVID-19 is not established. However, it is known that the virus attaches itself to angiotensin-converting enzyme-2 (ACE2) receptor on target host cells, which leads to the virus being internalized and able to replicate. ACE2 receptors are highly prevalent in upper and lower respiratory

tract cells but are also expressed in other cells, such as myocardial and renal cells, which may explain how COVID-19 can cause extrapulmonary symptoms.

## Clinical features

Like influenza viruses, transmission of COVID-19 is predominantly by inhaling large droplets or small aerosols from an infected person who coughs, sneezes, talks, sings or breathes heavily. Close proximity can allow viral transmission via the nose, eyes or mouth.

COVID-19 is highly infectious, with the initial variant having an incubation period of 1–14 days, which, when compared to influenza's period of 2–3 days, is evidence of how COVID-19 could quickly spread. However, with the newer variants the incubation period has reduced. During the pandemic, the UK government would often release information regarding the reproduction number (R), which represents the average number of secondary infections that result from a single infected person. For example, if R is 2, then for every one infected person, they will infect two people on average.

The most common symptoms that patients present with are fever, dyspnoea and cough. In the beginning of the pandemic, altered sense of smell (anosmia)/taste were common symptoms, however, it is much less prevalent in the newer variants. Other symptoms comprise of:

- Myalgia
- Fatigue
- Headache
- Sore throat
- Confusion (especially in elderly patients).

In some cases, patients had GI symptoms such as nausea, abdominal pain, vomiting or diarrhoea but this is more common in children.

Risk factors for more severe disease in patients include:

- Older age, especially over 70
- Male
- Having a comorbidity such as diabetes, cardiovascular disease or chronic respiratory/kidney disease
- Obesity
- Smokers
- Immunocompromised patients
- Dementia
- Disabilities such as Down syndrome, cerebral palsy or learning disabilities.

## Investigation and management

In healthcare settings, COVID-19 is often diagnosed with reverse transcription polymerase chain reaction (RT-PCR). This is done by obtaining a sample from the patient, usually from their nose, and then using a reverse transcriptase to turn the patient's +/− viral

RNA into DNA. This DNA is then combined with fluorescent fragments that only attach to the viral DNA and so when analyzed by a machine, it will return as positive.

Rapid antigen testing is also available and is used more in the community such as in care homes.

A CXR may be performed with classic features including ground-glass opacification and consolidation, typically bilaterally and peripherally.

Management is usually conservative like with influenza, requiring antipyretics, rest and lots of fluids. However, for patients with severe infection requiring oxygen, NICE recommends corticosteroids (such as dexamethasone or prednisolone) for up to 10 days. Tocilizumab (Il-6 blocker) can also be given in patients who are having systemic steroids and require oxygen or mechanical ventilation.

In patients without an oxygen requirement but who have an increased risk of severe illness from COVID-19 or are 70+ years old, have heart failure, diabetes or a BMI ≥35 then nirmatrelvir plus ritonavir is recommended.

## Complications

In severe disease, COVID-19 can lead to hypercoagulable states, manifesting as venous or arterial thromboembolism. Cardiovascular complications include arrhythmias, acute coronary syndromes or heart failure. Acute kidney injury is a common complication which may be due to haemodynamic changes, hypovolaemia or viral infection directly causing kidney tubular injury. Most people with COVID-19 make a full recovery within 12 weeks; however, if symptoms persist past this, then they may have long COVID with most common symptoms including fatigue, brain fog, feeling short of breath and palpitations.

## FUNGAL RESPIRATORY INFECTIONS

## Aspergillus and the lung

Aspergillus is a type of environmental fungus found in the air and soil worldwide, especially in the autumn and winter in the Northern Hemisphere. *Aspergillus fumigatus* is the most common type.

---

**HINTS AND TIPS**

Aspergillus causes different types of lung disease through two main pathological processes:

1. An allergy-type process where damage occurs owing to overactivation of the host's immune response mechanisms, e.g., allergic bronchopulmonary aspergillosis – see Asthma chapter for further information.
2. An infective process where damage occurs caused by fungal protease release, e.g., invasive aspergillosis and aspergilloma.

---

## Fungal infection in the immunocompetent patient

### Aspergilloma

An aspergilloma is a ball of fungal hyphae that forms within a pre-existing lung cavity (Fig. 18.6). Common reasons for cavity formation in the lung include postinfectious cavities (TB – typically apical, pneumonia), cancer and sarcoidosis. Aspergillomas are often asymptomatic but when symptomatic they commonly present with haemoptysis. Chest imaging may show a cavity with a fungal ball within. Initial treatment is management of the haemoptysis with resuscitation, transfusion, tranexamic acid and, in some cases, arterial embolization if significant haemoptysis is present. If systemic features such as fever and malaise are present, a trial of antifungal medication such as voriconazole may be considered. Surgical resection is considered if there is an ongoing haemoptysis risk.

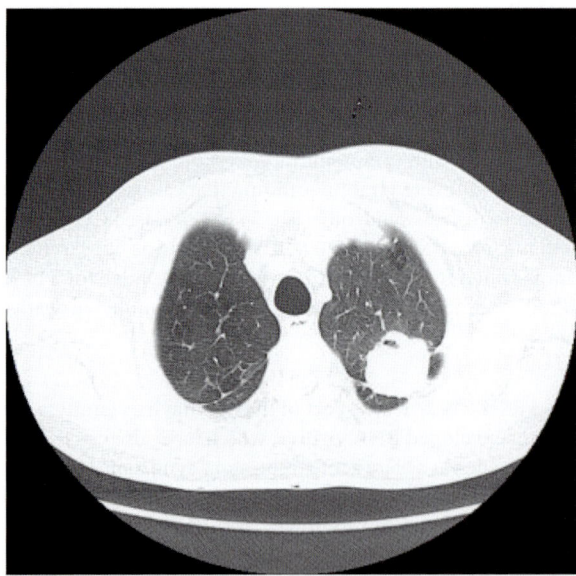

**Fig. 18.6** Computed tomography chest scan showing an aspergilloma within a lung cavity. (From Sagan D, Goździuk K, Korobowicz E. Predictive and prognostic value of preoperative symptoms in the surgical treatment of pulmonary aspergilloma. *J Surg Res*. 2010;163:e35–43.)

# Fungal infection in the immunocompromised patient

## Invasive aspergillosis

This occurs when Aspergillus hyphae invade the lung tissue. It occurs in patients who are immunocompromised, particularly as a cause of neutropenic sepsis following chemotherapy. Symptoms include cough, fever, chest pain and haemoptysis, and the diagnosis should be considered in immunocompromised patients who are not responding to broad-spectrum antibiotics. Treatment is with intravenous antifungals such as voriconazole or amphotericin B. It carries a high mortality.

## Pneumocystis pneumonia

*Pneumocystis jirovecii* (formerly *Pneumocystis carinii* and still referred to as 'PCP' occasionally) is a common environmental fungus. Risk factors for infection include HIV infection with a CD4 cell count $<200 \times 10^6$/L, steroid use and recent chemotherapy. Patients present with symptoms of breathlessness on exertion and a dry cough. Hypoxia and desaturation on exertion are common findings. Treatment includes high-dose cotrimoxazole (Septrin) and supplemental oxygen. High-dose steroids are given too if respiratory failure is present. A patient should always be offered an HIV test and the HIV team should be involved in diagnosis and treatment.

---

## ● Chapter Summary

- Pneumonia is a common condition defined as an acute infection of the lung parenchyma. Common risk factors include increasing age, diabetes, alcohol excess and chronic aspiration.
- The commonest causative organism in community-acquired pneumonia is *Streptococcus pneumoniae*. Atypical pathogens include Legionella, *Mycoplasma pneumoniae* and *Staphylococcus aureus.*
- Tuberculosis (TB) arises as a result of infection with *Mycobacterium tuberculosis*.
- TB typically presents with symptoms of breathlessness, cough and haemoptysis, and systemic features such as night sweats and weight loss. Risk factors include close contact with an infected individual, untreated human immunodeficiency virus infection and immunosuppression.
- Treatment of TB is with quadruple antimicrobial therapy, commonly rifampicin, isoniazid, pyrazinamide and ethambutol for the initial 2 months followed by 4 further months of dual therapy with rifampicin and isoniazid only.
- Influenza is an acute viral infection affecting the respiratory tract that occurs in annual seasonal epidemics during the winter months. Influenza viruses are unstable and therefore constantly change through antigenic drift and shift.
- COVID-19 is an infectious viral respiratory infection that caused a pandemic in 2020. Management may be supportive but can include steroids or antivirals.

### MLA Conditions
COVID-19
Influenza
Lower respiratory tract infections
Pneumonia
Tuberculosis
Upper respiratory tract infections

### MLA Presentations
Anosmia
Breathlessness
Chest pain
Confusion
Cough
Fatigue
Fever
Haemoptysis
Sore throat

## BRONCHIECTASIS

## Definition

Bronchiectasis is defined as abnormal dilatation of the bronchi and bronchioles caused by repeated cycles of airway infection and inflammation. Around 212,000 people were estimated to be living with bronchiectasis in the United Kingdom in 2019.

## Pathogenesis

The initial insult is usually infective, leading to airway damage. This allows persistent bacterial colonization of the bronchi and bronchioles, and a chronic inflammatory response develops. The resultant mucosal oedema damages the mucociliary clearance mechanisms, leading to mucus plugging of the terminal bronchioles and distal volume loss. As a consequence, bacterial clearance is further prevented and therefore a 'vicious cycle' develops of recurrent infection and thick respiratory secretions (Fig. 19.1).

## Aetiology

The causes of bronchiectasis are multiple and varied – they are summarized in Table 19.1 Broadly, bronchiectasis develops following a single infective insult resulting in distorted anatomy or secondary to a defect in the immune system. It can be focal and isolated to a single lobe (common if postobstructive) or diffuse throughout the lungs. Approximately 50% of cases of bronchiectasis are currently classed as idiopathic. Bronchiectasis can either be acquired (e.g., following a severe pulmonary infection) or have a genetic cause, most commonly cystic fibrosis (CF), which is discussed in detail later in this chapter. Rare causes include:

*Allergic bronchopulmonary aspergillosis (ABPA)* – an overactive IgG and IgE immune response to the fungus *Aspergillus fumigatus*, leading to inflammatory damage and bronchiectasis. It is usually associated with a long history of asthma and occurs in 1%–2% of asthmatics. It causes central bronchiectasis.

*Primary ciliary dyskinesia (PCD)* – an autosomal-recessive genetic defect causing a defect in the cilia making them unable to beat. In the lung this leads to loss of mucociliary clearance and bronchiectasis. It is associated with situs inversus in 30% of those diagnosed with bronchiectasis, chronic sinusitis, recurrent otitis media and male infertility.

*Kartagener syndrome* – the triad of PCD, dextrocardia and situs inversus, found in 50% of cases.

*Young syndrome* – the triad of bronchiectasis, sinusitis and azoospermia. It is characterized by excessively thick mucus

**Table 19.1** Displaying causes of bronchiectasis

| Causes of bronchiectasis | |
| --- | --- |
| Postinfectious | Tuberculosis<br>Measles<br>Whooping cough<br>Pertussis<br>Severe pneumonia |
| Postobstructive | Intraluminal: foreign body, chronic aspiration<br>Luminal: lung tumour, obstructive airways disease<br>Extraluminal: compression from mediastinal lymphadenopathy |
| Mucociliary defects | Cystic fibrosis<br>Primary ciliary dyskinesia<br>Kartagener syndrome<br>Young syndrome |
| Immunodeficiency | Acquired or congenital hypogammaglobulinaemia<br>Acquired immunodeficiency syndrome |
| Excessive immune response | Allergic bronchopulmonary aspergillosis |
| Systemic disorders | Rheumatoid arthritis<br>Connective tissue disorders such as systemic lupus erythematosus and Sjögren syndrome<br>Inflammatory bowel disease<br>Marfan syndrome<br>Yellow nail syndrome |
| Chronic aspiration | Impaired swallow<br>Reflux disease |

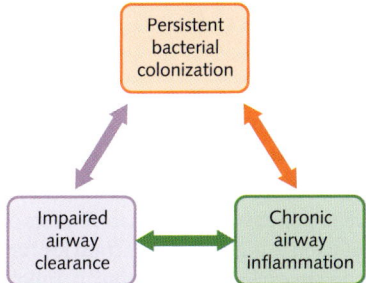

**Fig. 19.1** Pathogenesis of bronchiectasis – the 'vicious cycle'.

with normal ciliary function. The cause is unclear. As presentation is similar, always check for CF.

## Clinical features

Persistent cough productive of sputum is the most common symptom. This can be chronic, or intermittent and associated with symptoms of respiratory infection. Expectorated sputum may be mucopurulent and copious. Associated respiratory symptoms such as dyspnoea, chest pain and haemoptysis can occur. With disease progression, cor pulmonale and respiratory failure develop.

## Physical examination

Patients with bronchiectasis may appear breathless at rest and be cyanosed. Patients with severe disease may require supplementary oxygen. The patient may be malnourished from chronic respiratory disease or associated malabsorption. They may have sputum pots, inhalers or nebulizers at their bedside. Examination of the hands may reveal clubbing. Classically, coarse inspiratory crepitations that alter with coughing are heard on chest auscultation over areas of diseased lung. Scattered wheeze may be present due to airway obstruction caused by secretions. Patients may develop signs of right heart failure secondary to respiratory disease such as peripheral oedema, and a raised JVP. Patients may also have signs of the underlying disease such as:

- Insulin injection sites from CF-related diabetes
- Symmetrical polyarthropathy consistent with rheumatoid arthritis
- Dextrocardia related to Kartagener syndrome
- Abdominal surgery scars related to inflammatory bowel disease.

## Investigations

Investigations for bronchiectasis should be targeted at identifying the underlying cause. They should be considered in the following patients:

### Children

- Chronic productive cough, especially if culture-positive for an associated organism (e.g., *Staphylococcus aureus*, *Haemophilus influenzae* or *Pseudomonas aeruginosa*).
- Symptoms of asthma not responsive to standard treatment.
- Severe or recurrent pneumonia.
- Respiratory symptoms in those at high risk of aspiration.
- Unexplained haemoptysis.

### Adults

- Persistent productive cough, especially if onset at a young age or associated with haemoptysis.
- Patients with recurrent exacerbations of chronic obstructive pulmonary disease (COPD) or who are nonsmokers.

## Essential investigations

The following are basic investigations in the working diagnosis of bronchiectasis:

- Radiology – chest radiograph may be normal or show bronchial wall thickening and consolidation. High-resolution computed tomography is the investigation of choice (see Hints and Tips Box: CT scan in bronchiectasis).
- Sputum microbiology – sputum microscopy, culture and sensitivity to screen for atypical pathogens such as *S. aureus* and *H. influenzae*, *P. aeruginosa*, *M. tuberculosis* or nontuberculous mycobacterial disease and fungi such as Aspergillus.
- Lung function – spirometry may show airflow obstruction.
- Blood tests – immunoglobulin (Ig) A, M and G levels may demonstrate a specific deficiency. Aspergillus-specific IgE, Aspergillus precipitin (IgG) levels and total IgE levels should be sent if ABPA is considered.
- Functional antibodies to tetanus, *H. influenza* and pneumococcus if immunosuppression suspected.

---

**HINTS AND TIPS**

**COMPUTED TOMOGRAPHY SCAN IN BRONCHIECTASIS**

Computed tomography (CT) is a useful diagnostic tool in bronchiectasis and can help diagnose the underlying cause. Three signs to look for on CT that indicate bronchiectasis are:

1. 'Tram track sign' – the thickened bronchiolar walls do not taper as normal and become parallel, giving an appearance similar to tram tracks.
2. 'Signet ring sign' – each bronchus and its adjacent pulmonary artery should normally have an almost equivalent diameter when seen on cross-section on a CT. In bronchiectasis the bronchus is dilated and therefore gives an appearance of a signet ring with its adjacent artery (Fig. 19.2 demonstrates this on a chest X-ray and Fig. 19.3 demonstrates this on CT imaging).
3. 'Bunch of grapes sign' – the cross-sectional appearance of adjacent bronchi in cystic bronchiectasis.

---

## Additional investigations

The following are further investigations that should be considered if clinically relevant:

- Tests for CF in patients younger than 40 years old or where clinical suspicion is high (see CF section for further details).
- Bronchoscopy to exclude foreign body if unilobular disease or to obtain microbiological specimens in unusual presentations.

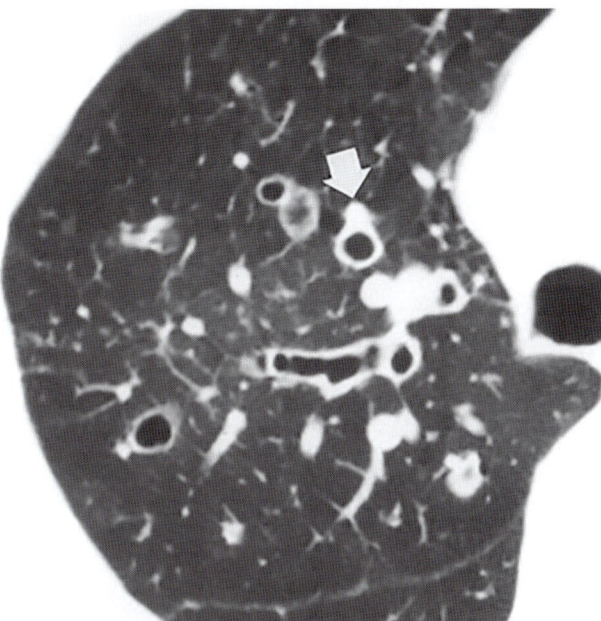

**Fig. 19.2** Chest X-ray image of signet ring sign. Note the thickened airway wall and the dilated airway and adjacent vessel demonstrating the 'signet ring' sign. (From Amarnath C, Irodi A, Jagia P, et al., eds. *Comprehensive Textbook of Clinical Radiology: Volume III: Chest and Cardiovascular System*. 1st ed. Bengaluru, India: Elsevier; 2023.)

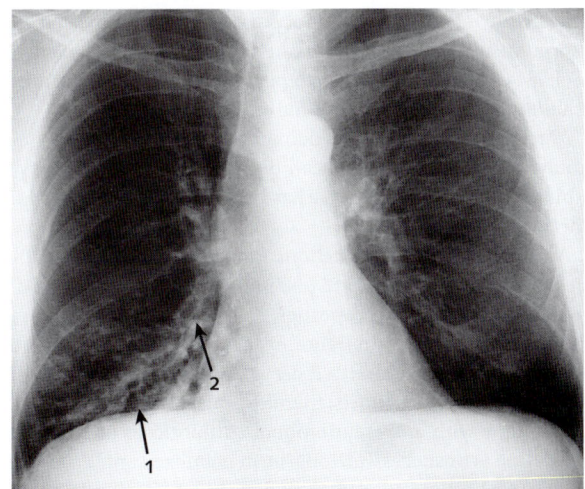

**Fig. 19.3** High-resolution computed tomography scan of a patient with bronchiectasis.

- Immunological studies if immunodeficiency is suggested. This should take place in conjunction with an immunologist and includes neutrophil and lymphocyte functional studies.

- Ciliary function testing – nasal brushings/biopsy at a tertiary centre.

## Treatment

Aims of treatment include:

1. Assessment
   - Identify and treat the underlying cause of bronchiectasis
   - Consider comorbidities
   - Assess for disease progression
   - Reassess pathogens
2. Optimization
   - Promote compliance with airways clearance with focus on reducing exacerbation frequency
   - Ensure exacerbations are treated with appropriate antibiotics and for appropriate duration
   - Ensure patient does not need intravenous antibiotic therapy
3. Further management
   - Screen and treat for respiratory failure with long-term oxygen therapy, noninvasive therapy if indicated, and further management with surgical, transplantation considered if appropriate

Physiotherapy:

This is key to maintaining good airway clearance and lung function and reducing exacerbations. Patients should meet with a physiotherapist to learn active cycle breathing techniques (ACBT) – a process in which respiratory secretions are cleared by using a combination of small and deep breaths that move secretions up the bronchial tree. If ACBT is not effective or demonstrates poor adherence, adjuncts including oscillating positive expiratory pressure devices (e.g., an Acapella device) and forced expiration technique should be considered. When patients are exacerbating, the recommendation is to increase airway clearance with postural drainage in conjunction. Pulmonary rehabilitation courses may also be helpful for bronchiectasis patients, especially patients who also have COPD. If airway clearance is not effective, then nebulized isotonic (0.9%) or hypertonic (3%) saline can be trialled to review if this aids airway clearance (especially in patients with viscous secretions or where there is evidence of sputum plugging). Drug treatments include:

$\beta_2$-agonist inhalers may be of benefit if a patient has airflow obstruction.

- Mucolytics such as carbocisteine are commonly used in practice to aid sputum expectoration; however, the evidence base for their use is limited. Nebulized normal saline is helpful for some patients.
- Nebulized antibiotic and or inhaled steroids if applicable.
- Trial of nasal irrigation and steroids for symptoms of rhinosinusitis.
- Ensure patients are vaccinated for influenza, pneumococcal and COVID-19.

- Short courses of antibiotics (10–14 days) are used to treat acute infective exacerbations and should be prescribed with reference to organisms previously grown on sputum culture. Amoxicillin is commonly used as first-line therapy if no previous colonizing organism has been identified. Local antibiotic guidelines should be consulted.
- Long-term antibiotics are considered in patients with three or more exacerbations a year. These can be nebulized antibiotics or oral macrolides (e.g., azithromycin).

## CYSTIC FIBROSIS

### Definition and pathophysiology

CF is a multisystem disorder caused by a genetic defect in the genes encoding the CF transmembrane conductance regulator (CFTR). The CFTR is a transmembrane regulator protein involved in chloride transport across epithelial cells via a complex channel. Loss of function causes excessively viscous mucus secretions and subsequent multiorgan dysfunction.

### Prevalence and aetiology

CF is the commonest genetically transmitted disease in whites. It is an autosomal recessive condition occurring in 1/2000 live births. Multiple genetic mutations have been identified as causing six distinct classes of CFTR defect. The commonest mutation is a specific gene deletion in the codon for phenylalanine at position 508 in the amino acid sequence (ΔF508). In part, the different genetic mutations contribute to the range of phenotypic presentation of CF from severe to milder presentations.

### Diagnosis and clinical features

Diagnosis is usually made during the neonatal and childhood period; however, milder phenotypes are being increasingly recognized in adulthood. In the United Kingdom, all neonates are screened with the heel prick test for immunoreactive trypsinogen, prompting further investigation if positive. Childhood symptoms include failure to thrive, meconium ileus, cough and recurrent chest infections. Diagnostic tests include:

1. Sweat chloride test – a result of >60 mmol/L is suggestive of CF.
2. CFTR genetic mutation testing.

As CF is a multisystem disorder, multiple organs are affected, as summarized in Fig. 19.4.

### Treatment

Patients with CF are managed using a multidisciplinary approach at specialist CF centres with access to respiratory physicians, physiotherapists, dieticians, pharmacists, psychologists, gastroenterologists

and endocrinologists (see Box: Burden of Treatment in CF). Within CF clinics, infection control is key and patients are segregated to avoid close contact leading to transfer of colonized bacteria.

Physiotherapy – patients usually require twice-daily physiotherapy and postural drainage to aid secretion management. Active cycle of breathing techniques and adjuncts including high-frequency chest wall oscillation devices (e.g., the Vest) can be used. General fitness and exercise are also encouraged.

**HINTS AND TIPS**

**BURDEN OF TREATMENT IN CYSTIC FIBROSIS**

Patients with cystic fibrosis (CF) require multiple different treatments daily throughout their life and this can be time consuming and severely impact on a patient's quality of life. Patients need support to help them comply with their treatment. On a daily basis, each patient may require:

- Two hours of physiotherapy
- Fifty tablets including pancreatic enzymes, vitamin supplements and antibiotics
- Nebulized therapy up to four times a day
- Intravenous antibiotics for exacerbations
- Subcutaneous insulin for CF-related diabetes.

Nutritional support – patients with CF have increased nutritional demands, owing to their respiratory disease and to CF-related malabsorption and diabetes. They therefore require involvement of a specialist dietician who can help plan a diet to meet their needs, including supplements and enzyme replacement.

Mucolytics – nebulized deoxyribonuclease (DNAse) and nebulized hypertonic saline can both decrease the viscosity of respiratory secretions. DNAse has been shown to improve lung function in studies.

Antiinflammatory medications – long-term macrolide antibiotics (e.g., azithromycin) are useful in some patients, owing to their antiinflammatory properties.

Antibiotics – used in acute exacerbations as documented later. Patients colonized with *P. aeruginosa* have more severe disease and a poorer prognosis; therefore, once colonized, eradication therapy with antipseudomonal antibiotics is attempted. If eradication is unsuccessful, long-term nebulized antibiotics may be used (e.g., colomycin). Intravenous antibiotics should be used for treating acute exacerbations in people who are severely unwell, not responding to or unable to take oral antibiotics.

CFTR potentiators – there is good evidence that patients with a specific mutation (G551D) benefit from ivacaftor, a drug that keeps the CFTR channel open, therefore decreasing secretion viscosity and improving lung function. Work is ongoing to develop other drugs to target other defects, but as yet none are licensed.

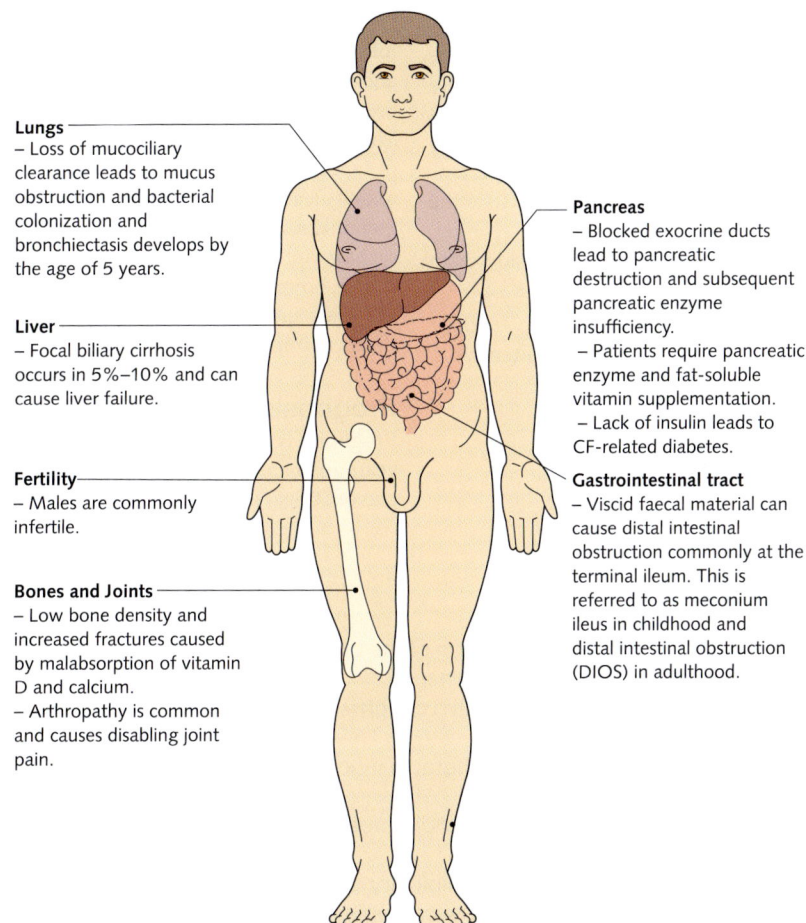

**Lungs**
– Loss of mucociliary clearance leads to mucus obstruction and bacterial colonization and bronchiectasis develops by the age of 5 years.

**Liver**
– Focal biliary cirrhosis occurs in 5%–10% and can cause liver failure.

**Fertility**
– Males are commonly infertile.

**Bones and Joints**
– Low bone density and increased fractures caused by malabsorption of vitamin D and calcium.
– Arthropathy is common and causes disabling joint pain.

**Pancreas**
– Blocked exocrine ducts lead to pancreatic destruction and subsequent pancreatic enzyme insufficiency.
 – Patients require pancreatic enzyme and fat-soluble vitamin supplementation.
 – Lack of insulin leads to CF-related diabetes.

**Gastrointestinal tract**
– Viscid faecal material can cause distal intestinal obstruction commonly at the terminal ileum. This is referred to as meconium ileus in childhood and distal intestinal obstruction (DIOS) in adulthood.

**Fig. 19.4** Multiple organs are affected by cystic fibrosis *(CF)*.

## Acute exacerbation

Signs of a pulmonary exacerbation can be symptoms of worsening cough, change in sputum production or worsened dyspnoea; however, the presentation may be more insidious with just weight loss and tiredness. A fall in forced expiratory volume ($FEV_1$) >10% may be indicative of an exacerbation. Treatment of an acute exacerbation includes:

1. Antibiotics (see Box: Organisms in cystic fibrosis)
2. Nutritional support
3. Regular physiotherapy with sputum clearance techniques
4. Respiratory support – oxygen and, if severe, ventilator support.

When prescribing antibiotics, reference should be made to previous culture results, local guidelines and the patient's allergy status. Patients with CF commonly need longer courses (typically 14 days) with higher doses. Intravenous antibiotics may be needed if severe or if oral options fail. Treatment with intravenous antibiotics at home may be an option and requires venous access devices such as a peripherally inserted central catheter line.

> **CLINICAL NOTES**
>
> ### ORGANISMS IN CYSTIC FIBROSIS
>
> As a cystic fibrosis patient gets older, the organisms that colonize the respiratory tract change. Some, for example, Pseudomonas or certain resistant bacteria, are associated with a worse prognosis. Key organisms in time order include:
>
> Increasing age
>
> 1. *Staphylococcus aureus*
> 2. *Haemophilus influenza* type b (Hib)
> 3. *Pseudomonas aeruginosa*
> 4. *Burkholderia cepacia*.

## Surgical management – lung transplant

There are currently five lung transplant centres in England, carrying out approximately 200 lung transplants a year. There are three main types – single lung, double lung and heart and lung transplant. CF is a common indication for transplant but others include COPD, pulmonary fibrosis and pulmonary hypertension. Currently the demand for organs continues to outstrip the supply.

In CF, referral to a transplant centre should be considered in the following situations:

1. $FEV_1$ <30% (or rapid decline)
2. Exacerbation requiring high dependency unit or intensive therapy unit
3. Pneumothorax in advanced disease
4. Haemoptysis requiring embolization
5. Progressive increase in medical therapy required.

In addition to the risks of the operation itself, the main risks following lung transplant are rejection (both acute and chronic) and side effects from immunosuppression. Lifelong immunosuppression is required to prevent rejection of the transplanted lung. The side effects of immunosuppression include an increased risk of cancer, particularly skin and haematological cancer, nephrotoxicity leading to renal failure and infection, both bacterial and viral including cytomegalovirus.

Survival following lung transplant differs depending on the centre; however, it is currently approximately 80% at 1 year, 50% at 5 years and 35% at 10 years, although long-term survival continues to improve.

## Prognosis of cystic fibrosis

Prognosis is improving: currently, mean survival is around 40 years and babies diagnosed with CF today have a predicted lifespan of 50 years. Death is mainly from respiratory complications.

---

● **Chapter Summary**

- Bronchiectasis is defined as abnormal dilatation of the bronchi and bronchioles caused by repeated cycles of airway infection and inflammation.
- Bronchiectasis presents as a chronic productive cough with recurrent infections and is caused by multiple underlying disorders.
- Treatment of bronchiectasis includes physiotherapy, mucolytics to aid airway clearance and antibiotics to treat infection.
- Cystic fibrosis is a genetic multisystem disorder characterized by excessively viscous mucus secretions.
- Treatment of cystic fibrosis requires a multidisciplinary approach with input from physicians, dieticians, physiotherapists and psychologists at a specialist centre.

**MLA Conditions**
Bronchiectasis
Cystic fibrosis
Whooping cough

### Further reading

Cystic Fibrosis Trust. www.cysticfibrosis.org.uk.
Pasteur MC, Bilton D, Hill AT. British Thoracic Society Bronchiectasis non-CF Guideline Group. British Thoracic Society guideline for non-CF bronchiectasis. *Thorax*. 2010;65(Suppl 1):i1–58.

## PLEURAL EFFUSION

### Introduction

A pleural effusion is the presence of fluid between the visceral and parietal pleura. Effusions can be categorized as transudative or exudative, depending on the protein concentration (Table 20.1). Transudative pleural effusions (<25 g/L of protein) occur as a result of increased hydrostatic pressure or decreased osmotic pressure in the microvascular circulation, caused by hypoproteinaemia. Exudative pleural effusions (>35 g/L of protein) occur when local factors influencing pleural fluid formation and reabsorption are altered, through injury or inflammation. Effusions of 25–35 g/L protein must be analyzed using Light's criteria (see next section). Common causes of each type of effusion are shown in Table 20.1.

### Light's criteria

These state that the effusion is an **exudate** if one or more of the following criteria are met:

- Fluid/serum protein ratio of >0.5
- Fluid/serum lactate dehydrogenase (LDH) ratio >0.6
- Fluid LDH greater than two-thirds of the upper limit of normal serum.

### Clinical features

Pleural effusions are typically asymptomatic until >500 mL of fluid is present. Breathlessness, dry cough and pleuritic pain suggesting pleural inflammation are common symptoms. Constitutional symptoms related to the underlying cause (e.g., weight loss, night sweats and fevers) may be present.

Signs on examination of the affected side include decreased expansion, a stony dull percussion note, reduced or absent breath sounds and reduced vocal resonance over the area of effusion. Bronchial breathing is often present above an effusion and a pleural rub may be heard with pleural inflammation.

### Diagnosis and investigations

Key questions when trying to identify the cause of an effusion include:

1. Is it unilateral or bilateral?
2. Is it transudative or exudative?

The first steps in making a diagnosis should be to take a careful history, perform an examination and perform a chest radiograph. In the presence of a strong clinical suspicion of transudative and bilateral pleural effusions, for example, in a patient with suspected left ventricular failure, pleural fluid aspiration should **not** be performed. Initial treatment of the underlying illness followed by clinical reassessment should take place.

The diagnostic process for a unilateral effusion is summarized in Fig. 20.1. Classically, pleural effusion appears on a chest X-ray (CXR) as a basal opacity obscuring the hemidiaphragm, with a concave meniscus at its upper border (Fig. 20.2). Fluid can be seen on a posteroanterior CXR at volumes of >200 mL.

Ultrasound imaging can assist with the differentiation between pleural fluid and solid mass as well as the identification of septations within the effusion, and in guiding pleural aspiration. Diagnostic pleural aspiration is performed under ultrasound guidance using a 21-gauge needle and 50 mL syringe. The aspiration site should be just above a rib to avoid the neurovascular bundle that runs just below each rib. Pleural fluid should be examined for gross appearance (Table 20.2) and for pH, protein, glucose and LDH levels; microscopy, culture and sensitivity (MC&S) and cytology testing should also be performed. Paired serum LDH and protein should be tested. Cytology is positive in 60% of malignant effusions.

A computed tomography (CT) scan of the chest with pleural enhancement should be arranged in all undiagnosed exudative pleural effusions and in cases of complex pleural infection that are not resolving with antibiotics and drainage. If malignancy is suspected but aspiration has not confirmed diagnosis, thoracoscopy under local anaesthetic to obtain pleural biopsies, proceeding to pleurodesis if appropriate, may be considered (see Chapter 10 for further information). Imaging-guided percutaneous pleural biopsy is an alternative if pleural nodularity is seen on CT.

### Treatment

Treatment is dependent on the underlying disease. Treatment of transudates should focus on the underlying cause and they do not routinely require drainage.

#### Malignant effusion

If asymptomatic, the effusion should be observed, and treated only if symptoms arise. Effusions can arise from many types of malignancy; however, they are most commonly secondary to lung cancer, breast cancer or lymphoma. Therapeutic aspiration of 500–1500 mL can help with symptom relief in patients with a

**Table 20.1** BTS guidelines 2023 – type of pleural effusions by cause and frequency

| Effusion type | Frequency | Cause | Notes |
|---|---|---|---|
| Transudative (protein < 25 g/L) | Common | Heart failure | Commonly bilateral effusions |
| | | Hepatic failure/liver cirrhosis | |
| | | Nephrotic syndrome | |
| | | Hypoalbuminaemia | |
| | Less common | Chronic hypothyroidism | |
| | | Mitral stenosis | |
| Exudative (protein > 35 g/L) | Common | Malignancy | Commonest cause in over 60 year olds |
| | | Pleural infection | |
| | | Pulmonary embolism | Often small effusions with high symptom burden |
| | Less common | Drugs | Many drugs including nitrofurantoin, amiodarone, methotrexate and phenytoin |
| | | Meigs syndrome | Right pleural effusion and ovarian fibroma |

very poor life expectancy. Insertion of a small bore (10–14 French) chest drain and controlled drainage is preferable to repeated therapeutic aspiration. Pleurodesis with graded talc introduced into the pleural cavity via the chest drain causes sterile inflammation and adhesion of the visceral and parietal pleura and prevents fluid reaccumulation. Alternatively, ambulatory indwelling pleural catheters can be used in recurrent symptomatic effusions.

## Empyema

This is defined as pus within the pleural space. Formation of empyema is a progressive process with three recognized

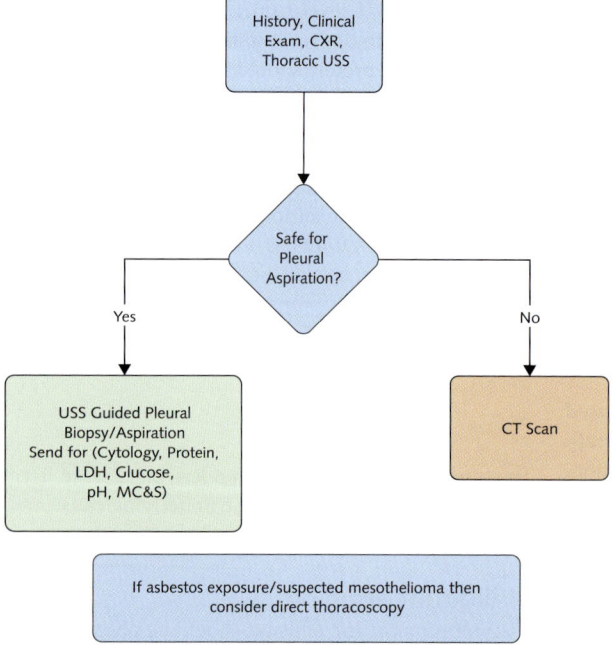

**Fig. 20.1** Unilateral pleural effusion diagnostic pathway. *CXR*, Chest X-ray; *FBC*, full blood count; *LDH*, lactate dehydrogenase; *NT-proBNP*, N-terminal prohormone brain natriuretic peptide; *PE*, pulmonary embolism; *TB*, tuberculosis; *TUS*, thoracic ultrasound. (From Roberts ME, Rahman NM, Maskell NA, et al. British Thoracic Society guideline for pleural disease. *Thorax*. 2023;78:s1–s42.)

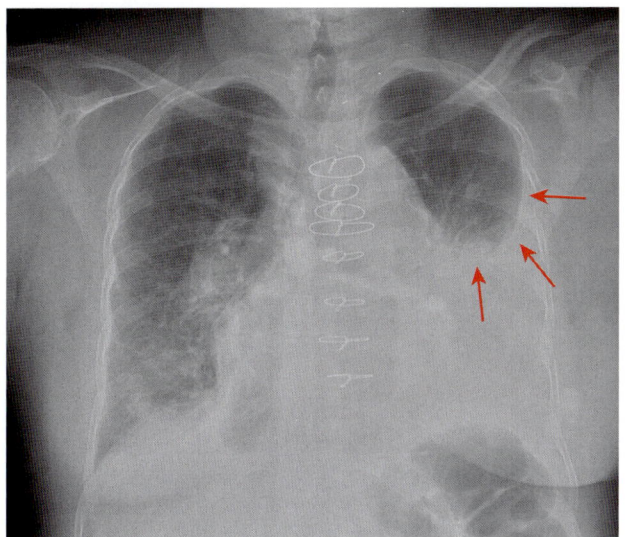

**Fig. 20.2** Chest X-ray image of left-sided pleural effusion. (From Stoller JK, Heuer AJ, Chatburn RL, Mireles-Cabodevila E, Vines DL, eds. *Egan's fundamentals of respiratory care*. 13th ed. St. Louis, Missouri: Elsevier; 2024.)

stages, starting with a simple parapneumonic effusion that progresses to a complicated fibrinopurulent stage and a final organizing stage with formation of a pleural peel. Clinical features are similar to the presentation of pneumonia (fever, sputum, breathlessness). Anaerobic empyema may present insidiously with only weight loss and decreased appetite, especially in elderly patients. Treatment is with antibiotics that penetrate the pleural space, commonly penicillin and β-lactamase inhibitors. Refer to local microbiological guidelines for guidance here. Supportive treatment with nutrition is important. High suspicion of a complex parapneumonic effusion or empyema and therefore indications for chest drain insertion are:

1. Aspiration of frank pus/turbid fluid
2. Organisms cultured from the pleural fluid or on Gram stain
3. Pleural fluid pH <7.2.

The BTS guidelines recommend the use of RAPID scoring (Renal, Age, Purulence, Infection Source, Dietary factors) to risk stratify patients with confirmed pleural infection to predict mortality.

> **RED FLAG** ▨
>
> **THINK EMPYEMA**
>
> Empyema often presents as pneumonia, which is poorly responsive to appropriate antibiotics – watch for a failure of the C-reactive protein level to drop by >50% in 72 hours or ongoing fevers. Consider empyema in these patients and investigate.

If infection persists despite adequate antibiotic treatment and drainage, surgical treatment may be required and referral to the thoracic surgeons is indicated.

## HAEMOTHORAX

Haemothorax refers to blood in the pleural cavity. It is common in both penetrating and nonpenetrating injuries of the chest and may cause hypovolaemic shock and reduced vital capacity through compression.

Blood may originate from the lungs, internal mammary artery, mediastinal great vessels, heart or abdominal structures via the diaphragm.

Haemothoraces can be classified as either massive (estimated blood volume >1.5 L) or small (<1.5 L). Massive haemothoraces usually require thoracotomy, whereas smaller ones can be treated expectantly with chest drains and medical management.

## CHYLOTHORAX

A chylothorax is an accumulation of lymph in the pleural space. Commonest causes are rupture or obstruction of the thoracic duct caused by surgical trauma or neoplasm, for example, lymphoma. A latent period of 2–10 days occurs between injury and onset. The pleural fluid is high in lipid content and is

**Table 20.2** Pleural fluid appearances and possible diagnoses

| Fluid appearance | Suspected disease |
| --- | --- |
| Straw-coloured serous fluid | Commonest appearance |
| Blood-stained | Malignant effusion<br>Pulmonary embolism with infarction<br>Haemothorax (check haematocrit level – if >50% of the patient's blood is haemocrit, then diagnostic) |
| Frank pus or purulent fluid | Empyema |
| Milky fluid | Chylothorax |
| 'Anchovy sauce'-like | Ruptured amoebic abscess |

characteristically milky in appearance. If suspected, pleural fluid should be tested for cholesterol crystals, chylomicrons, and triglyceride and cholesterol levels to help differentiate from a pseudochylothorax. Levels of triglyceride and chylomicrons will be high in true chylothorax, while levels of cholesterol are high in pseudochylothorax.

## CHEST DRAIN INSERTION

Chest drains can be used for the drainage of air, pus or liquid (effusion or blood) from the pleural space.

### Indications

- Pneumothorax:
  - Ventilated patients
  - Tension pneumothorax (after initial needle relief)
  - Persistent or recurrent pneumothorax
  - Large secondary spontaneous pneumothorax
- Malignant pleural effusions for pleurodesis
- Empyema
- Traumatic haemopneumothorax
- Postsurgical procedures, especially cardiothoracic.

Chest drain insertion should be performed by a competent practitioner under ultrasound guidance in a sterile environment. Two methods of insertion are used – the 'Seldinger' technique involving insertion of the drain over a guide wire and the 'surgical' technique involving blunt dissection down to the pleural cavity. Where possible, drains should be inserted in the 'triangle of safety' as shown in Fig. 20.3. Drains are available in several different sizes based on their diameter and sized by the French gauge system, from small '6 French' drains to large '24 French' drains. The size of drain used depends on the reason for insertion, for example, larger 18 French drains are used for empyema to prevent thick pus from blocking the drain. Once inserted, the drain should be connected to a chest drain bottle with an underwater seal to prevent air entry into the pleural cavity. Unless during an emergency, chest drains should not be inserted out of hours. Full guidelines for insertion are available in the British Thoracic Society (BTS) guidelines 2023.

### Basic chest drain management

Fluid should not be drained too quickly and the drain should be clamped if draining >1.5 L in an hour. This is to prevent the development of re-expansion pulmonary oedema, symptoms of which include chest pain and breathlessness. CXR should be obtained after insertion to check the drain position. The drain should be reviewed daily for:

1. Insertion site – check for surgical emphysema (air in the subcutaneous tissue, when palpated it can cause crepitus, an unusual 'crackling' sound as air is pushed through the tissue) and evidence of drain site infection.

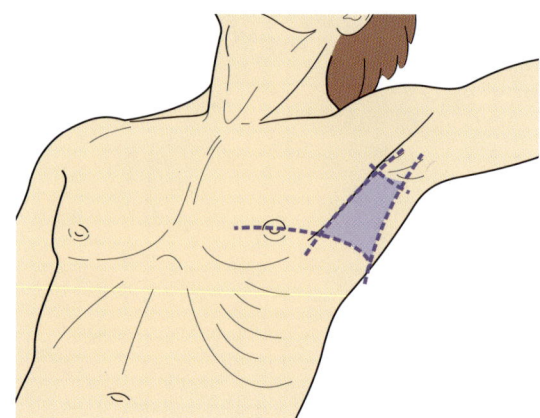

**Fig. 20.3** The triangle of safety for chest drain insertion is bounded by three landmarks: the lateral border of pectoralis major, the 5th intercostal space (roughly the level of the nipple) and the anterior border of latissimus dorsi. (From Laws D, Neville E, Duffy J, et al. BTS guidelines for the insertion of a chest drain. *Thorax*. 2003;58:ii53–ii59.)

2. Drain fluid output – a drain output chart should be kept with cumulative fluid output.
3. Evidence of 'swinging' – fluid movement with respiration as intrapleural pressures change. This suggests the drain is correctly positioned and patent. Ask the patient to take a big breath in and out while observing the drain.
4. Evidence of 'bubbling' – suggestive of persistent air leak from the lung into the pleural cavity. Ask the patient to cough to check for air leak. **A bubbling chest drain should never be clamped as this may lead to tension pneumothorax**.

If the drain is no longer swinging or bubbling, a repeat CXR to evaluate the effusion or pneumothorax should be considered. Normal saline 'flushes' into the pleural cavity can be used to check drain patency and are frequently prescribed to be performed regularly to avoid drain blockage in empyema. In pneumothorax the drain can be removed once the air leak has stopped and the lung can be seen fully reinflated on CXR. In pleural effusion or empyema, the drain can be removed once fluid drainage is complete. If drainage is complete in pleural infection but a residual pleural collection remains, then treatment with combination tissue plasminogen activator and DNAse should be considered to break down septations and reduce fluid viscosity to allow for complete drainage.

## PNEUMOTHORAX

### Definition

Pneumothorax is air within the pleural space between the lungs and the chest wall. It is classified as 'spontaneous', traumatic or iatrogenic (commonly following lung biopsy).

Primary spontaneous pneumothorax (PSP) occurs in people with apparently healthy lungs. Secondary spontaneous pneumothorax (SSP) occurs in patients with underlying lung disease. SSP is associated with a higher morbidity and mortality than PSP and its management is often more complex.

## Aetiology

### Primary spontaneous pneumothorax

Anatomical abnormalities such as subpleural blebs and apical bullae have been found in people with PSP and are thought to predispose to an air leak. Small airway inflammation is also present and may contribute to an increase in airway resistance causing 'emphysema-like changes'.

Patients are typically:

- Tall, thin young males (age range 20–40 years).
- Male:female ratio is 5:1.
- Smoking is a significant risk factor for developing PSP. It is associated with a 12% risk in healthy smoking men compared with 0.1% in nonsmoking men.
- PSP is more common in patients with Marfan syndrome and homocystinuria.
- Rarely, PSP is familial: Birt–Hogg–Dube syndrome is an autosomal-dominant mutation in the folliculin gene that predisposes to spontaneous pneumothorax following pulmonary cyst rupture.

Recurrence risk within 4 years is approximately 50% and is highest in smokers, with increasing age and with tall height.

### Secondary spontaneous pneumothorax

This is most commonly caused by chronic obstructive pulmonary disease (COPD) but can be caused by any underlying lung disease. When first described, tuberculosis (TB) was the most common cause. SSP may be the first presentation of an undiagnosed lung disease. Rare causes to consider include catamenial pneumothorax (pneumothorax occurring at the same time as menstruation), pneumocystis pneumonia (PCP) infection, especially in patients diagnosed with HIV infection, Langerhans cell histiocytosis and lymphangioleiomyomatosis.

## Clinical features

Common symptoms include:

- Sudden-onset unilateral pleuritic chest pain
- Dyspnoea
- Rapid deterioration in existing lung condition (e.g., COPD).

Many patients present with only minimal symptoms, especially patients with PSP who may not present for several days. In general, symptoms are more severe for those with SSP than PSP. Correlation between symptom burden and pneumothorax size is not reliable in SSP. **If cardiorespiratory distress is present, tension pneumothorax must be considered and dealt with as a medical emergency (see Tension pneumothorax section).**

Examination may reveal the following signs on the side of the pneumothorax:

- Reduced chest expansion
- Hyperresonance to percussion
- Diminished breath sounds.

## Investigations

### Chest X-ray

A standard erect CXR in inspiration is recommended for diagnosis. Characteristically, displacement of the pleural line with absent lung markings peripherally can be seen (Fig. 20.4). CXR tends to underestimate the size of pneumothorax.

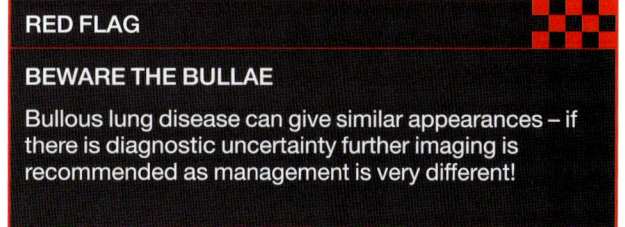

RED FLAG

**BEWARE THE BULLAE**

Bullous lung disease can give similar appearances – if there is diagnostic uncertainty further imaging is recommended as management is very different!

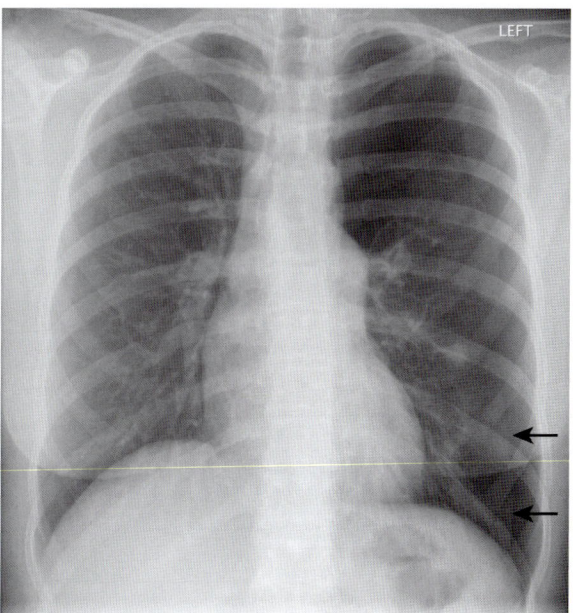

**Fig. 20.4** Left-sided pneumothorax. (From Corne J, Pointon K. *Chest X-ray made easy*. 3rd ed. Churchill Livingstone, London UK, Elsevier; 2009.)

## Chest computed tomography

This is regarded as the gold standard for detection of small pneumothoraces and size estimation. It has the added advantage of identifying additional lung pathology; however, because of cost and availability constraints, it is not the first-line investigation.

## Ultrasound Scan (USS)

This has recently emerged as a tool in diagnosing pneumothoraces in critically ill or trauma patients where erect CXR is not available. The sonographer looks for the loss of 'lung sliding' and the presence of the 'stratosphere sign'.

## Management

The aim of treatment is to relieve symptoms and resolve the pneumothorax by allowing the pleural air leak to close. As per BTS pleural guidelines 2023, management of pneumothoraces depends upon whether the pneumothorax is:

- Asymptomatic or symptomatic.
- If high-risk characteristics are present: Haemodynamic compromise (tension pneumothorax), significant hypoxia, bilateral pneumothorax, underlying lung disease, ≥50 years of age with significant smoking history or haemothorax.
- If it is safe to intervene (≥2 cm laterally or apically on CXR or any size on CT scan that can be safely accessed

with radiological support) and consideration of the patient's priority (procedure avoidance, rapid symptomatic relief).

Initial treatment options include observation, high-flow oxygen, needle aspiration and small bore (<14 French) intercostal chest drain insertion with connection to an underwater drain. As well as correcting hypoxaemia, high-flow oxygen increases the rate of pneumothorax resolution. The BTS guidelines provide a useful treatment algorithm for pneumothorax (see Fig. 20.5).

In PSP, if the patient is asymptomatic or minimally symptomatic (no significant pain or breathlessness and no haemodynamic compromise), then conservative management can be considered regardless of the size. Therapeutic aspiration is recommended if the interpleural distance is >2 cm at the level of the hilum when measured on CXR and if the patient's priority is for rapid symptom relief. If successful, the patient may be discharged with outpatient follow-up in 2–4 weeks; however, if the pneumothorax does not decrease in size with aspiration, a chest drain is likely required.

SSP carries a mortality of 10% and therefore more aggressive treatment is recommended. If high-risk characteristics are present, such as bilateral pneumothoraces and tension pneumothoraces, then chest drain insertion is always required. However, if the patient is asymptomatic and the interpleural distance is <2 cm, then conservative care can be adopted with the patient admitted.

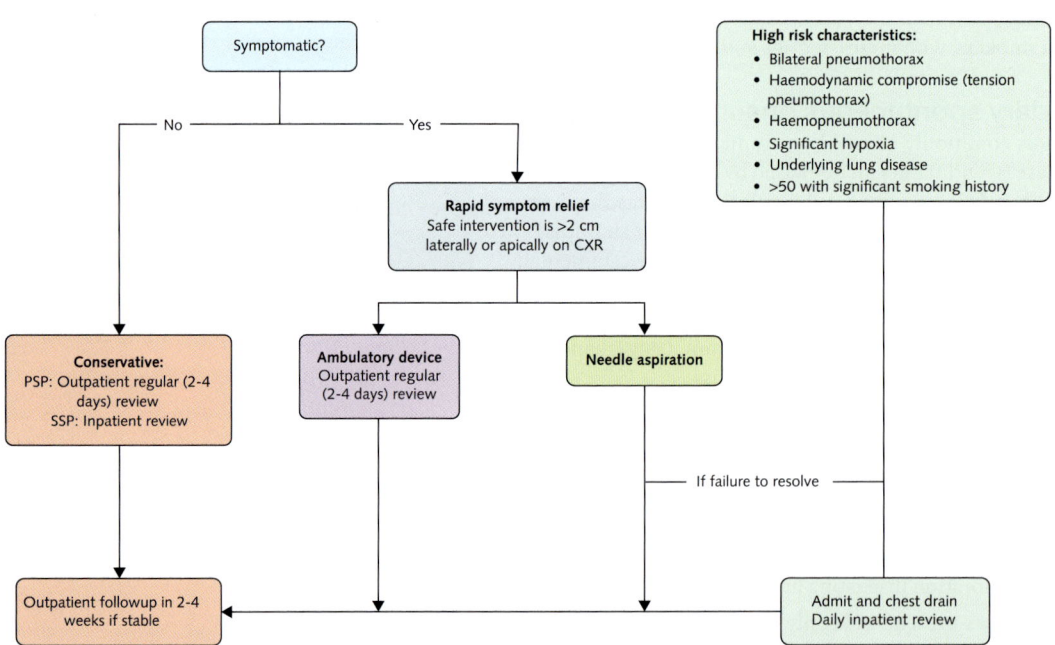

**Fig. 20.5** BTS pneumothorax pathway. *CXR*, Chest X-ray; *COPD*, chronic obstructive pulmonary disease; *OPD*, outpatient department; *PSP*, primary spontaneous pneumothorax; *SSP*, secondary spontaneous pneumothorax. (From Roberts ME, Rahman NM, Maskell NA, et al. British Thoracic Society guideline for pleural disease. *Thorax*. 2023;78:s1–s42.)

## Persistent air leak

This is defined as the persistent bubbling of air through a correctly placed chest drain after 48 hours. Low-pressure suction (−10 to −20 cm $H_2O$) can be applied to encourage apposition of the pleura and closure of the air leak. This risks re-expansion pulmonary oedema (RPO) that manifests as cough and chest tightness. RPO is more common in PSP and with early suction (<48 hours postdrain insertion).

## Surgical management

In cases with persistent air leak at 3–5 days post drain insertion or where the lung fails to re-expand, as viewed on CXR, a thoracic surgery opinion should be sought. Surgical management options include:

- Video-assisted thoracoscopic surgery (VATS) for surgical pleurodesis.
- Open thoracotomy and pleurectomy.

Surgery can also be considered for pneumothorax treatment in adults at first presentation if recurrence prevention is deemed important (e.g., tension pneumothorax or patient is in a high-risk occupation).

Recurrence rates are slightly higher with VATS than with open thoracotomy; however, recovery is much quicker following VATS.

## Chemical pleurodesis

For patients with recurrent or difficult pneumothoraces who are not fit for surgical management, chemical pleurodesis to prevent recurrence can be considered. A sclerosing agent such as tetracycline or sterile-graded talc is instilled via the intercostal drain to cause aseptic pleural inflammation and adhesion of the visceral and parietal pleura. Recurrence rates remain significant so surgical methods are preferred, if possible.

---

**HINTS AND TIPS**

**AIR TRAVEL AND DIVING**

Air travel: Avoid for at least a week after full resolution of the pneumothorax, as confirmed by chest X-ray. However, the British Thoracic Society advises that the risk of recurrence remains increased for a year following the pneumothorax and therefore patients may want to minimize air travel during this time.

Diving: Advise patients with pneumothoraces **never to dive again** unless a very secure definitive prevention strategy has been performed.

---

## TENSION PNEUMOTHORAX

**Tension pneumothorax is a medical emergency that can lead to cardiac arrest.** It can arise from a variety of clinical situations in both ventilated and nonventilated patients but most often occurs following trauma or in patients with known pneumothoraces.

## Pathogenesis

It occurs when a one-way valve system is formed at the site of the pleural membrane tear. Air is able to move into the pleural cavity during inspiration but not out during expiration. As a result, intrapleural pressure exceeds atmospheric pressure. This puts pressure on the heart, impairing venous return to it and reducing cardiac output, thus leading to haemodynamic compromise.

## Clinical features

- Agitation and respiratory distress
- Tracheal deviation away from the pneumothorax side
- Decreased breath sounds and hyperresonance on the affected side
- Raised jugular venous pressure, hypotension and tachycardia
- Cardiac arrest – commonly pulseless electrical activity arrest.

## Investigation

These are rarely useful in tension pneumothorax as there is usually insufficient time to obtain a CXR. Do not wait for a CXR if the diagnosis is clinically certain or the patient is significantly compromised, as you risk cardiac arrest. Traditionally, a CXR showing a tension should never be obtained.

## Management

Immediate management should be the insertion of a large-bore cannula (the biggest you can find) into the second intercostal space, midclavicular line, on the side of the pneumothorax – see Fig. 20.6 for the anatomical landmarks. An audible 'hiss' can be heard on successful insertion that corresponds to the air escaping the intrapleural space. Once the immediate pressure has been relieved and the patient stabilized, a chest drain should be inserted.

---

## NEOPLASMS OF THE PLEURA: MALIGNANT MESOTHELIOMA

Malignant mesothelioma is a tumour of mesothelial surfaces, most commonly affecting the pleura. There are approximately 2700 new cases of mesothelioma each year in the UK, but it accounts for <1% of all new cancer cases. It is associated with occupational exposure to asbestos in 85% of cases, especially fibres less than 0.25 μm in diameter (e.g., crocidolite and amosite). The median latent period between exposure and

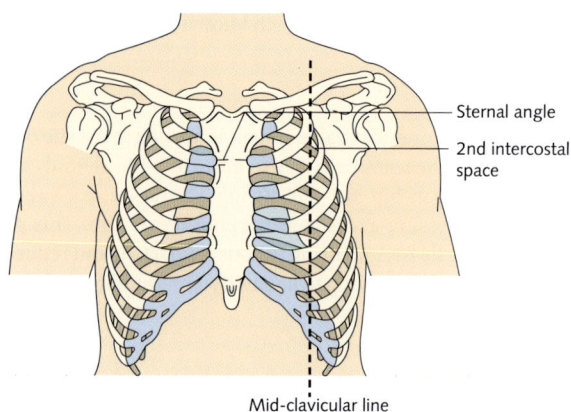

**Fig. 20.6** Diagram showing anatomical landmarks for needle decompression in a tension pneumothorax.

disease is 40 years. Mesothelioma has heterogenous histology; however, the three main subtypes are:

1. Epithelioid (associated with a better prognosis)
2. Sarcomatoid
3. Biphasic.

The tumour begins as nodules in the pleura and goes on to obliterate the pleural cavity.

## Clinical features

Initial symptoms are commonly chest pain and breathlessness related to pleural effusion. Systemic features such as weight loss may be present. It rarely presents with symptomatic metastases. A detailed occupational exposure is key with particular references to occupations with known asbestos exposure including asbestos manufacture, shipbuilding and building maintenance. Consider mesothelioma in all patients with pleural effusion or pleural thickening.

## Investigations

Features of the chest radiograph are:

- Pleural effusions
- Unilateral pleural thickening
- Nodular pleural appearance.

If pleural effusion is present, investigations should proceed as detailed previously. Pleural biopsy via thoracoscopy or guided by imaging can provide tissue diagnosis.

## Treatment and prognosis

Currently treatment involves a multidisciplinary approach to symptom control and palliation through chemotherapy and radiotherapy. No curative treatment is currently available. For patients with a good performance status at diagnosis (PS 0–2), systemic chemotherapy with two agents, commonly cisplatin and pemetrexed, can extend life by 2–3 months. Palliative radiotherapy to the chest wall can be considered to alleviate pain. Specialist nurses should be involved in patient care from diagnosis and early referral to palliative care services for symptom control is important. Prognosis is very poor, with a median survival of 8–14 months.

## Compensation and mesothelioma

It is important when making a diagnosis of mesothelioma to supply the patient with medicolegal advice about compensation, and the physician making the diagnosis and specialist nurses are often best placed to do this. Patients are entitled to claim compensation via two avenues:

1. Industrial Injuries Disablement Benefit via the government Department for Work and Pensions.
2. A civil law claim via the courts for compensation from the employer or their insurance company. Any claim must be brought within 3 years of diagnosis.

---

**HINTS AND TIPS**

**ASBESTOS-RELATED LUNG DISEASE**

In addition to mesothelioma, asbestos can cause other lung diseases:

1. Benign – pleural plaques, benign effusion, diffuse pleural thickening
2. Asbestosis – interstitial fibrosis related to asbestos inhalation
3. Lung cancer.

---

## Chapter Summary

- Pleural effusions can be categorized as transudative or exudative based on their protein and lactate dehydrogenase content. Knowing these helps to diagnose the cause of the effusion and guide management.
- Empyema is defined as pus within the pleural space and is suggested by a pH <7.2 on pleural aspiration. It requires prompt drainage.
- While admitted to the ward, patients with chest drains inserted should be reviewed daily for drain position, fluid output and evidence of 'swinging' or 'bubbling'.
- Management of a pneumothorax depends on whether it is traumatic or spontaneous, the presence or absence of underlying lung disease, the size of the pneumothorax and the patient's symptoms.
- A tension pneumothorax is a medical emergency that needs to be treated with urgent needle decompression using a large-bore cannula inserted into the second intercostal space at the midclavicular line.
- Mesothelioma is a cancer affecting the pleura that presents with chest pain. It is related to previous asbestos exposure and has a very poor prognosis.

**MLA Conditions**
Asbestos-related lung disease
Breast cancer
Chronic obstructive pulmonary disease
Human immunodeficiency virus
Lung cancer
Lymphoma
Occupational lung disease
Pneumonia
Pneumothorax
Tuberculosis

**MLA Presentations**
Breathlessness
Cardiac/cardiorespiratory arrest
Cardiac failure
Chest pain
Cough
End-of-life care/symptoms of terminal illness
Fever
Pain on inspiration
Pleural effusion
Shock
Trauma

### Further reading
Roberts ME, Rahman NM, Maskell NA On behalf of the BTS Pleural Guideline Development Group, et al. British Thoracic Society Guideline for pleural disease. *Thorax* 2023;78:s1-s42.
BTS statement on malignant mesothelioma in the UK, 2007. *Thorax* 2007;62:ii1-ii19.

Baas P, Fennell D, Kerr KM, et al. ESMO Guidelines Committee. Malignant pleural mesothelioma: ESMO Clinical Practice Guidelines for diagnosis, treatment and follow-up. *Ann Oncol.* 2015;26 (Suppl 5):v31-9.

# Thromboembolic disease and pulmonary hypertension

## PULMONARY EMBOLISM

### Definition

A pulmonary embolus (PE) arises when an embolus derived from a venous thrombus is transported in the bloodstream and obstructs the pulmonary vascular tree.

### Epidemiology

PE is a common condition among the general population. The incidence of pulmonary embolism in epidemiological studies ranges from 35 to 115 per 100,000 inhabitants. The incidence of acute PE is difficult to define due to its range of presentations from an asymptomatic incidental finding to sudden death.

### Aetiology

PE most commonly arises from thrombi originating in the deep venous system of the lower limb. Venous ultrasonography demonstrates the presence of DVT in 30%–50% of patients with acute PE, and DVT has been found by venography in 70% of those with proven PE. There are multiple predisposing factors for VTE and these are summarized in Table 21.1. They can be split into patient-related risk factors, usually permanent, and setting-related risk factors that are usually temporary. PE is considered 'provoked' if temporary risk factors are present within the preceding 3 months. These are important to identify as their presence can affect anticoagulation duration. In acute PE, 30% of cases have no identifiable risk factors.

### Clinical features

The presentation of acute PE is variable, from asymptomatic to sudden death. Common symptoms include:

- Sudden-onset pleuritic chest pain
- Dyspnoea (which can be acute or acute on chronic dyspnoea)
- Haemoptysis
- Syncope or presyncope.

Clinical features can include signs of a lower limb DVT – a swollen or tender calf.

Hypotension and features of shock are rare but indicate haemodynamic instability from acute PE and should be identified and treated as a medical emergency (see later for more details).

### Investigations

Chest X-ray (CXR) is not sensitive or specific in the diagnosis of PE but is a valuable tool for excluding other causes of symptoms, for example, pneumothorax.

---

**HINTS AND TIPS**

**CHEST X-RAY SIGNS OF PULMONARY EMBOLUS**

Chest X-ray in pulmonary embolus is frequently normal. When present, chest X-ray abnormalities include an enlarged pulmonary artery and a peripheral wedge-shaped airspace opacity that often implies lung infarction.

---

Arterial blood gas sampling – to assess for a relative hypoxia. The A-a gradient can be a useful tool here (see Chapter 12, Acute respiratory failure).

Electrocardiogram (ECG) – the most common abnormality is a sinus tachycardia. In severe cases the ECG may show signs of

---

**Table 21.1** Predisposing risk factors for venous thromboembolism

| Strong risk factors | | Moderate risk factors | | Weak risk factors | |
|---|---|---|---|---|---|
| **Setting related** | **Patient related** | **Setting related** | **Patient related** | **Setting related** | **Patient related** |
| Lower limb fracture Hip or knee replacement Major trauma Myocardial infarction | Previous VTE | Central venous lines Chemotherapy HRT and OCP Infection Postpartum | Inflammatory bowel disease Heart failure Thrombophilia Malignancy | Bed rest >3 days Pregnancy | Obesity Increasing age Diabetes Immobility |

*HRT, Hormone replacement therapy; OCP, oral contraceptive pill; VTE, venous thromboembolism.*

**Table 21.2** The Wells score aids stratification of the likelihood that a patient has a pulmonary embolism

| Sign/symptom | Score |
| --- | --- |
| Clinical signs and symptoms of DVT? | Yes + 3 |
| PE is no. 1 diagnosis, or equally likely | Yes + 3 |
| Heart rate >100 bpm? | Yes + 1.5 |
| Immobilization at least 3 days, or surgery in the previous 4 weeks? | Yes + 1.5 |
| Previous, objectively diagnosed PE or DVT? | Yes + 1.5 |
| Haemoptysis? | Yes + 1 |
| Malignancy with treatment within 6 months, or palliative? | Yes + 1 |
| Patient has none of these: score 0 = low probability, 1–2 = moderate probability, >3 = high probability. | |

*bpm, Beats per minute; DVT, deep vein thrombosis; PE, pulmonary embolism.*

right ventricular strain (T-wave inversion V1–4 and the inferior leads and right bundle branch block). Classically, the ECG shows S1-Q3-T3; however, this is rare in practice. Atrial tachycardias, particularly atrial fibrillation, can be associated with PE.

A D-dimer test should only be performed where there is a low probability of a PE. The index of suspicion for a PE can be determined clinically using the Wells score (Table 21.2). D-dimer is a fibrin degradation product that is present in the blood following fibrinolysis. It can be elevated in other situations, including infection, renal failure and postsurgery. A negative test result makes the presence of an acute PE very unlikely in low-probability individuals but does not exclude PE in higher-risk patients.

A computed tomography pulmonary angiogram (CTPA) allows direct imaging of the clot, and thus accurate assessment of clot size, number and location. It is now the preferred method of diagnostic imaging.

Radioisotope ventilation:perfusion (*V/Q*) scans demonstrate ventilated areas of lung and filling defects on the corresponding perfusion scans. They are useful in patients who are unable to have contrast (e.g., in renal failure or contrast allergy) or where avoiding radiation is important, such as in pregnant women. See Box 21.1 for further information. They are not helpful if the CXR is abnormal.

Echocardiography may be useful in the acute setting to examine for acute right ventricular failure and may help guide thrombolysis decisions if a patient is too unwell for CTPA.

A diagnostic algorithm for suspected PE in a haemodynamically stable patient is shown in Fig. 21.1.

## Management

Management of acute PE starts with the assessment of whether the patient is in cardiogenic shock secondary to the PE.

### BOX 21.1 VENOUS THROMBOEMBOLISM IN PREGNANCY AND THE PUERPERIUM

**Diagnosis**
Initial investigations should include an electrocardiogram and chest X-ray (CXR). D-dimer will be raised owing to pregnancy and therefore should not be performed as a diagnostic test. Ultrasound Doppler of the lower limbs should be performed if deep vein thrombosis is suspected and, if a clot is found, treatment is initiated with no further investigation needed. If the initial CXR is abnormal and there is a clinical suspicion of pulmonary embolus, then computed tomography pulmonary angiogram (CTPA) should be performed in preference to *V/Q* scanning. If the CXR is normal, either CTPA or low-dose perfusion (Q) scan can be performed – reference should be made to local guidelines. CTPA and low-dose perfusion scans both confer a small radiation dose risk to the foetus (approximately 0.1 milligray [mGy] with CTPA and 0.5 mGy with *V/Q* scans). The advantages of CTPA imaging are that it is usually more readily available and delivers a low radiation dose to the foetus alongside identifying other pathology. *V/Q* compared to CT imaging delivers a lower radiation dose to pregnant breast tissue and is therefore associated with a lesser risk of breast cancer. Pregnant women should therefore give consent prior to proceeding with any imaging.

**Management**
Low-molecular-weight heparin is safe during pregnancy as it does not cross the placenta. The maternal booking body weight should be used to calculate the therapeutic dose in the treatment of a nonmassive pulmonary embolus (PE). Warfarin is teratogenic, therefore should not be used. Systemic thrombolysis can be administered in massive PE; however, in high-risk patients, surgical embolectomy and lower-dose catheter-directed thrombolysis should be considered, if available.

## Hypotensive/shocked patients

This is defined as a systolic blood pressure of <90 mmHg or a drop of >40 mmHg persisting after 15 minutes of appropriate fluid resuscitation and in the absence of an alternative cause (e.g., sepsis). If shock is present, primary reperfusion through either catheter-directed thrombolysis or systemic thrombolysis with a 'clot-busting' drug recombinant tissue-type plasminogen activator (e.g., alteplase) may be indicated providing there are no contraindications, which include intracranial haemorrhage, suspected aortic dissection or ischaemic stroke within 3 months.

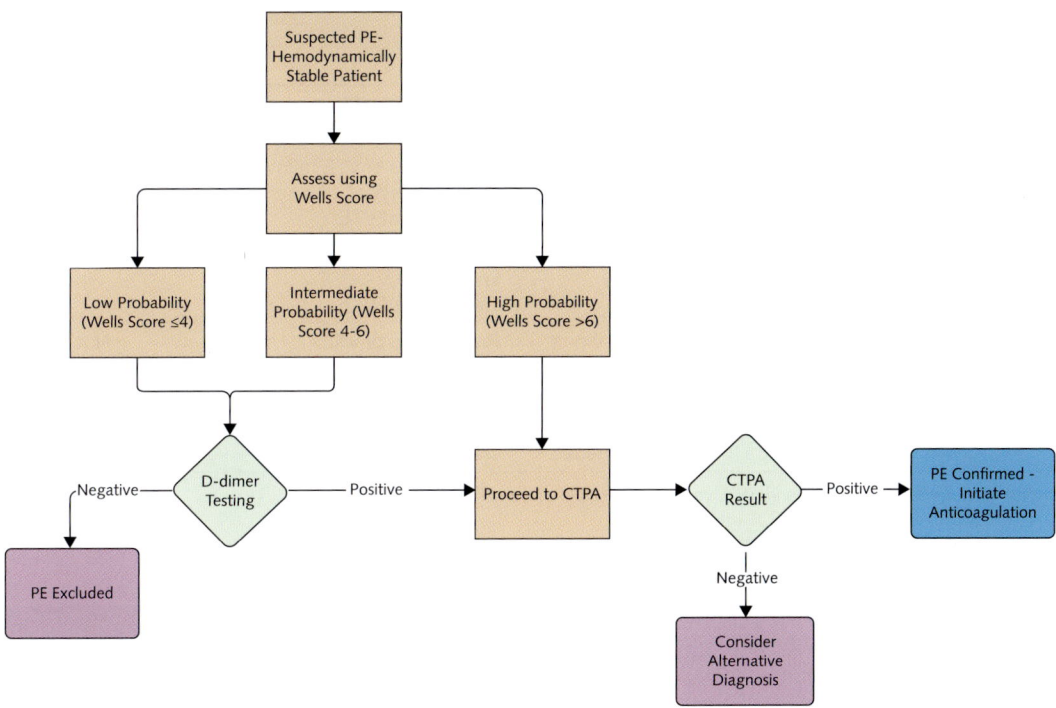

**Fig. 21.1** Diagnostic algorithm for suspected pulmonary embolism. *CT,* Computed tomography; *PE,* pulmonary embolism. (From Konstantinides SV, Torbicki A, Agnelli G, et al. 2014 ESC guidelines on the diagnosis and management of acute pulmonary embolism. *Eur Heart J.* 2014;35:3033–3069, 3069a–3069k.)

## Stable patients

If the patient is stable, treatment is based on clinical risk. Risk stratification can be based on either the pulmonary embolism severity index score or simplified pulmonary embolism severity index score (sPESI). These tools have been developed for use following acute PE to predict prognosis by looking at these risk factors (age >80 years old, history of cancer, history of chronic cardiopulmonary disease, heart rate ≥110 beats per minute, systolic blood pressure <100 mmHg, oxygen saturation <90%). A score of one or more points on the sPESI indicates a high risk and conveys a 30-day mortality risk of 8.9%.

Furthermore, with a score of ≥1 on the sPESI, the European Society of Cardiology recommends this group should be considered as intermediate risk with recommendation to perform both CT imaging and echocardiography to look for right ventricular function. If both CT and echo are positive, then rescue perfusion can be considered, but if one positive or both negative, commencing inpatient anticoagulation is recommended.

Treatment in hospital includes anticoagulation and supportive management (oxygen and analgesia). Local hospital trust guidelines should be checked as to first line for the treatment of PE (which is usually low-molecular-weight heparin (LMWH). LMWH should be given subcutaneously if renal function allows,

and is considered as preferable to unfractionated heparin (UFH) which is delivered by intravenous infusion. UFH is used in patients with a high risk of bleeding or in severe renal failure. If diagnostic scanning is likely to be delayed for over 4 hours, anticoagulation should be started while awaiting confirmation of diagnosis. Once confirmed, the patient can be initiated on a vitamin K antagonist (warfarin) or a direct oral anticoagulant, and treatment should continue for at least 3 months; see Table 21.3 for further details on anticoagulation in VTE. A clinical history and full examination including breast examination in women and a urine dipstick, should be performed to assess for occult malignancy as a predisposing risk factor. Further investigations can be guided by examination findings. Anticoagulation treatment may be extended to lifelong if the patient has had multiple embolic events or no clear precipitating reversible cause was identified. Patients are often seen in a VTE clinic to review this at 3 months.

## Prevention

Hospital inpatients are at high risk of developing VTE. All hospital inpatients must have VTE forms completed on admission to assess their risk. Methods to decrease risk include:

**Table 21.3** Anticoagulation in venous thromboembolism

| Group | Example | Route | Use | Monitoring required |
|---|---|---|---|---|
| Vitamin K antagonist | Warfarin | Oral | Treatment of VTE | INR monitoring required |
| Direct thrombin inhibitor | Dabigatran | Oral | Prophylaxis of VTE following hip and knee surgery Treatment of VTE | Not required |
| Direct inhibitors of factor X | Apixaban Rivaroxaban | Oral | Prophylaxis of VTE following hip and knee surgery Treatment of VTE | Not required |
| Low-molecular-weight heparin | Dalteparin Enoxaparin | Subcutaneous | Prophylaxis of VTE Treatment of VTE (especially initial treatment) | Not required |
| Unfractionated heparin | Heparin | Intravenous Subcutaneous | Prophylaxis of VTE Treatment of VTE | APTT monitoring required if given IV |

*IV, Intravenous; UFH, unfractionated heparin; VTE, venous thromboembolism.*

- Early mobilization of patients after operations
- Use of tight elastic stockings (TED stockings)
- Prophylactic anticoagulation for hospital inpatients at risk.

## Chronic thromboembolic pulmonary hypertension

Chronic thromboembolic disease develops in 0.5%–4% of patients following acute PE with an increased risk in those with large, unprovoked or recurrent clots. If suspected, patients should undergo echocardiogram to look for evidence of pulmonary hypertension, and a repeat CTPA to assess for chronic clot formation. Lifelong anticoagulation should be continued in this case. If a surgical candidate, patients can undergo pulmonary endarterectomy to remove the chronic thrombus with the aim of improving symptoms (Fig. 21.2).

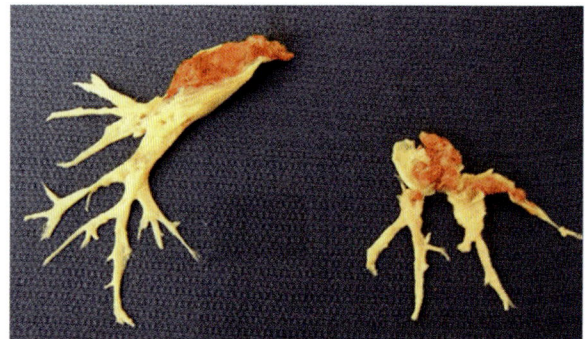

**Fig. 21.2** Chronic thrombus removed at pulmonary endarterectomy. (From Medscape Pulmonary Medicine. Chronic thromboembolic pulmonary hypertension: Treatment. Medscape; 2007.)

## PULMONARY HYPERTENSION

### Definition and pathophysiology

Pulmonary hypertension (PH) is defined as a mean pulmonary artery pressure of >25 mmHg at rest, as assessed by right heart catheterization. The normal range for pulmonary artery pressure is 14 ± 3 mmHg. There are multiple different mechanisms of disease leading to elevated pulmonary artery pressure. They are broadly divided into five groups (Table 21.4).

In pulmonary artery hypertension (PAH) (group 1), an imbalance of vasoactive mediators leads to a progressive narrowing of the pulmonary arterial bed and, consequently,

raised pulmonary artery pressures. In chronic thromboembolic pulmonary hypertension (CTEPH) (group 4), the pressure increases owing to mechanical obstruction by the thrombus within the pulmonary arterial system. Chronic hypoxia caused by lung disease (group 3) leads to vascular destruction and vasoconstriction and, eventually, raised pulmonary artery pressures. Thus the disease processes are heterogenous; however, the end physiological result is the same. Classification is important as it helps guide treatment and prognosis.

### Epidemiology

The reported prevalence of PH in the United Kingdom is 97 cases per million population. Data showing comparative prevalence between different classification groups is poor; however, PH

**Table 21.4** Mechanisms of pulmonary hypertension

| Group | Mechanism of PH | Examples of disease |
|---|---|---|
| 1 | PAH (multifactorial pathogenesis involving vasoconstriction, cell proliferation, fibrosis and thrombosis) | Idiopathic PAH<br>Heritable PAH<br>PAH secondary to drugs<br>PAH secondary to systemic disease, e.g., HIV or connective tissue disorders such as scleroderma |
| 2 | PH due to left heart disease (results from backpressure from the left heart to the pulmonary vasculature and may involve increases in vascular tone and remodelling) | Left ventricular systolic dysfunction<br>Left ventricular diastolic dysfunction<br>Valvular disease |
| 3 | PH due to lung disease (arises from hypoxic vasoconstriction, loss of pulmonary capillaries and possible vascular remodelling) | COPD<br>ILD<br>OSA<br>Other causes of chronic hypoxia |
| 4 | Mechanical pulmonary artery obstruction (results from obstruction of pulmonary arteries by pulmonary emboli, followed by more diffuse vascular remodelling) | Chronic thromboembolic pulmonary hypertension |
| 5 | PH with unclear or multifactorial mechanisms | Haematological disorders such as myeloproliferative disease, sickle cell disease<br>Systemic disorders, e.g., sarcoidosis and thyroid disease<br>Metabolic disorders |

COPD, Chronic obstructive pulmonary disease; ILD, interstitial lung disease; PAH, pulmonary artery hypertension; PH, pulmonary hypertension.

secondary to left heart disease is accepted as the most common cause.

Idiopathic PAH is rare in the general population; however, within certain population groups the prevalence is high, for example, it is 9% in those with systemic sclerosis. Mutations in the bone morphogenetic receptor 2 (*BMPR2*) gene are implicated in 75% of familial PAH.

## Presentation

Patients initially have nonspecific insidious symptoms with few clinical signs, and as such the condition is often diagnosed late. The commonest symptom is progressive exertional dyspnoea. Signs are usually owing to heart failure secondary to raised pulmonary pressures (e.g., raised JVP, accentuated P2 of the second heart sound, a third heart sound, right ventricular parasternal heave, tricuspid regurgitation, pedal oedema and ascites) but may be indicative of the underlying disease (e.g., connective tissue disease).

## Investigation

Investigation focuses on diagnosing PH and assessing for underlying causes. Common investigations include an ECG, looking for signs of right ventricular hypertrophy; a CXR to look for evidence of cardiac failure and any underlying respiratory pathology; and full pulmonary function tests, including transfer factor (a measure of the capacity of the lung to transfer gas from the air to the blood). CTPA may be considered to look for CTEPH, especially if there is known previous thromboembolic disease. Echocardiography can be used to estimate systolic pulmonary artery pressure and therefore predict the risk of PH. Diagnosis can only be confirmed using right heart catheterization, where further measurements such as the pulmonary arterial wedge pressure can be obtained and help differentiate the cause. A raised pulmonary arterial wedge pressure may suggest PH secondary to left heart disease.

## Management

Treatment is specific to diagnostic group. If left heart disease or pulmonary disease is the underlying cause, treatment should focus on these. Supportive measures for all patients include diuretics to treat the symptoms of right heart failure, flu vaccination and long-term oxygen therapy. Maternal mortality remains high in women with PH during pregnancy and therefore women should be counselled and offered contraceptive therapy. Anticoagulation and pulmonary endarterectomy are considered as specific treatments for CTEPH. However, not all patients are deemed operable and up to one-third may have persistent or recurrent CTEPH following surgery. Riociguat (a soluble guanylate cyclase stimulator) is approved for the treatment of inoperable or persistent/recurrent CTEPH.

Further medical treatment options exist for PAH. High-dose calcium channel blockers such as diltiazem are of benefit in a small proportion of patients with idiopathic PAH. Prediction of response to calcium channel blockers can be assessed with vaso-active testing during right heart catheterization. Several other vasodilator drugs have been shown to improve exercise capacity and these are summarized in Table 21.5. Lung transplant may be considered in severe end-stage disease.

**Table 21.5** Drugs licensed in the treatment of pulmonary hypertension

| Drug class | Examples | Route |
| --- | --- | --- |
| Prostanoids | Prostacyclin Iloprost | IV infusion Nebulized and IV |
| Endothelin receptor antagonists | Bosentan Ambrisentan | Oral |
| Phosphodiesterase 5 inhibitors | Sildenafil | Oral |

*IV, Intravenous.*

## Prognosis

This is poor, as disease is often detected late, can be rapidly progressive and response to treatment is variable. Mean survival is 2–3 years from diagnosis. Death is usually secondary to right heart failure.

● **Chapter Summary**

- Pulmonary embolus (PE) is a common condition that presents with chest pain and breathlessness, and it can carry a high mortality if left untreated.
- Key diagnostic tests for PE include a D-dimer test based on a patient's Wells score, and subsequent computed tomography pulmonary angiogram or *V/Q* scanning.
- PE can be subdivided into 'massive' or 'nonmassive' depending on whether the patient is haemodynamically stable. Acute treatment is guided by this distinction.
- Diagnosis and management of PE in pregnant women differs from the nonpregnant population and specialist advice should be sought.
- Pulmonary hypertension is the end result of multiple different pathologies and is defined as a mean pulmonary artery pressure of >25 mmHg at right heart catheterization.
- Pulmonary hypertension presents with exertional dyspnoea and, latterly, signs of right heart failure.

**MLA Conditions**
Pulmonary embolism
Pulmonary hypertension

**MLA Presentation**
Shock

### Further reading

European Society of Cardiology. Clinical practical guidelines, 2009. Pulmonary hypertension (Guidelines on Diagnosis and Treatment of). http://www.escardio.org/guidelines-surveys/esc-guidelines/Pages/pulmonary-arterial-hypertension.aspx.

Kiely DG, Elliot CA, Sabroe I, Condliffe R. Pulmonary hypertension: diagnosis and management. *BMJ.* 2013;346:f2028.

Konstantinides SV, Meyer G, Becattini C, et al. 2019 ESC guidelines for the diagnosis and management of acute pulmonary embolism developed in collaboration with the European Respiratory Society (ERS): The Task Force for the diagnosis and management of acute pulmonary embolism of the European Society of Cardiology (ESC). *Eur Heart J.* 2020;41(4):543–603.

NICE. Venous thromboembolic diseases: diagnosis, management and thrombophilia testing. 2020.

Royal College of Obstetricians and Gynaecologists. *Thromboembolic Disease in Pregnancy and the Puerperium: Acute Management. Green-top Guideline No. 37b.* London: RCOG; 2015.

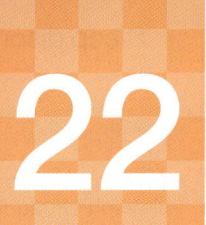
## SLEEP APNOEA

Sleep apnoea is the temporary cessation of breathing during sleep. There are two recognized forms: obstructive sleep apnoea (OSA) and central sleep apnoea. While both share the common apnoeic episodes – suspension of breathing for short periods – the pathogenesis is quite different for each condition. While OSA is becoming an increasingly common condition, central sleep apnoea remains rare.

## OBSTRUCTIVE SLEEP APNOEA

In OSA, there is either partial (hypopnoea) or total (apnoea) collapse of the pharyngeal airway during sleep, leading to a reduction in flow and causing arousal and partial wakening. This phenomenon occurs multiple times during the night, resulting in interrupted, nonrestorative sleep.

### Prevalence

OSA affects roughly 1 billion people worldwide and 1.5 million people in the United Kingdom. However, about 85% of patients in the United Kingdom remain undiagnosed. Although OSA can affect anyone, it is more common in those who are overweight and obese, affecting up to 70% of morbidly obese individuals. While true figures are unknown, it is estimated that half of all OSA cases are in overweight individuals. With the current obesity crisis in the developed world, the prevalence is increasing, and while awareness of the condition is improving, it is thought that many cases remain undiagnosed.

### Pathogenesis

OSA results from occlusion of the upper airway and is common in overweight, middle-aged men. On inspiration upper-airway pressure becomes negative, but airway patency is maintained by upper-airway muscle (e.g., genioglossus) tone. During deep sleep, these muscles relax causing narrowing of the upper airways, even in normal subjects. However, if the airway is already narrowed, for example, by the weight of adipose tissue in obese patients or because of a small jaw (micrognathia), the airway collapses and OSA results. Other risk factors include:

- Down syndrome
- Adenotonsillar hypertrophy
- Soft tissue deposition seen in hypothyroidism or amyloidosis

- Macroglossia – enlarged tongue (seen in acromegaly)
- Nasal obstruction (as in rhinitis)
- Alcohol (which reduces the arousal response and has been shown to reduce muscle tone).

A cycle is generated during sleep in which:

- The upper-airway dilating muscles lose tone (usually accompanied by loud snoring)
- The airway is occluded
- The patient wakes (often not completely, patients are not consciously aware of the waking process)
- The airway reopens.

As a consequence of this cycle, sleep is unrefreshing and daytime sleepiness is common, particularly during monotonous situations such as motorway driving. Each arousal also causes a transient rise in blood pressure through a burst of sympathetic activity and catecholamine release, which in combination with hypoxaemia may lead to sustained hypertension, pulmonary hypertension, cor pulmonale, ischaemic heart disease and stroke.

### Clinical features

- Chronic snoring, with pauses in breathing, followed by a choking or gasping sound (often noticed by partners rather than the patient themselves)
- Daytime somnolence
- Morning headaches
- Difficulty concentrating
- Mood swings
- Dry throat
- Loss of libido
- Nocturia
- Difficulties with memory

In addition to the above, the patient may appear obese and have a wide neck or small jaw, enlarged tonsils or nasal obstruction (polyps, deviated septum).

### Investigations

Patients can have the severity of their daytime sleepiness assessed using the Epworth Sleepiness Scale (see http://epworthsleepinessscale.com/ and Box 22.1), a scale used to assess daytime somnolence. A score of 10 or less is normal. Between 11 and 15 indicates likely mild-to-moderate disease, and specialist medical advice should be sought. A score of 16 or over is indicative of severe sleepiness.

hypopnoea index (AHI). An apnoea is defined as a >90% reduction in nasal flow for at least 10 seconds, while a hypopnoea is defined as a >30% reduction in nasal flow for at least 10 seconds followed by a 3% or 4% desaturation. If there is the presence of respiratory/abdominal movement, this is classified as an obstructive event. If there is an absence of effort, then it is a central event. An AHI of ≥5/hour is diagnostic of sleep apnoea. Sleep apnoea severity is categorized based on the AHI, as mild OSA (AHI 5–14/hour), moderate (AHI 15–29/hour) and severe (AHI ≥30/hour).

A full polysomnography measures brain activity via an electroencephalogram (EEG) but usually patients have a limited multichannel study in their own home, without EEG. Recently novel wearable devices have been validated to ease the diagnosis of OSA.

## Treatment

Weight loss is a key treatment for those who are overweight, not just for the apnoea but also for the other metabolic syndrome-associated risks. This is often challenging and can require significant support to maintain, with more extreme measures such as bariatric surgery an option in select cases. Other conservative measures, such as avoiding alcohol and sedatives that relax the upper airway, can be effective.

Despite these measures, for most patients nightly continuous positive airway pressure (CPAP) is recommended. With CPAP, respiratory support is given via the patient's upper airway. The patient breathes spontaneously and the lungs are

Patients are subsequently referred to a sleep or respiratory specialist for overnight sleep studies and polysomnography (Fig. 22.1). During the sleep study, the total number of apnoeas and hypopnoeas occurring every hour results in the apnoea/

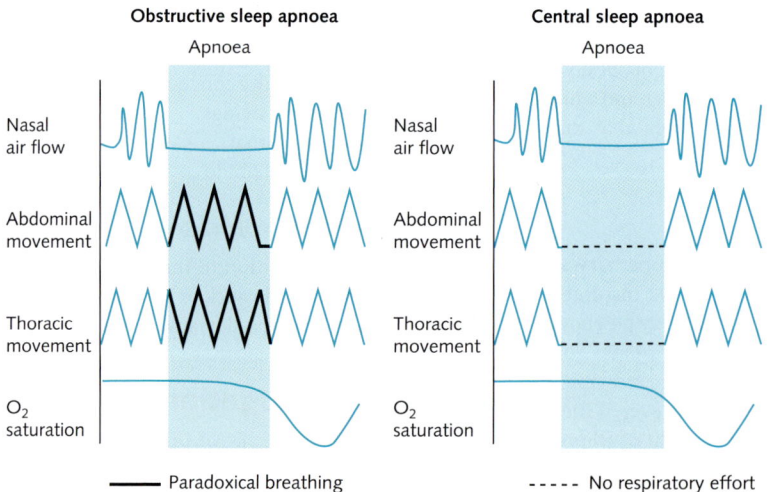

**Fig. 22.1** Example results of polysomnographs showing the two types of sleep apnoea. Sleep apnoea can be detected by reduced air flow and a delayed desaturation following the apnoea. Normally, the thorax and abdomen move in the same direction; however, in obstructive sleep apnoea the thorax and abdomen move in opposite directions to each other – an abnormal pattern called paradoxical breathing. Conversely, in central sleep apnoea, there is neither thoracic nor abdominal movement because the respiratory centre in the brain has stopped instructing the respiratory muscles to move.

expanded by a volume of gas delivered at a positive pressure. This decreases the work of the respiratory muscles, particularly the diaphragm. As the name implies, CPAP delivers a continuous positive air pressure throughout the respiratory cycle, and is used to keep the upper airway open in OSA. The results can be remarkable and it is recommended for those with moderate or severe symptoms.

However, there are downsides to CPAP. The equipment requires specialist training to use and set up. For many, using a CPAP machine becomes a lifelong commitment, bringing a burdensome piece of equipment wherever the patient goes. Some patients find CPAP difficult to use because the mask is uncomfortable, as is the sensation of having air forced in through the mouth and nose. CPAP exists in many forms, with whole airway and nasal masks available. Patients also often complain that the machine is noisy and cumbersome, thus affecting their relationship with their partner. However, this should be balanced against the increased health risks associated with sleep apnoea, as well as the noise from snoring! (Fig. 22.2).

Other treatments include a mandibular assessment device (Fig. 22.3). This is either first-line treatment in minimally symptomatic mild OSA patients or in patients who have not tolerated CPAP therapy. This is a dental device worn in the mouth while sleeping and is recommended to be fitted by a dental practitioner with an interest in dental sleep medicine, following a dental assessment. The device moves the mandible forward and increases the area of the oropharynx. These have been shown to be effective and may be a useful alternative in less severe cases. Other treatments may include tonsillectomy with tonsil enlargement, or nasal polypectomy in certain instances.

## Complications

Sleep apnoea can have many serious consequences on various aspects of a patient's life. On a personal level, the constant snoring can put a major strain on the relationship between a patient and his or her partner. Furthermore, it can have more widespread

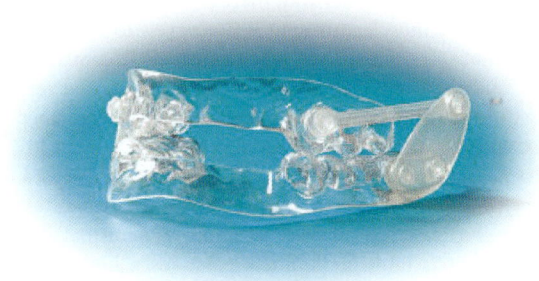

**Fig. 22.3** Mandibular repositioning device. (From Vecchierini MF, Léger D, Laaban JP, et al. Efficacy and compliance of mandibular repositioning device in obstructive sleep apnea syndrome under a patient-driven protocol of care. *Sleep Med*. 2008;9:762–769.)

consequences for patients who drive, as daytime somnolence significantly increases the risk of falling asleep at the wheel, a dangerous consequence for both the patient and anyone else on the road. It is important to tell patients that they must inform the Driver and Vehicle Licensing Agency of their diagnosis if they are symptomatic and have daytime somnolence.

Sleep apnoea is also dangerous for the physical health of the patient. As most patients are overweight or obese, they are already at increased risk of heart disease, diabetes and associated complications. However, even taking that into account, these patients are at increased risk for developing hypertension, heart disease and stroke.

## CENTRAL SLEEP APNOEA

Central sleep apnoea is a rarer condition causing an irregular breathing pattern during sleep. In central sleep apnoea, either the airway remains patent but there is no efferent output from the respiratory centres in the brain, or there is a primary weakness of the

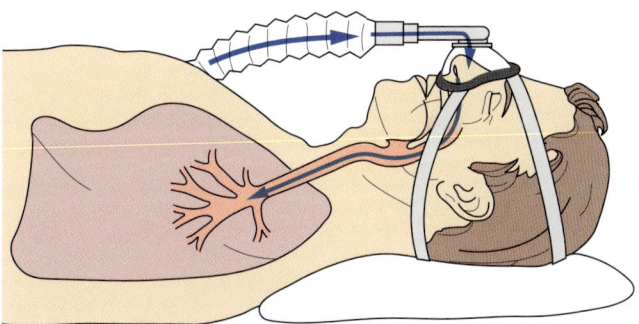

**Fig. 22.2** Continuous positive airway pressure machine for obstructive sleep apnoea in position.

respiratory muscles. Either way, there is no respiratory effort by the respiratory muscles, causing $P_aCO_2$ levels to rise. The high $P_aCO_2$ arouses the patient, who then rebreathes to normalize the $P_aCO_2$ and then falls asleep again. This cycle can be repeated many times during the night and leads to a disruptive sleep pattern. Central sleep apnoea is more common in patients with congestive heart failure and patients with neurological diseases (e.g., strokes). It can also be seen in people with no abnormalities, such as those who live at high altitude, or simply be a normal variant.

The result is multiple apnoeic episodes a night, some of which the patient may or may not be aware of, again causing unrefreshing sleep and daytime somnolence. In certain instances, there is a predictability of the regular cyclical timings of apnoeic episodes followed by hyperventilation, resulting in a pattern known as Cheyne–Stokes respiration. The pattern of pauses is also described in polysomnography in Fig. 22.1 and is investigated with sleep studies in the same way as OSA.

Given that central sleep apnoea can be a normal variant or suggest a significant underlying pathological process, the treatments vary considerably. If separate underlying pathology is present, detecting and treating it may resolve the apnoeic episodes. If there are no underlying problems and the patient is not symptomatic, reassurance can be given that nothing is wrong. Sometimes CPAP, or noninvasive ventilation (NIV) with bilevel positive pressures if carbon dioxide retention is occurring, can play a role in more complex central sleep apnoea management (see Chapter 12, Acute respiratory failure).

## OBESITY HYPOVENTILATION SYNDROME

Obesity hypoventilation syndrome, or Pickwickian syndrome, is a disorder of breathing commonly associated with OSA, characterized by a high body mass index (BMI ≥30 kg/m²),

sleep disturbance and daytime hypercapnia, in the absence of parenchymal lung disease. However, comorbid conditions do occur (e.g., COPD and OHS). The exact underlying mechanisms are not known but it is thought to be a combination of a lack of stimulation from the brainstem combined with a large volume of excess weight compressing the chest and upper airways.

The condition presents in a similar way to sleep apnoea, with daytime somnolence, depression and headaches (from hypercapnia). In fact, as patients often have the two conditions, it can be very difficult to distinguish them.

Diagnosis is through a combination of clinical findings (obese patient, cyanosis) and arterial blood gas results, which reveal the characteristic hypoxia and hypercapnia pattern of type II respiratory failure. Other diagnostic criteria include the demonstration of a sleep disorder (overnight oximetry or polysomnography) with absence of other causes of hypoventilation.

### CLINICAL NOTES

**DIAGNOSTIC CRITERIA FOR OBESITY HYPOVENTILATION SYNDROME**

Body mass index ≥30 kg/m²
Daytime $P_aCO_2$ >45 mmHg
Associated sleep apnoea syndrome/other sleep-
   disordered breathing
Absence of other causes of hypoventilation

Treatment, as with OSA, initially involves conservative measures such as weight loss. Nocturnal noninvasive ventilation (NIV) using bilevel positive airway pressure, in order to blow off excess carbon dioxide) is the primary treatment of choice (see Chapter 12 for more details).

## ● Chapter Summary

- Obstructive sleep apnoea (OSA) causes collapse of the pharyngeal airway during sleep, resulting in partial wakening during the night and subsequent interrupted, nonrestorative sleep. Clinical features include snoring and daytime somnolence.
- Screening for OSA is performed with a sleepiness score to assess symptom severity. Overnight sleep studies measure the duration and frequency of apnoeic episodes, as well as associated desaturations.
- Management for OSA includes weight loss and avoidance of sedatives, and overnight continuous positive airway pressure (CPAP) to splint open the airway at night.
- Central sleep apnoea is a complex phenomenon caused by central nervous system pathology, resulting in multiple apnoeic episodes at night. Management is by treating the underlying cause, with nocturnal CPAP or bilevel positive airway pressure (BiPAP) used if symptomatic.
- Obesity hypoventilation syndrome is a related extension of OSA with associated hypercapnia and type II respiratory failure. It is managed with weight loss and nocturnal NIV.

**MLA Condition**
Obstructive sleep apnoea

**MLA Presentations**
Sleep problems
Snoring

### Useful links

http://sleepmed.com.au/bariatric1.pdf.
http://www.nhlbi.nih.gov/health/health-topics/topics/sleepapnea/atrisk.html.

https://www.sleepsociety.org.uk/wp-content/uploads/2015/07/OSA-Toolkit-2015-FINAL.pdf.

# Respiratory manifestations of systemic disease 23

## INTRODUCTION

Respiratory symptoms are common to many disorders. There are many disease processes that, while not having a primary lung pathology, often present to respiratory clinics or wards. While the breadth of conditions with respiratory manifestations is too vast to cover, here is an overview of several key conditions not to be missed, including:

- Sarcoidosis
- Vasculitis
- Rheumatological diseases
- HIV-related lung disease.

## SARCOIDOSIS

### Definition and epidemiology

Sarcoidosis is a multisystem granulomatous disorder of unknown aetiology. Pulmonary involvement is common and noncaseating granulomas form within the lung.

Sarcoidosis is a relatively rare condition and prevalence in the United Kingdom is estimated to be 19 per 100,000 population. It is more common in women and the peak age of incidence is 20–40 years. Women of black African origin are more likely to suffer with severe disease.

### Pathology

Sarcoidosis is characterized by the formation of noncaseating (nonnecrotizing) granulomas. These granulomas are infiltrated by Th1 lymphocytes (a subset of CD4 cells) and macrophages, which fuse to form multinucleated giant epithelioid cells.

Often these granulomas resolve, leading to spontaneous remission; however, up to 20% of cases have persistent inflammation, which results in interstitial fibrosis of the affected tissue.

### Clinical features

The clinical presentation of sarcoidosis is dependent on the organ involved. Often patients are asymptomatic, and the diagnosis is made after an incidental finding on chest radiograph. The majority of patients (>90%) have pulmonary involvement, which may cause:

- Dyspnoea
- Chest pain
- Dry cough.

Other nonspecific constitutional features include:

- Lymphadenopathy
- Fever
- Fatigue
- Loss.

Common extrapulmonary features include:

- Erythema nodosum/lupus pernio of the skin (Fig. 23.1). Note lupus pernio is rare but pathognomonic of sarcoidosis.
- Arthralgia.
- Uveitis.
- Cranial nerve palsies (in neurosarcoid).
- Cardiomyopathies (rare).

### CLINICAL NOTES

#### LOFGREN SYNDROME

This is a subtype of acute sarcoidosis with a common constellation of symptoms:

- Hilar lymphadenopathy
- Erythema nodosum
- Joint symptoms (arthralgia, commonly of the ankles)
- Fever.

Patients with Lofgren syndrome tend to have a good prognosis, with most patients achieving spontaneous remission.

### Investigation

Table 23.1 demonstrates useful investigations in a patient with suspected sarcoidosis. The Global Initiative for Obstructive Lung Disease (GOLD) standard diagnostic method for sarcoidosis remains biopsy, showing epithelioid noncaseating granulomas on histology.

Chest radiographs can be useful in staging disease and determining prognosis (Fig. 23.2), often classically showing bilateral hilar lymphadenopathy. It is important to remember that staging disease in sarcoidosis does not reflect disease progression, that is, stage III disease can develop with a patient never having developed stage I.

### Management

If the patient has hilar lymphadenopathy and no lung involvement, then no treatment is required.

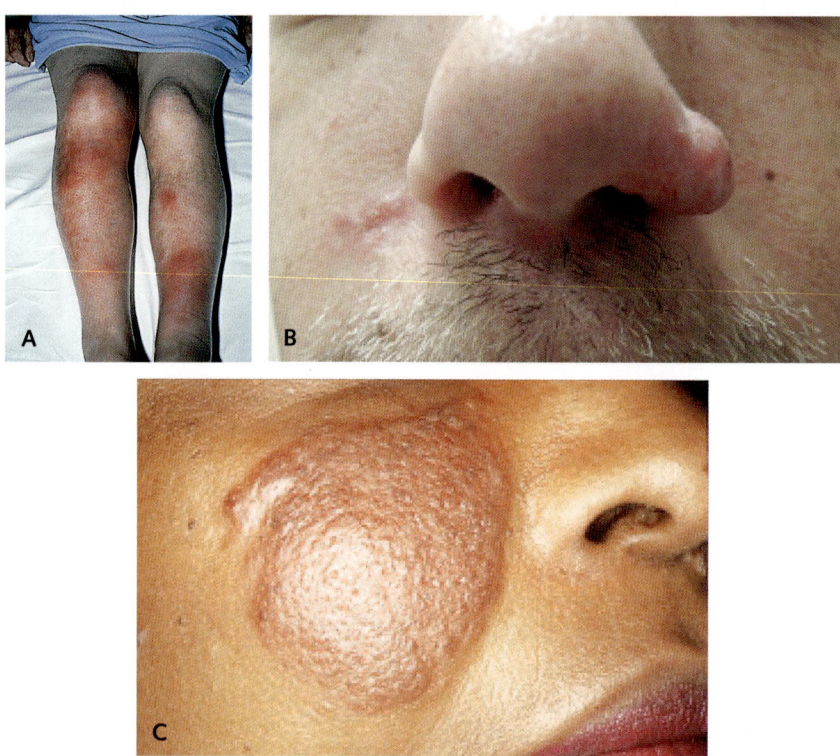

**Fig. 23.1** Skin manifestations of sarcoidosis. (A) Erythema nodosum. (B) Lupus pernio. (C) Sarcoid nodules. (With permission from Weller R, Hunter JAA, Savin J, Dah M. *Clinical dermatology*. 4th ed. Hoboken, New Jersey. Wiley-Blackwell; 2009; Wanat KA, Rosenbach M. Cutaneous sarcoidosis. *Clin Chest Med*. 2015;36:685–702; and Freund KB, Sarraf D, Mieler WF, Yannuzzi L. *The retinal atlas*. 2nd ed. Amsterdam, Netherlands: Elsevier; 2017.)

**Table 23.1** Useful investigations in sarcoidosis

| Test | Use |
|---|---|
| Full blood count | May show a normochromic normocytic anaemia |
| Erythrocyte sedimentation rate | Often raised; can be used to monitor disease activity |
| Serum calcium | Granulomas secrete vitamin D, causing hypercalcaemia |
| Serum ACE | Granulomas secrete ACE. Can be twice normal levels. Used to monitor disease activity |
| Chest X-ray | Typical features. Useful in staging disease |
| High-resolution computed tomography | Disease staging, identifying pulmonary fibrosis |
| Biopsy | GOLD standard for diagnosis |

*ACE, Angiotensin-converting enzyme; GOLD, Global Initiative for Obstructive Lung Disease.*

If infiltration has occurred for more than 6 weeks, treat with corticosteroids (prednisolone 20–40 mg/day typically for 1–3 months, then a reduced maintenance dose).

Prognosis is dependent on disease stage. In the UK, mortality is less than 5% in the white population and approximately 10% in Afro-Americans. If shadowing is present on chest radiographs for more than 2 years, the risk of fibrosis increases.

## VASCULITIS

Vasculitis is a broad term incorporating a heterogeneous group of disorders that share a common underlying feature – inflammation of blood vessels.

They tend to be multiorgan diseases primarily affecting the kidneys, lungs, joints and skin. This section will consider three vasculitides with well-described pulmonary manifestations:

- Goodpasture syndrome
- Granulomatosis with polyangiitis (previously Wegener granulomatosis)

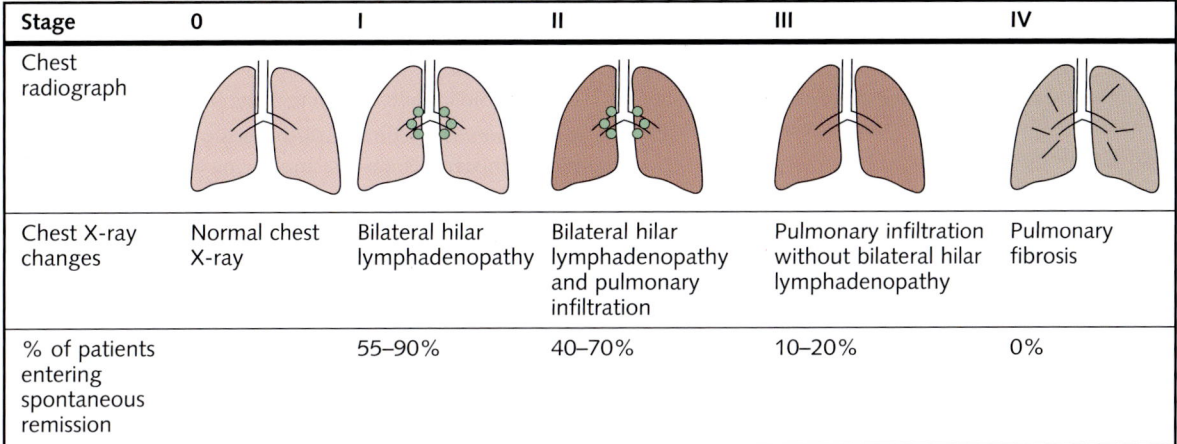

| Stage | 0 | I | II | III | IV |
|---|---|---|---|---|---|
| Chest radiograph | | | | | |
| Chest X-ray changes | Normal chest X-ray | Bilateral hilar lymphadenopathy | Bilateral hilar lymphadenopathy and pulmonary infiltration | Pulmonary infiltration without bilateral hilar lymphadenopathy | Pulmonary fibrosis |
| % of patients entering spontaneous remission | | 55–90% | 40–70% | 10–20% | 0% |

**Fig. 23.2** The staging of sarcoidosis by chest radiographs.

- Eosinophilic granulomatosis with polyangiitis (EGPA) (previously Churg–Strauss disease).

## Goodpasture syndrome

Goodpasture syndrome is a small-vessel vasculitis characterized by glomerulonephritis and respiratory symptoms. The syndrome is driven by a type II hypersensitivity reaction whereby immunoglobulin (IgG) autoantibodies to the glomerular basement membrane (anti-GBM) attach to the glomerulus, causing glomerulonephritis. In the lung, anti-GBM antibodies cross-react with the alveolar basement membrane, causing diffuse pulmonary haemorrhage.

Patients present with haemoptysis, haematuria and oedema. Serum anti-GBM antibodies are diagnostic but not always present, with patterns of anaemia, acute renal failure and reduced urine output also seen. A full autoimmune screen should be performed and a renal biopsy may be required in the absence of anti-GBM antibodies. Chest radiography is variable but typically shows bilateral patchy consolidation. Treatment is by corticosteroids or plasmapheresis to remove antibodies. The course of the disease is variable: some patients resolve completely, whereas others proceed to renal failure, where supportive care is adopted.

## Granulomatosis with polyangiitis

Granulomatosis with polyangiitis (formerly Wegener granulomatosis) is a rare, necrotizing vasculitis of unknown aetiology affecting small blood vessels. It classically involves midline structures, including the nose (Fig. 23.3) – causing epistaxis, lungs – causing haemoptysis and kidneys, where it causes glomerulonephritis – causing oedema. Other areas of the body, such as joints, eyes and skin, are less commonly affected.

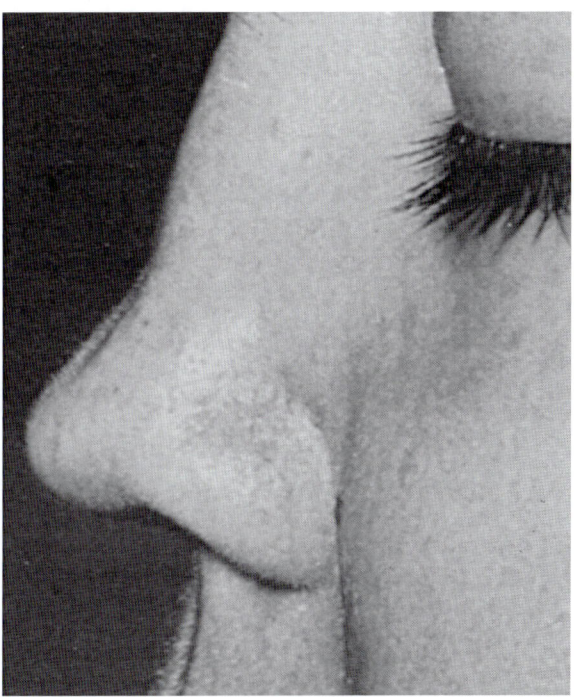

**Fig. 23.3** Features of granulomatosis with polyangiitis. Classical saddle-shaped nose deformity.

Symptoms often begin as a flu-like illness with fevers, rhinorrhoea and cough. In the lung, mucosal thickening and ulceration occur, producing the clinical features of cough, haemoptysis and dyspnoea. Granulomatosis with polyangiitis can be suggested by an autoantibody screen with the presence of cytoplasmic anti-neutrophil cytoplasmic antibodies (cANCA), although this is not positive in approximately 10%–15% of patients. The GOLD standard of diagnosis remains biopsy (renal, nasal mucosa or affected area).

If untreated, mortality after 2 years is 93%, but the disease responds well to a combination of high-dose prednisolone and cyclophosphamide. Other immunosuppressant treatments include methotrexate or rituximab.

## Eosinophilic granulomatosis with polyangiitis

- Eosinophilic granulomatosis with polyangiitis (formerly known as Churg–Strauss disease) is a small-vessel vasculitis, typically presenting with late-onset asthma. It is characterized by the pathological triad of:
  - Granulomatous inflammation
  - Eosinophilia (seen on full blood count)
  - Small-vessel vasculitis (purpura may be seen).

As per Watts et al., the first stage typically includes late-onset asthma and sinusitis. The second stage is when eosinophilic infiltrates and thus pulmonary infiltrates develop. The third stage is when vasculitis occurs. Vasospasm is also a common feature and patients are at risk of developing myocardial infarction. Investigations demonstrate eosinophilia, positive cANCA in 40%, raised inflammatory markers, infiltrates on chest imaging and a characteristic lung biopsy. Treatment is usually with high-dose corticosteroids or monoclonal antibodies.

## SYSTEMIC RHEUMATOLOGICAL DISEASES

Respiratory involvement is often a cause of high morbidity and a sign of poor prognosis in patients with autoimmune diseases, such as:

- Rheumatoid arthritis
- Systemic lupus erythematosus (SLE)
- Systemic sclerosis
- Ankylosing spondylitis.

## Rheumatoid arthritis

Rheumatoid arthritis is a chronic inflammatory condition characterized by a symmetrical deforming polyarthropathy. It has many extraarticular features, including manifestations in the lung.

In all, 10%–15% of patients with rheumatoid arthritis have lung involvement and usually these patients have severe disease. Patients can develop:

- Diffuse pulmonary fibrosis
- Bronchiolitis obliterans: causing severe airflow obstruction

- Follicular bronchiolitis
- Pleural fibrosis
- Pleural effusions
- Rheumatoid nodules within the lung (rare).

Management of rheumatoid arthritis is with immunosuppression through steroids, disease-modifying antirheumatic drugs and biological treatments. Note that the immunosuppressive treatments predispose to infection (including atypical or fungal infections) and rare but significant side effects of methotrexate treatment are pneumonitis or pulmonary fibrosis.

**CLINICAL NOTES**

**CAPLAN SYNDROME**

Caplan syndrome is the combination of rheumatoid arthritis and pneumoconiosis, characterized by well-defined intrapulmonary nodules seen on chest radiography. Patients present with cough, shortness of breath and arthropathy with early morning stiffness of inflammatory arthritis. The condition occurs in miners working with fine dusts (coal, silica, asbestos). Management is as per rheumatoid arthritis, with an important differential being tuberculosis.

## Systemic lupus erythematosus

SLE is a multisystem autoimmune disease in which multiple autoantibodies form immune complexes, which deposit in a variety of organs, including the skin, joints, kidneys and lungs.

Respiratory involvement is usually in the form of pleurisy, with or without an effusion, and pulmonary fibrosis is rare. Investigation is with autoimmune profiling of antinuclear antibodies, a highly sensitive test, and anti–double-stranded DNA, a highly specific test, with multiple other autoantibody variants. Again, treatment is with immunosuppression and the risk of respiratory infection remains.

## Systemic sclerosis

Systemic sclerosis is a severe autoimmune connective tissue disorder where there is increased fibroblast activity resulting in the abnormal growth of connective tissue. It exists in two forms, limited cutaneous or diffuse cutaneous, with the latter being more aggressive and with a higher mortality. Pulmonary involvement is common but often asymptomatic. If symptomatic, it is a sign of severe disease and is associated with a poor prognosis. Patients typically develop pulmonary fibrosis presenting as progressive exertional dyspnoea and cough. In severe forms, rapidly progressive pulmonary hypertension develops, which leads to cor pulmonale. There are a number of autoantibodies associated with systemic sclerosis,

**Table 23.2** Summary table to compare Goodpasture syndrome, GPA and EGPA

| Goodpasture syndrome | GPA | EGPA |
|---|---|---|
| Immune complex-mediated, anti-GBM antibodies are diagnostic | ANCA associated | Eosinophilia (+ often ANCA associated) |
| Presents with haemoptysis, glomerulonephritis and acute renal failure | Affects upper airways (epistaxis), lower airways (haemoptysis) and kidneys (glomerulonephritis) | Stage 1: late-onset asthma, allergic rhinitis<br>Stage 2: eosinophilic pulmonary infiltrates<br>Stage 3: small vessel vasculitis (where ANCA is often associated) |

with anti-topoisomerase 1 (anti-Scl 70) strongly associated with lung and renal disease (and thus diffuse sclerosis). Broad-spectrum immunosuppressants are used in management.

## Ankylosing spondylitis

Ankylosing spondylitis is a chronic inflammatory condition of the spine and sacroiliac joints, which predominantly affects men. It has several extraarticular manifestations, including:

- Acute iritis
- Aortic regurgitation
- Apical lung fibrosis.

It is classed as a seronegative arthropathy. Diagnosis is clinical and should be managed by a rheumatologist. The presence of lung fibrosis is a marker of disease severity and patients should monitor for symptoms of breathlessness, prompting further investigation.

## HIV-RELATED LUNG DISEASE

HIV is a blood-borne retrovirus that produces suppression of the host immune system by binding to CD4 receptors on lymphocytes, monocytes, macrophages and neural cells. As the disease progresses the number of CD4 cells reduces, creating immunosuppression and opportunity for infection. Once the CD4 count lowers significantly (CD4 < 200 cells/μL), an acquired immune deficiency syndrome (AIDS) develops, allowing life-threatening opportunistic infections and neoplasms to develop. There are several opportunistic infections known as AIDS-defining illnesses that can occur, indicating AIDS regardless of the CD4 count.

In respiratory medicine, there are many ways that HIV-related illnesses can present. A patient's CD4 count can effectively predict the risk of developing certain conditions, with different illnesses presenting at certain thresholds of CD4 count (Table 23.2). Knowledge of the different illnesses that can present at differing CD4 counts (Table 23.3) can prove vital in diagnosing the complicating illness, meaning specialist testing such as high-resolution computed tomography, serology and cultures can be performed appropriately.

Diagnosis is often difficult in HIV infection, and a high index of suspicion should be present in any patient presenting with recurrent pneumonia or atypical infection. Management requires specialist input from genitourinary and infectious disease specialists once the diagnosis is confirmed. Management is with antiretroviral therapy, meaning few patients progress to AIDS. The disease is monitored by assessing the viral load of HIV and monitoring the CD4 count. Management of complicating respiratory conditions is discussed in Chapter 18.

**Table 23.3** CD4 count and respiratory presentations in HIV infection

| CD4 count | Respiratory conditions in HIV infection |
|---|---|
| <500 cells/μL | Recurrent bacterial pneumonia<br>Mycobacterium infections (other than TB) |
| <200 cells/μL | Bacterial pneumonia with bacteraemia<br>*Pneumocystis jirovecii* pneumonia<br>*Cryptococcus neoformans* pneumonitis |
| <100 cells/μL | *Staphylococcus aureus* or *Pseudomonas* pneumonia<br>*Toxoplasma gondii*<br>Kaposi sarcoma with pulmonary involvement |
| <50 cells/μL | Endemic fungi<br>CMV lung disease<br>*Mycobacterium avium*<br>Aspergillus |

*CMV, Cytomegalovirus; TB, tuberculosis.*

## ● Chapter Summary

- Sarcoidosis is a condition of infiltrative noncaseating granulomas which form in multiple organs, with lung involvement in >90% of cases. Typically, hilar lymphadenopathy is a defining characteristic, with diagnosis made on granuloma biopsy.
- Vasculitis is an inflammation of blood vessels that can affect small, medium and large vessels. The three vasculitides most commonly affecting the lung are granulomatosis with polyangiitis, Goodpasture syndrome and eosinophilic granulomatosis with polyangiitis.
- Connective tissue diseases can cause lung pathology, either through the disease process itself or through complications of their treatment.
- Lung involvement of rheumatoid arthritis can involve diffuse pulmonary fibrosis, bronchiolitis obliterans and pleural effusions.
- Human immunodeficiency virus–related lung disease involves atypical infections secondary to immunosuppression and even rare malignancies. Knowledge of the patient's CD4 count can assist in predicting the type of pathology likely to affect the patient, with a greater number of atypical infections occurring the more immunosuppressed the patient is. Several respiratory infections are known as AIDS-defining illnesses.

**MLA Conditions**
Ankylosing spondylitis
HIV
Rheumatoid arthritis
Sarcoidosis
Systemic lupus erythematosus

**MLA Presentations**
Acute joint pain
Acute kidney injury
Anaemia
Breathlessness
Chest pain
Cough
Epistaxis
Fever
Haematuria
Haemoptysis
Lymphadenopathy
Peripheral oedema and ankle swelling
Purpura
Rhinosinusitis
Skin or subcutaneous lump (erythema nodosum)
Uveitis
Weight loss

# SELF-ASSESSMENT

# MLA High Yield Association Table

| Diagnoses (key labs) | Key findings |
|---|---|
| Salbutamol side effects | Fine resting tremor |
| Horner syndrome | Partial ptosis, miosis, anhydrosis, enophthalmos |
| High $CO_2$ retention | Bounding pulse, retention flap |
| Pancoast tumour | Unilateral muscle wasting of hands (particularly T1 distribution), ipsilateral Horner syndrome |
| Systemic sclerosis | Sclerodactyly |
| Rheumatoid arthritis | Swan neck, ulnar deviation, Z thumb, Boutonniere |
| Pectus excavatum | Depressed sternum |
| Pleural effusion | Stony dull percussion note |
| Pneumothorax | Hyperresonant percussion note, trachea central or deviated away |
| Pneumonia | Bronchial breathing |
| Lobar collapse | Dull percussion note, trachea deviated towards affected side |
| Bilateral hilar lymphadenopathy | TB, sarcoidosis, lymphoma |
| Eosinophilic granulomatosis with polyangiitis (EGPA) | Vasculitis (small-medium vessels), asthma, eosinophilia, sinusitis |
| Kartagener's | Sinusitis, bronchiectasis, otitis media, dextrocardia |
| Epiglottitis | Drooling, sudden onset, bacterial – group B *Haemophilus influenzae* |
| Croup | Gradual, barking cough, hoarse voice, viral – RSV/parainfluenza |
| Asthma | Variable symptoms, diurnal variation in $FEV_1$, wheeze, cough, eosinophilia |
| Allergic bronchopulmonary aspergillosis | Positive IgE and IgG precipitants to *Aspergillus fumigatus*, bronchiectasis, eosinophilia |
| Moderate asthma exacerbation | >50% of predicted peak flow, able to complete sentences |
| Severe asthma exacerbation | 33%–50% of predicted peak flow, unable to complete sentences in one breath, RR $\geq25$, HR $\geq110$ |
| Life-threatening asthma exacerbation | <33% of predicted peak flow, unable to speak, $P_aO_2$ <8 kPa, $P_aCO_2$ normal or raised, silent chest |
| COPD | Persistent airflow limitation from airway +/– alveolar abnormalities due to noxious particles/gases |
| Cor pulmonale | Right ventricular failure secondary to disorders affecting the lung (peripheral oedema, raised JVP, tricuspid regurgitation, right ventricular heave) |
| Centrilobular emphysema | Septal destruction and dilatation limited to centre of acinus and terminal bronchiole (upper lobe dominant) |
| Panlobular emphysema | Destruction of acinus distal to terminal bronchioles (lower lobe dominant) |
| Systemic sclerosis | Raynaud disease, dysphagia |
| Sarcoidosis | Erythema nodosum, bilateral hilar lymphadenopathy |
| Dermatomyositis | Gottron's papules |

*Continued*

| Diagnoses (key labs) | Key findings |
| --- | --- |
| Hypersensitivity pneumonitis | Immunological reaction caused by inhalation of an antigen (acute, chronic, subacute) |
| Bird fancier's lung | Bird feathers/droppings, causative antigens: bird proteins |
| Farmer's lung | Mouldy hay, grain, causative antigens: thermophilic actinomycete, *Aspergillus* species |
| Silicosis | Sandblasting stoneworkers, quarry workers |
| Acute/chronic berylliosis | Miners, electrical equipment manufacturers |
| Siderosis | Welders |
| Caplan syndrome | Coal workers pneumoconiosis, seropositive rheumatoid arthritis, cavitating lesions on CXR |
| Asbestos | Serpentine fibres (white asbestos), amphibole fibres – crocidolite (blue asbestos) |
| Asbestosis | Clubbing, bi-basal late inspiratory crackles, pleural plaques, honeycombing on HRCT |
| Interstitial lung disease | HRCT – UIP (usual interstitial pneumonitis) pattern, NSIP (nonspecific usual interstitial pneumonitis) pattern |
| Small cell carcinoma | Usually located close to the hilar, neuroendocrine tumour – paraneoplastic syndrome (ACTH, SIADH, calcitonin), rapid spread |
| Squamous cell carcinoma | Pancoast's tumour, cavitation, hypercalcaemia |
| Adenocarcinoma | Usually located in lung periphery, metastasize late, EGFR mutations for targeted treatment |
| Carcinoid | Rare, facial flushing, diarrhoea, wheeze, palpitations, majority arise in the GI system and <5% are bronchial tumours |
| Hoarse voice | Mediastinal node compression or tumour invasion on recurrent laryngeal nerve |
| Superior vena cava obstruction | Headache, breathlessness, swollen oedematous face and upper limbs, venous congestion in neck (Sx exaggerated by lying down/bending over) |
| SIADH | Low total body sodium, low serum osmolality, high serum osmolality |
| Legionella | Multisystem disease, abnormal liver enzymes, travel (Mediterranean), hyponatraemia, gram-negative bacillus, dry cough |
| *Mycoplasma pneumonia* | Erythema multiforme, haemolysis, hepatitis, cold agglutinins (blood slightly precipitates in cold temp), dry cough |
| *Chlamydophila psittaci* pneumonia | Zoonotic infections commonly from parrots, fevers, joint pain, nose bleeds |
| *Coxiella burnetii* pneumonia | Zoonotic infections commonly from sheep/goats, 'Q fever' – fever, myalgia, headache, hepatitis |
| TB | Cavitating lung disease (upper lobe predominant), hilar lymphadenopathy, pleural effusion, miliary TB (disseminated small nodules) |
| Extrapulmonary TB | Erythema nodosum, spinal TB, meningitis, SOL |
| Influenza | High fever, dry cough, myalgia, URTI |
| Aspergilloma | Aspergillosis, fungal hyphae ball in lung cavity, often asymptomatic or present with haemoptysis |
| Invasive aspergillosis | Immunocompromised (neutropenic), cough, fever, haemoptysis |
| *Pneumocystis jirovecii* | Immunosuppressed (HIV with CD4 <200), steroid use, recent chemotherapy, hypoxia and desaturation on exercise |
| Kartagener syndrome triad | Primary ciliary dyskinesia (PCD), dextrocardia and situs inversus |
| Young syndrome triad | Bronchiectasis, sinusitis and azoospermia (causing infertility) |
| CT findings of bronchiectasis | Signet ring sign, Tram track sign, Bunch of grapes sign |

| Diagnoses (key labs) | Key findings |
|---|---|
| Childhood symptoms of cystic fibrosis | Failure to thrive, meconium ileus, cough and recurrent chest infections |
| Light's criteria for an exudative effusion | Fluid/serum protein ratio >0.5, fluid/serum lactate dehydrogenase ratio >0.6, fluid lactate dehydrogenase >two-thirds the upper limit of normal serum |
| Chest drain insertion | Safety triangle (the lateral border of pectoralis major, the 5th intercostal space [roughly the level of the nipple] and the anterior border of latissimus dorsi) |
| Obesity hypoventilation syndrome | BMI >30, daytime $P_aCO_2$ >45 mmHg/6 kPa, sleep-disordered breathing, absence of other causes of hypoventilation |
| Goodpasture syndrome | Haemoptysis, glomerulonephritis and acute renal failure |
| Granulomatosis with polyangiitis | Affects upper airways (epistaxis), lower airways (haemoptysis) and kidneys (glomerulonephritis) |
| Eosinophilic granulomatosis with polyangiitis | Stage one: late-onset asthma, allergic rhinitis<br>Stage two: eosinophilic pulmonary infiltrates<br>Stage 3: small vessel vasculitis; associated with ANCA positivity |

# MLA Single Best Answer (SBA) Questions

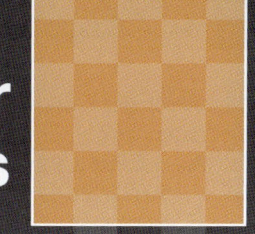

## Chapter 1  Overview of the respiratory system

1. Which of the following is a *restrictive* lung disorder?
   A. Asthma.
   B. Chronic bronchitis.
   C. Pulmonary fibrosis.
   D. Chronic obstructive pulmonary disease (COPD).
   E. Bronchiectasis.

2. Which of these abbreviations represents the partial pressure of alveolar oxygen tension?
   A. $PO_2$.
   B. $P_aO_2$.
   C. $P_vO_2$.
   D. $P_AO_2$.
   E. $P_aCO_2$.

3. Which of these terms describes the movement of air in and out of the respiratory system?
   A. Diffusion.
   B. Expiration.
   C. Tidal volume.
   D. Obstructive disorder.
   E. Ventilation.

4. Which of the following is an obstructive lung disorder?
   A. Pneumonia.
   B. Pleural effusion.
   C. Pulmonary fibrosis
   D. COPD.
   E. Sarcoidosis.

## Chapter 2  Organization of the respiratory tract

5. Which of the following is true of the larynx?
   A. It is a structure discontinuous with the trachea.
   B. It protects the trachea and bronchi during swallowing.
   C. It contains multiple external muscles.
   D. It is innervated by the pharyngeal plexus.
   E. It is unimportant in phonation.

6. The hilum of the lung contains which of the following?
   A. The vagus nerve.
   B. The pulmonary ligament.
   C. The recurrent laryngeal nerve.

   D. Mucosa-associated lymphoid tissue (MALT).
   E. The bronchial circulation.

7. Which of the following is true of the nasal cavity?
   A. It contains Clara cells.
   B. It is lined with columnar epithelium in the upper region.
   C. It is important in gas exchange.
   D. It is covered in olfactory epithelium in the lower region.
   E. It is important in defence against infection.

8. Which of the following is true of the lower respiratory tract?
   A. The trachea is encircled by rings of cartilage.
   B. The left main bronchus is more acutely angled than the right.
   C. Both type I and type II pneumocytes exist.
   D. It contains respiratory bronchioles where the majority of gas exchange occurs.
   E. It lacks mucosa-associated lymphoid tissue (MALT).

9. Which of the following is true of alveolar macrophages?
   A. They are neutrophil-derived blood cells.
   B. They circulate in the blood in macrophage form.
   C. They phagocytose foreign material.
   D. They are a prominent physical defence against infection.
   E. They exist mainly outside the respiratory zone.

10. Which of the following comments about the respiratory tree is most accurate?
    A. The main bronchi turn to segmental bronchi at the carina.
    B. Bronchioles contain no cartilage in their walls.
    C. There are approximately 12–14 divisions of the respiratory tree.
    D. Three main airway zones are described.
    E. Approximately 500 mL of the respiratory tree by volume is described as anatomical dead space in a 75-kg man.

11. Which of the following is true about physical airway defences?
    A. S-fibres are the main irritant airway receptor stimulated by infective material.
    B. Filtering of air by the nasopharynx removes fine particulate matter from inspired air.
    C. Coughing involves a high-velocity expiration against a closed glottis.
    D. Mucociliary clearance removes the majority of large particulate matter.
    E. Cilia beat at around 10,000 strokes per minute.

12. The components of cellular and humoral lung defences include which of the following?
    A. A predominance of IgG antibody.
    B. Surfactant produced by type I pneumocytes.
    C. A predominant basophilic response to bacterial infection.
    D. Filtration of air by the nasopharynx.
    E. Antiproteases, including hepatic $\alpha_1$-antitrypsin

## Chapter 3 Pulmonary circulation

13. Which of the following best describes the pulmonary circulation?
    A. A high-pressure, high-resistance system.
    B. A high-pressure, low-resistance system.
    C. A low-pressure, high-resistance system.
    D. A low-pressure, low-resistance system.
    E. A negative-pressure, low-resistance system.

14. Which one of the following statements is true?
    A. Blood vessels at the lung bases are subjected to a lower hydrostatic pressure than those at the apices.
    B. Blood flow is greater at the apices of the lungs.
    C. Blood flow is greater at the bases of the lungs.
    D. The pressure in the pulmonary circulation is normally equal to that of the systemic circulation.
    E. The pressure in the pulmonary circulation is normally greater than that of the systemic circulation.

15. An 80-year-old woman with severe pneumonia and extensive consolidation of the right lung desaturates whenever nurses turn her on to her right side. Why is this?
    A. Increased ventilation of the right lung increasing ventilation:perfusion mismatch.
    B. Reduced ventilation of the right lung reducing ventilation:perfusion mismatch.
    C. Reduced blood flow to the right lung increasing ventilation:perfusion mismatch.
    D. Increased blood flow to the right lung increasing ventilation:perfusion mismatch.
    E. Increased blood flow to the right lung reducing ventilation:perfusion mismatch.

## Chapter 4 Physiology, ventilation and gas exchange

16. The functional residual capacity (FRC) is defined as which of the following?
    A. Volume of air remaining in lungs at the end of a normal expiration.
    B. Volume of air that can be breathed in by a maximum inspiration following a maximum expiration.
    C. Volume of air remaining in lungs at the end of a maximum expiration.
    D. Volume of air that can be expelled by a maximum effort at the end of a normal expiration.
    E. Volume of air breathed in by a maximum inspiration at the end of a normal expiration.

17. A patient with chronic obstructive pulmonary disease (COPD) has become increasingly breathless and tachypnoeic over the past 6 months. On examination, the patient is hyperexpanded and has a barrel chest. Which of the following answers best accounts for these findings?
    A. Increased functional residual capacity.
    B. Increased inspiratory capacity.
    C. Increased tidal volumes.
    D. Increased residual volume.
    E. Reduced inspiratory capacity.

18. An elderly man attends the outpatient clinic complaining of breathlessness on exertion and weight loss. On examination, he has clubbing, is cyanosed and has fine inspiratory crackles. The patient is sent for spirometry. Which of the following is most likely?
    A. Reduced forced expiratory volume in 1 second ($FEV_1$) and normal forced vital capacity (FVC).
    B. Reduced $FEV_1$ and FVC.
    C. Normal $FEV_1$ and reduced FVC.
    D. Normal $FEV_1$ and FVC.
    E. Increased $FEV_1$ and FVC.

19. Tidal volume can be defined as which of the following?
    A. The volume of air remaining in the lungs following maximal expiration.
    B. The volume of air that can be breathed following maximal expiration.
    C. The volume of air breathed in and out in a single normal breath.
    D. The volume of air that can be expelled by a maximal effort at the end of normal expiration.
    E. The volume of air remaining at the end of normal expiration.

## Chapter 5  Perfusion and gas transport

20. Which of the following is true of the ventilation:perfusion ($V$:$Q$) ratio?
    A. Ventilation increases towards the apex of the lung.
    B. Perfusion decreases towards the base of the lung.
    C. VA/Q is dependent on lung volume and posture.
    D. VA/Q is uniform throughout the lung in the healthy patient.
    E. Perfusion is increased to those areas of the lung that are underventilated.

21. Which of the following best describes gas transport in the blood?
    A. Once oxygen is bound to the haem group of haemoglobin, the ferrous ($Fe2+$) ion changes to the ferric state ($Fe3+$).
    B. Myoglobin has a lower affinity for oxygen than haemoglobin A.
    C. Carbon dioxide and oxygen have similar diffusing capacity in the lung.
    D. During exercise an individual will hyperventilate in order to blow off carbon dioxide.
    E. Increase in carbon dioxide and decrease in pH enhance dissociation of oxygen from oxyhaemoglobin.

22. A 50-year-old gentleman presented to the GP with dyspnoea and a productive chronic cough of clear phlegm. He also has a 30-pack-year history of smoking. An ABG performed on room air shows pH 7.41; $PO_2$ 12.5 kPa; $PCO_2$ 6.3 kPa; $C[HCO_3^-]$ 35 mmol/L. What does this ABG show?
    A. Compensated respiratory acidosis.
    B. Compensated respiratory alkalosis.
    C. Compensated metabolic acidosis.
    D. Compensated metabolic alkalosis.
    E. Respiratory acidosis.

## Chapter 6  Control of respiratory function

23. Which of these factors do not affect ventilator response to $P_aCO_2$?
    A. $PaO2$.
    B. Psychiatric state.
    C. Genetics.
    D. Pulmonary disease.
    E. Fitness.

24. With regards to respiratory regulation, where do peripheral chemoreceptors typically lie?
    A. Alveoli.
    B. Carotid sinus and aortic arch.
    C. Brainstem.
    D. Cerebral cortex.
    E. Laryngopharynx.

25. Which of the following, when stimulated, induces bradycardia and hypotension?
    A. Chemoreceptors.
    B. C-fibres.
    C. Rapidly adapting receptors.
    D. Pontine neurones.
    E. Carotid bodies.

26. What are carotid bodies?
    A. Neurones
    B. Location of the Bötzinger complex
    C. Chemoreceptors
    D. Where peripheral chemoreceptors are located
    E. Slowly adapting receptors

## Chapter 7  Basic pharmacology

27. Which of the following regarding salbutamol is correct?
    A. It is used predominantly in the treatment of allergic rhinitis.
    B. It has a short duration of action.
    C. It exerts its action via $\beta1$-receptors.
    D. It is highly receptor specific.
    E. It commonly causes a bradycardic response.

28. Which of the following statements on formoterol is correct?
    A. It is a partial receptor agonist.
    B. It is a full receptor agonist.
    C. It has near identical pharmacokinetics to salmeterol.
    D. It is unsuitable for use in single maintenance and reliever therapy (MART).
    E. It causes a greater change in heart rate than salmeterol.

29. Which of the following makes the use of theophyllines challenging?
    A. They exert effects in a similar manner to $\beta2$-agonists.
    B. Both oral and intravenous formulations exist.
    C. Hepatic enzyme activity varies markedly between patients.
    D. Their complete mechanism of action is not understood.
    E. They are only useful in severe asthma attacks.

30. Which of the following therapies are not used to aid smoking cessation?
    A. Varenicline
    B. Bupropion.
    C. Nicotine replacement therapy.
    D. Chlordiazepoxide.
    E. Motivational interviewing.

## Chapter 8  Taking a respiratory history

31. A 50-year-old male presents with a chronic dry cough for 3 months. He is a nonsmoker and has a past medical history of ischaemic heart disease. Which of the following medication is the most likely potential cause?
    A. Statin.
    B. β-blocker.
    C. Sildenafil.
    D. Angiotensin-converting enzyme (ACE) inhibitor.
    E. Aspirin.

32. A patient with severe chronic obstructive pulmonary disease (COPD) attends a respiratory clinic complaining of bilateral ankle swelling. Which complication of COPD does this symptom suggest?
    A. Deep vein thrombosis (DVT).
    B. Cor pulmonale.
    C. Bronchial carcinoma.
    D. Tuberculosis.
    E. *Pseudomonas* colonization.

33. A 27-year-old man presents with a 5-month history of purulent sputum. He has never smoked and tells you that he had whooping cough as a child. What is the most likely diagnosis?
    A. Asthma.
    B. Bronchiectasis.
    C. Cystic fibrosis.
    D. COPD.
    E. Pulmonary embolism.

## Chapter 9  Examination of the respiratory system

34. A 60-year-old woman with a new diagnosis of metastatic breast cancer attends the A&E unit with a 4-day history of increasing shortness of breath. On examination, there is markedly reduced chest expansion on the left side with stony dull percussion and absent breath sounds at the left base. Vocal resonance is reduced at the left base. What is the most likely diagnosis?
    A. Pleural effusion.
    B. Lung collapse.
    C. Lung fibrosis.
    D. Consolidation.
    E. Pneumothorax.

35. Which of the following best describes the four typical characteristics of Horner syndrome?
    A. Unilateral ptosis, mydriasis, anhidrosis, exophthalmos.
    B. Unilateral ptosis, mydriasis, anhidrosis, enophthalmos.
    C. Bilateral ptosis, miosis, anhidrosis, exophthalmos.
    D. Unilateral ptosis, miosis, anhidrosis, enophthalmos.
    E. Neck engorgement, cyanosis, facial swelling, arm swelling.

36. Which of the following is NOT a respiratory cause of clubbing?
    A. Cystic fibrosis.
    B. COPD.
    C. Lung cancer.
    D. Empyema.
    E. Bronchiectasis.

37. A 73-year-old gentleman has been diagnosed with a left lower zone CAP in the A&E department. Given that his chest X-ray shows only left lower zone consolidation, which of the following would you expect to find on examination of his chest?
    A. Increased breath sounds (bronchial).
    B. Hyperresonant percussion note.
    C. Tracheal deviation.
    D. Decreased tactile fremitus.
    E. Reduced breath sounds.

## Chapter 10  The respiratory patient: clinical investigations

38. What is a normal value for peak expiratory flow rate (PEFR) in a healthy adult?
    A. 50–150 L/min.
    B. 150–250 L/min.
    C. 250–350 L/min.
    D. 350–450 L/min.
    E. 450–600 L/min.

39. Which of these tests assesses breathlessness by asking the patient to walk a 10-metre distance during increasingly short time intervals?
    A. Six-minute walk test.
    B. Exercise electrocardiograph.
    C. Shuttle test.
    D. Cardiopulmonary exercise testing.
    E. Sit-to-stand test.

40. Which of the following tests is useful to provide information about diurnal variation that could aid an asthma diagnosis?
    A. Peak flow diary.
    B. Body plethysmography.
    C. Spirometry.
    D. Fraction of exhaled nitric oxide.
    E. Bronchial challenge test.

# Chapter 11 The respiratory patient: imaging investigations

41. A 60-year-old smoker with a 6-week history of a nonproductive cough, weight loss and a single episode of haemoptysis has a chest radiograph performed that demonstrates a 4-cm mass at the right hilum, when he comes to see you in clinic. What is the next most appropriate investigation in this patient's management?
    A. Repeat the chest radiograph in 6 weeks to assess for resolution.
    B. Order a high-resolution computed tomography (CT) chest scan.
    C. Order a chest magnetic resonance image (MRI).
    D. Perform bronchoscopy.
    E. Order a CT chest and abdomen with liver and adrenal views.

42. You see a 40-year-old female presenting with acute shortness of breath following a recent long-haul flight. She is tachypnoeic, requiring 40% oxygen to maintain saturations. Which of these is the most appropriate initial imaging investigation for the patient?
    A. Erect chest radiograph.
    B. Chest ultrasound.
    C. Computed tomography pulmonary angiogram (CTPA).
    D. Ventilation/perfusion (V/Q) scan.
    E. High-resolution CT.

43. A 30-year-old man presents with a 1-week history of pleuritic chest pain, high temperatures and raised inflammatory markers. A plain chest radiograph shows a left-sided pleural effusion. Which of the following is the investigation of choice for a suspected empyema?
    A. High-resolution CT chest.
    B. MRI chest.
    C. Lateral chest X-ray.
    D. Thoracic ultrasound.
    E. Positron emission tomography (PET) scan.

# Chapter 12 Acute respiratory failure

44. Which of these is not a typical management strategy for airway obstruction?
    A. Head tilt and chin lift.
    B. Laryngeal mask airway.
    C. Nasopharyngeal airway.
    D. Thyroidectomy.
    E. Jaw thrust.

45. Which of the following oxygen delivery devices is most appropriate to use in the initial assessment of a severe asthma attack?
    A. Nasal oxygen.
    B. Nonrebreather reservoir mask.
    C. Venturi mask.
    D. Continuous positive airway pressure (CPAP).
    E. Noninvasive ventilation (NIV).

46. An arterial blood gas (ABG) reading was taken from a patient with an infective exacerbation of chronic obstructive pulmonary disease (COPD) on air. The ABG analysis gives the following readings:

| Parameter | Reading | Normal range |
|---|---|---|
| pH | 7.28 | 7.35–7.45 |
| $pO_2$ | 7.4 | 10–14 kPa |
| $pCO_2$ | 9.3 | 4.5–6 kPa |
| $HCO_3$ | 38 | 22–26 mmol/L |

Which of the following options best describes this ABG result?
    A. Respiratory alkalosis with metabolic compensation.
    B. Decompensated metabolic acidosis.
    C. Type I respiratory failure with a compensated metabolic acidosis.
    D. Type II respiratory failure with a decompensated respiratory acidosis.
    E. Type II respiratory failure with a fully compensated respiratory acidosis.

47. An arterial blood gas (ABG) reading was taken from a patient with a severe pneumonia requiring 35% oxygen. The ABG analysis gives the following readings:

| Parameter | Reading | Normal range |
|---|---|---|
| pH | 7.30 | 7.35–7.45 |
| $pO_2$ | 9.6 | 10–14 kPa |
| $pCO_2$ | 3.0 | 4.5–6 kPa |
| $HCO_3$ | 18 | 22–26 mmol/L |

Which of these phrases below best describes the ABG result?
    A. Respiratory acidosis.
    B. Respiratory alkalosis.
    C. Metabolic acidosis.
    D. Metabolic alkalosis.
    E. Respiratory alkalosis with metabolic compensation.

48. Which of the following is a common complication of invasive mechanical ventilation?
    A. Pulmonary embolism.
    B. Diaphragm paralysis.
    C. Ventilator-associated pneumonia.
    D. Confusion.
    E. Obstructive sleep apnoea.

## Chapter 13 The upper respiratory tract

49. An anxious mother brings her 2-year-old son to the GP surgery with a 3-day history of cough and fevers. The child's cough is particularly bad at night and as a result he has not been sleeping. On examination, the child is irritable and has a characteristic barking cough. What is the most likely diagnosis?
    A. Asthma.
    B. Epiglottitis.
    C. Croup.
    D. Bronchiolitis.
    E. Viral-induced wheeze.

50. Which of the following is the appropriate dose of adrenaline to give in adult anaphylaxis?
    A. 0.5 mL of 1:1000 intravenous (IV) adrenaline.
    B. 0.5 mL of 1:10,000 IV adrenaline.
    C. 1 mL of 1:1000 intramuscular (IM) adrenaline.
    D. 0.5 mL of 1:1000 IM adrenaline.
    E. 1 mL of 1:1000 IV adrenaline.

51. Which of the following organisms is a typical cause for epiglottis?
    A. *Haemophilus influenza.*
    B. *Streptococcus pneumonia.*
    C. *Staphylococcus aureus.*
    D. *Escherichia coli.*
    E. *Clostridioides difficile.*

## Chapter 14 Asthma

52. You are working as junior doctor in a GP surgery when an 18-year-old young woman presents with an intermittently tight chest. Symptoms come on while she is playing football. Respiratory and cardiovascular examinations are normal. A peak expiratory flow rate diary shows diurnal variation. Which of these symptoms would prompt you to investigate for an alternative diagnosis?
    A. Wheeze.
    B. Chest tightness.
    C. Cough.
    D. Breathlessness.
    E. Weight loss.

53. Which of these is not a symptom of life-threatening acute asthma?
    A. Peak expiratory flow rate (PEFR) of 45% predicted.
    B. $P_aO_2$ <8 kPa.
    C. Silent chest.
    D. Confusion.
    E. Bradycardia.

54. Which of the following is NOT consistent with a diagnosis of asthma in adults?
    A. Nocturnal coughing.
    B. An improvement in FEV1 of 8% after bronchodilator administration.
    C. FeNO of 50 ppb.
    D. Raised eosinophils.
    E. An improvement in $FEV_1$ of 20% after bronchodilator administration.

55. Which of the following should be done when a patient presents to A&E/hospital with an asthma attack?
    A. Give prednisolone 40 mg orally for at least 5 days.
    B. Give prednisolone 30 mg orally for at least 5 days.
    C. Inform the GP of the asthma attack within 24 hours of discharge.
    D. Options A and C.
    E. Options B and C.

## Chapter 15 Chronic obstructive pulmonary disease

56. A 75-year-old man with a 50-pack-year smoking history attends the GP surgery complaining of shortness of breath and a productive cough every day for the past 6 months. Which of the following investigations would be most helpful in making a diagnosis of chronic obstructive pulmonary disease (COPD)?
    A. Erect chest radiograph.
    B. Spirometry.
    C. Echocardiogram.
    D. Full blood count.
    E. Sputum culture.

57. A 70-year-old woman has been admitted to hospital with an acute exacerbation of chronic obstructive pulmonary disease (COPD). She is managed with 35% oxygen on facemask, nebulized bronchodilators, antibiotics and steroids. The patient develops type II respiratory failure and her most recent blood gas demonstrates pH 7.18, $PO_2$ 7.9 kPa and $PCO_2$ 11 kPa. What is the most appropriate next management step?
    A. Give 15 L oxygen through a nonrebreather mask.
    B. Reduce the level of oxygen.
    C. Refer to intensive care.
    D. Start patient on noninvasive ventilation (NIV) (bilevel positive airway pressure).
    E. Increase the dose of steroids.

58. What is the most cost-effective management in COPD?
    A. Starting on combination inhaled therapy.
    B. Smoking cessation.
    C. Influenza vaccination.
    D. Pulmonary rehabilitation.
    E. Oral steroids.

## Chapter 16 Disorders of the interstitium

59. Which of these is not a commonly recognized cause of hypersensitivity pneumonitis?
    A. Bird proteins.
    B. Mushroom spores.
    C. Asbestos.
    D. Mouldy hay.
    E. Sugar cane fibres.

60. A 70-year-old male nonsmoker presents to clinic with a 1-year history of breathlessness on exertion and a dry cough. He is clubbed and on chest auscultation he has bilateral fine inspiratory crackles. Which of the following investigation results would most support a diagnosis of idiopathic pulmonary fibrosis (IPF)?
    A. A high-resolution computed tomography (HRCT) scan with bilateral honeycomb change.
    B. An obstructive pattern on spirometry.
    C. A chest radiograph showing cardiomegaly and pulmonary oedema.
    D. A raised white cell count (WBC) and C-reactive protein (CRP) level on blood tests.
    E. An HRCT with consolidation and collapse of the right lower lobe.

61. Which of the following conditions is a disease seen in coal miners that causes symptoms of a productive cough and breathlessness?
    A. Simple pneumoconiosis.
    B. Sarcoidosis.
    C. Silicosis.
    D. Progressive massive fibrosis.
    E. Asbestosis.

## Chapter 17 Lung cancer

62. To which sites would you typically expect bronchial carcinomas to metastasize?
    A. Bone, brain, skin, thyroid, bowel.
    B. Bone, breast, adrenals, skin, bowel.
    C. Liver, bone, brain, adrenals, skin.
    D. Liver, breast, bone, kidney, thyroid.
    E. Liver, breast, brain, bone, bowel.

63. A squamous cell lung tumour is described as stage T2 N1 M0 by the tumour, node, metastasis (TNM) staging system. Which of these descriptions best fits this staging?
    A. A single 5-cm right-sided apical lung tumour with spread to contralateral hilar lymph nodes.
    B. A solitary 4-cm left-sided hilar lung tumour with involvement of two ipsilateral hilar lymph nodes but no distal metastases.
    C. Multiple lung masses seen throughout both lungs with a large mass seen in the right breast.
    D. A solitary peripheral 3-cm lung mass which has invaded into the pleural space. Five ipsilateral lymph nodes are seen and there are multiple nodular deposits in the liver.
    E. A single 5-mm peripheral lung mass is seen in the left lung with no nodal or metastatic disease seen.

64. A 62-year-old man is referred with a 3-month history of persistent dry cough, weight loss and anorexia. He is a lifelong smoker of 20 cigarettes/day and has recently returned from a week-long holiday in Spain. His wife has recently been diagnosed with Cushing disease. His chest X-ray shows a solitary 4-cm round mass near his right hilum. Routine blood tests, including full blood count, and renal function, observations and examination are otherwise unremarkable. Which of these is the most appropriate next investigative step?
    A. Request a lateral chest X-ray.
    B. Measure his 9.00 am cortisol level.
    C. Perform a Mantoux test.
    D. Arrange a staging computed tomography (CT) chest scan including the neck, liver and adrenals.
    E. Arrange for a high-resolution CT scan of the chest and start a course of oral steroids.

65. A 58-year-old woman with known small-cell lung cancer presents to the A&E department with severe headaches, facial swelling and breathlessness. She completed a course of chemotherapy 2 months ago and missed her last two follow-up appointments. On examination, she has a swollen, flushed face with venous engorgement of her neck. Which are the next most appropriate management steps?
    A. Give intramuscular (IM) adrenaline, intravenous (IV) hydrocortisone and antihistamines.
    B. Give her subcutaneous morphine and wait for her symptoms to settle.
    C. Arrange an urgent computed tomography (CT) scan of the chest and consider oral dexamethasone.
    D. Discharge her with paracetamol for her headaches.
    E. Start IV antibiotics and perform a set of blood cultures.

66. Which of the following statements is true?
    A. Small-cell lung cancer is the commonest form of lung cancer.
    B. All patients with lung cancer have haemoptysis.
    C. Finger clubbing is specific to lung cancer.
    D. Spinal cord compression is an example of a paraneoplastic syndrome.
    E. Stopping smoking improves life expectancy even after lung cancer diagnosis.

67. An 80-year-old lung cancer patient who has previously refused treatment presented with nausea, vomiting, tiredness, confusion and constipation. He is dehydrated and has a short QT interval on ECG. Which of the following complications of lung cancer does he have?
    A. Syndrome of inappropriate ADH secretion.
    B. Hypercalcaemia.
    C. Ectopic ACTH production.
    D. Pancoast tumour.
    E. Brain metastasis.

## Chapter 18 Respiratory infections

68. Which of the following is the most common causative organism in community-acquired pneumonia?
    A. *Staph*ylococcus aureus.
    B. Klebsiella pneumoniae.
    C. Streptococcus pneumoniae.
    D. Moraxella catarrhalis.
    E. Haemo*philus influenzae.*

69. A 75-year-old man with chronic obstructive pulmonary disease (COPD) is admitted to hospital following 1 week of flu-like symptoms. Over the past 2 days, he has developed a productive cough, fevers and progressive dyspnoea. Sequential chest X-rays show a rapidly progressive left-sided consolidation with evidence of cavitation. What is the most likely causative organism?
    A. *Staph*ylococcus aureus.
    B. Klebsiella pneumoniae.
    C. Streptococcus pneumoniae.
    D. Moraxella catarrhalis.
    E. Haemo*philus influenzae.*

70. A 25-year-old male is admitted to the A&E department with a dry cough and worsening dyspnoea over several weeks. He appears very cachectic and discloses that 6 months ago he was diagnosed with HIV infection but he has not attended any clinic appointments. What is the most likely causative organism?

A. *Moraxella catarrhalis.*
B. *Pneumocystis jirovecii.*
C. *Aspergillus fumigatus.*
D. Cytomegalovirus.
E. Influenza A.

71. Which stain is used to diagnose TB?
    A. Congo red.
    B. Haematoxylin.
    C. Eosin.
    D. Ziehl–Neelsen.
    E. Lugol's iodine.

72. Which of the following treatments is NOT used for COVID-19?
    A. Steroids.
    B. Oseltamivir.
    C. Tocilizumab.
    D. Nirmatrelvir.
    E. Ritonavir.

## Chapter 19 Bronchiectasis and cystic fibrosis

73. Which of these is not an acquired cause of bronchiectasis?
    A. Childhood measles.
    B. Foreign body.
    C. Obstructing tumour.
    D. Cystic fibrosis.
    E. Whooping cough.

74. An 80-year-old female nonsmoker with a history of childhood measles infection presents to the respiratory clinic with a chronic productive cough and recurrent infections over several years. You suspect a diagnosis of bronchiectasis. What would be the most useful diagnostic investigation?
    A. High-resolution computed tomography scan.
    B. Chest radiograph.
    C. Sweat test.
    D. Routine blood tests.
    E. Flexible bronchoscopy.

75. Which of the following is the most common mutation that causes cystic fibrosis?
    A. G551D.
    B. F508del.
    C. G542X.
    D. N1303K.
    E. W1282X.

## Chapter 20 Pleural disease

76. Which of the following is not a recognized cause of pleural effusion?
    A. Hepatic failure.
    B. Chronic kidney disease.
    C. Malnourishment.
    D. Leukaemia.
    E. Hypocalcaemia.

77. A 67-year-old smoker presenting with weight loss and malaise is found to have a unilateral pleural effusion on chest X-ray. A diagnostic tap drains bloody fluid. What is the most likely diagnosis?
    A. Bronchial carcinoma.
    B. Hepatitis C.
    C. Bronchiectasis.
    D. Cardiac failure.
    E. Sarcoidosis.

78. A 40-year-old male is brought into the A&E unit following a road traffic accident. He has sustained a chest wall injury and is in acute respiratory distress. ATLS assessment reveals that he is tachypnoeic, hypoxic and hypotensive. Chest examination reveals left-sided hyperresonance with absent breath sounds. What is the next most appropriate step?
    A. Administer high-flow oxygen, take a chest radiograph and arrange analysis of arterial blood gas.
    B. Insert a large bore cannula into the midclavicular line of the left second intercostal space.
    C. Arrange an urgent computed tomography (CT) pulmonary angiogram of the chest.
    D. Insert a chest drain into the left chest using the Seldinger technique under ultrasound guidance.
    E. Perform ultrasound-guided pleural fluid aspiration from the left side of the chest.

79. Which of the following features on pleural aspiration would indicate empyema?
    A. Pleural fluid pH of >7.2.
    B. Pleural fluid protein of 20 g/dL.
    C. Haemorrhagic appearance of pleural fluid.
    D. Pleural fluid microscopy showing no organisms.
    E. Appearance of pus on pleural aspirate.

80. Which of the following is NOT a high-risk characteristic in pneumothorax?
    A. Haemodynamic compromise (tension pneumothorax).
    B. Significant hypoxia.
    C. Unilateral pneumothorax in an otherwise healthy individual.
    D. Underlying lung disease.
    E. ≥50 years of age with significant smoking history.

## Chapter 21 Thromboembolic disease and pulmonary hypertension

81. A 60-year-old man presents to the A&E unit with sudden-onset chest pain, breathlessness and haemoptysis. He also has a 3-day history of a swollen and painful right calf. Given the likely diagnosis causing his breathlessness, which of the following investigations is the gold standard for diagnosis?
    A. D-dimer test.
    B. Computed tomography (CT) pulmonary angiogram.
    C. Pulmonary angiography.
    D. Chest radiograph.
    E. Spirometry.

82. A 25-year-old woman presents with pleuritic pain and breathlessness following a long-haul flight. Chest radiograph is normal. Which of these factors is not taken into account in the Wells scoring system?
    A. Previous pulmonary embolism.
    B. Oral contraceptive pill.
    C. Malignancy.
    D. Haemoptysis.
    E. Evidence of deep vein thrombosis.

83. You are the FY1 on the respiratory ward looking after a patient who has had a recent pulmonary embolism. Your consultant would like to start the patient on anticoagulation with a direct inhibitor of factor X. Which of the following medications would be appropriate to start?
    A. Warfarin.
    B. Rivaroxaban.
    C. Dabigatran.
    D. Enoxaparin.
    E. Unfractionated heparin.

84. Which of the following statements about pulmonary hypertension (PH) is false?
    A. PH is defined as a mean pulmonary artery pressure of >25 mmHg at rest, as assessed by right heart catheterization.
    B. The most common cause of PH in the United Kingdom is pulmonary artery hypertension.
    C. PH is associated with connective tissue disorders such as systemic sclerosis.
    D. Where appropriate, PH may be treated by vasodilators including prostanoids and phosphodiesterase 5 inhibitors.
    E. PH presents insidiously with progressive exertional dyspnoea.

## Chapter 22 Sleep disorders

85. Which of the following are risk factors for the development of obstructive sleep apnoea?
    A. Down syndrome.
    B. Obesity.
    C. Acromegaly.
    D. Amyloidosis.
    E. All of the above.

86. Which of the following is the best treatment for a patient who was diagnosed with severe obstructive sleep apnoea (AHI 35 events/hour) who has no evidence of nocturnal hypoxia?
    A. Continuous positive airway pressure therapy (CPAP).
    B. Noninvasive ventilation (NIV).
    C. Mandibular advancement device.
    D. Lifestyle measures alone.
    E. No treatment required.

87. A 65-year-old man presents to the sleep clinic and is given a diagnosis of mild sleep apnoea (AHI 10 events/hour). He is sleepy in the daytime with an Epworth Sleepiness Score of 20/24. He is a lorry driver. What advice would you give to him regarding driving?
    A. He cannot drive, must inform the DVLA immediately and stop working.
    B. He cannot drive, but he does not have to inform the DVLA for 3 months.
    C. He can continue to drive as he has mild OSA.
    D. He can continue to drive as long as he has built-in breaks.
    E. He can continue to drive but does need to inform the DVLA.

## Chapter 23 Respiratory manifestations of systemic disease

88. Which of these descriptions best matches Lofgren syndrome?
    A. A triad of late-onset asthma, eosinophilia and small vessel vasculitis.
    B. A presentation of sarcoidosis combining hilar lymphadenopathy, erythema nodosum, joint symptoms and fever.
    C. A variant of Guillain–Barré syndrome, comprising ophthalmoplegia, ataxia and hyporeflexia.
    D. A combination of rheumatoid arthritis and pneumoconiosis, with well-defined pulmonary nodules on chest radiography.
    E. A combination of rheumatoid arthritis, neutropenia and splenomegaly.

89. Which of these rheumatological conditions classically causes apical lung fibrosis?
    A. Rheumatoid arthritis.
    B. Systemic sclerosis.
    C. Systemic lupus erythematosus.
    D. Sjögren syndrome.
    E. Ankylosing spondylitis.

90. Which condition presents with late-onset asthma and eosinophilia?
    A. Rheumatoid arthritis.
    B. Granulomatosis with polyangiitis.
    C. Eosinophilic granulomatosis with polyangiitis (EGPA).
    D. Goodpasture syndrome.
    E. Systemic lupus erythematosus.

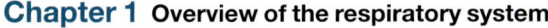

## Chapter 1 Overview of the respiratory system

1. C. Pulmonary fibrosis. While bronchiectasis and COPD can demonstrate restrictive components in certain instances, pulmonary fibrosis is the only restrictive disease available. The change to the lung tissue restricts adequate lung expansion. All other options are primarily obstructive conditions.
2. D. $P_AO_2$ represents the partial pressure of alveolar oxygen tension. The large 'A' represents *a*lveolar while the small 'a' represents *a*rterial; 'v' represents venous and carbon dioxide is represented in the same format.
3. E. Ventilation is defined as the movement of air in and out of the respiratory tract.
4. D. COPD is an obstructive lung disease while sarcoidosis and pulmonary fibrosis are both sometimes associated with traction bronchiectasis, they are largely restrictive lung diseases.

## Chapter 2 Organization of the respiratory tract

5. B. The larynx is continuous with the trachea, and moves back during swallowing to cover the trachea and direct food down the oesophagus, preventing aspiration. The larynx has one external muscle, the cricothyroid, and multiple internal muscles. Innervation is from the vagus nerve. It is crucial to phonation (speech).
6. B. The hilum of the lung contains the main bronchi, the pulmonary artery and vein, nerves, lymph nodes and the pulmonary ligament. The bronchial circulation delivers oxygenated blood to the lung parenchyma and does not pass through the hilum.
7. E. The nasal cavity comprises the nose and nasopharynx. The upper third of the nasal cavity is lined with olfactory, and the remainder with columnar, epithelium. It plays no role in gas exchange but is important in warming and humidifying air. Ciliated cells in the lower two-thirds trap particulate matter and prevent it from reaching the lower airways.
8. C. The trachea is surrounded by C-shaped cartilage rings and is not encircled. The right main bronchus is more acute than the left, and, as such, foreign bodies are more likely to lodge here than in the left bronchus. The majority of gas exchange occurs in the alveoli, although exchange does occur in the respiratory bronchioles. MALT is present in the walls of the lower respiratory tract.

9. C. Alveolar macrophages exist predominantly in the alveoli and are derived from circulating monocytes. They are a key cellular defence mechanism and phagocytose bacteria and foreign material.
10. B. Bronchioles are the first point in the tree to contain noncartilaginous walls. The carina describes the division of the trachea into left and right main bronchi. There are more than twenty divisions of the respiratory tree, with two main zones (the conducting zone and respiratory zone). The dead space consists of around 150 mL.
11. D. Large material is predominantly removed by mucociliary clearance, whether in the nasopharynx or lower down the respiratory tract. Cilia waft at approximately 1000 strokes per minute. Irritant C-fibres stimulate the cough reflex.
12. E. Antiproteases are a key humoral lung defence. IgA, not IgG, is the most prevalent antibody and neutrophils, not basophils, are the key cellular response to bacterial infection. Filtration of air is a physical defence. Surfactant is a cellular response but from type II pneumocytes.

## Chapter 3 Pulmonary circulation

13. D. The pulmonary circulation is a low-pressure, low-resistance system.
14. C. In the upright human, lung hydrostatic pressure is greater in the blood vessels that supply the lung bases than those supplying the apices. The greater hydrostatic pressure leads to distension of the capillaries and increased blood flow. Therefore, blood flow is greater at the lung bases compared with the apices.
15. D. Blood flow is gravity dependent. Therefore, when this patient is turned on to her right side, blood flow to the right lung is increased, and because this lung is poorly ventilated owing to extensive consolidation, ventilaton:perfusion mismatch is increased, causing the patient to desaturate.

## Chapter 4 Physiology, ventilation and gas exchange

16. A. The FRC is the volume of air remaining in lungs at the end of a normal expiration.
17. D. Increased residual volume. This occurs due to increased air-trapping which in turn leads to hyperexpansion.

18. B. This patient has symptoms and signs in keeping with pulmonary fibrosis. Such patients usually develop a restrictive lung disorder characterized by a reduced $FEV_1$ and FVC, with a preserved or increased $FEV_1$/FVC ratio.

19. C. Tidal volume is the volume of air that is breathed in and out in a single normal breath.

## Chapter 5 Perfusion and gas transport

20. C. $V_A/Q$ is dependent on lung volume and posture. Changes in posture do alter the $V{:}Q$ ratio. Ventilation and blood flow are decreased at the apices compared with the bases, and thus the $V{:}Q$ is not uniform across the lung, even in health. Perfusion is reduced to underventilated areas of the lung by hypoxic vasoconstriction.

21. E. Increase in carbon dioxide and decrease in pH enhance dissociation of oxygen from oxyhaemoglobin. This enhanced dissociation at high carbon dioxide levels is termed the Bohr effect. The association between oxygen and haemoglobin is not an oxidation; it is an oxygenation. Myoglobin accepts the oxygen molecule from oxyhaemoglobin and temporarily stores it for skeletal muscle. Carbon dioxide has a 20-fold greater diffusing capacity than oxygen. In exercise, there is increase in depth of breathing (hyperpnoea), not hyperventilation.

22. A. To interpret ABGs, start by looking at the pH value. Here, the pH value is normal. Then, by looking at the $CO_2$ levels, you can see this is raised and so there is an element of respiratory acidosis. Finally, looking at the bicarbonate levels, we can see this is also raised and so will compensate for the respiratory acidosis and return the blood pH levels back to normal.

## Chapter 6 Control of respiratory function

23. D. Pulmonary disease. Although this may affect levels of $P_aCO_2$, it does not affect the body's response to it.

24. B. Carotid sinus and aortic arch. The carotid sinus and aortic arch contain the carotid and aortic bodies, respectively, responsible for sensing $P_aO_2$, $P_aCO_2$, pH and temperature. Central chemoreceptors lie in the brainstem on the ventrolateral surface of the medulla. There are multiple different receptors within the lungs themselves, which respond to a variety of stimuli.

25. B. C-fibres, when stimulated, induce bradycardia and hypotension.

26. D. Carotid bodies are the site of peripheral chemoreceptors, which are sensitive to the following parameters: $P_aO_2$, $P_aCO_2$, pH, blood flow and

temperature. Of note, central chemoreceptors are NOT sensitive to $P_aO_2$, they are sensitive to $P_aCO_2$.

## Chapter 7 Basic pharmacology

27. B. It has a short duration of action. Salbutamol is a short-acting $\beta_2$-receptor agonist used to treat lower-airway disease. It has a degree of nonspecific receptor activity, and side effects such as headache, fine tremor and tachycardia result from cross-stimulation of $\beta_1$-receptors.

28. B. It is a full receptor agonist. Formoterol is a full agonist of the $\beta_2$-receptor, unlike salmeterol, which is a partial agonist. For this reason, formoterol can be used in SMART.

29. C. Hepatic enzyme activity varies markedly between patients. Wide variations in enzyme activity and thus breakdown across patient populations lead to varying levels of theophyllines in the blood. This is challenging as theophyllines have a narrow therapeutic window and, as such, therapeutic drug levels in the blood must be checked regularly.

30. D. Chlordiazepoxide. Chlordiazepoxide is a medication used in alcohol withdrawal, not smoking cessation.

## Chapter 8 Taking a respiratory history

31. D. ACE inhibitor. This is a common drug used in patients with hypertension and ischaemic heart disease, which can induce a dry cough as a side effect in around 10% of patients. The patient should be switched to an angiotensin-2 receptor blocker as an alternative agent. None of the other agents listed typically cause a chronic cough.

32. B. Cor pulmonale. This is right-sided heart failure secondary to pulmonary hypertension caused by severe chronic lung disease. Other features include a raised jugular venous pressure and palpable pulsatile liver edge secondary to hepatic congestion. DVT occurs unilaterally and bronchial carcinoma or infection are unlikely to present in this manner.

33. B. Whooping cough as a child is a possible cause of persistently dilated airways which leads to bronchiectasis. Bronchiectasis is characterized by excess mucous production. While cystic fibrosis remains a possibility, he is likely to have presented much earlier. The other diagnoses are far less likely.

## Chapter 9 Examination of the respiratory system

34. A. Pleural effusion. These are the classical features of a pleural effusion, likely malignant in origin. Consolidation may cause dull percussion but you would expect

bronchial breathing on auscultation, while collapse would not give such definitive signs or progressive symptoms. Lung fibrosis would cause fine inspiratory crepitations and pneumothorax would give a hyperresonant percussion note.

35. D. Unilateral ptosis, miosis, anhidrosis and enophthalmos. Remember a small pupil, sunken eyeball, drooping eyelid and no sweating, as the sympathetic innervation to the face is interrupted. Bilateral Horner syndrome is extremely rare. Answer E describes superior vena cava obstruction.

36. B. Remember that COPD is NOT a cause of clubbing and so if a patient with COPD has clubbing, then lung cancer must be excluded.

37. A. Consolidation is the presence of fluid in the alveoli and therefore, as fluid conducts sound better than air, you get increased breath sounds and increased tactile vocal fremitus. Due to the fluid being present, the percussion note is dull and there is no tracheal deviation.

## Chapter 10 The respiratory patient: clinical investigations

38. E. 450–600 L/min. The normal value for a patient's PEFR is altered depending on age, gender and height. The predicted normal for a patient can be calculated from PEFR charts.

39. C. Shuttle test. Spirometry is a lung function test done with the patient at rest. The 6-minute walk test measures the total distance that a patient can walk in a 6-minute time period. Cardiopulmonary exercise testing measures multiple variables during a period of incremental exercise, usually performed on an exercise bike.

40. A. A peak flow diary is very useful when done correctly. Ideally patients should record morning and afternoon/early evening measurements and take the best of three readings. This done over a 2-week period is useful to show evidence of diurnal variation which can be suggestive of asthma.

## Chapter 11 The respiratory patient: imaging investigations

41. E. Order a CT chest and abdomen with liver and adrenal views. The patient has a history in keeping with a lung cancer and a mass seen on chest radiograph. Repeating the radiograph would not add anything. A high-resolution CT chest may miss the mass as slices are taken further apart. MRI at present has no clearly defined role in lung cancer management.

Bronchoscopy may be needed at some stage; however, a CT should be performed first to give accurate guidance for staging and demonstrating the anatomy prior to bronchoscopy. There is enough information to suggest this is lung cancer, and so a staging CT including liver and adrenals at this stage would be appropriate.

42. A. Erect chest radiograph. The history is suggestive of pulmonary embolus, however other diagnoses such as pneumothorax, collapse or infection cannot be completely excluded at this stage. The most appropriate initial investigation therefore is simple chest radiography to exclude alternative causes of breathlessness. Once this has taken place and no other cause of breathlessness is identified (chest radiography is often normal in pulmonary embolism), further imaging should be considered such as CTPA or V/Q scan. This decision should be guided by renal function, pregnancy status, signs of deep vein thrombosis and degree of suspicion for the underlying pathology.

43. D. A thoracic ultrasound is the most sensitive marker for a suspected empyema. Visualizing loculations or septations on ultrasound is highly suggestive of a complex pleural infection that needs drainage. Ultrasound also enables safe pleural drainage to be performed. While a CT chest with pleural phase contrast is helpful, ultrasound is still the investigation of choice.

## Chapter 12 Acute respiratory failure

44. D. Thyroidectomy. A cricothyroidotomy may be an extreme solution to managing a compromised airway, but simply removing their thyroid gland would not help at all.

45. B. Nonrebreather reservoir mask. While A, B and C may all provide adequate oxygenation, in the initial assessment of an acutely unwell patient, the highest readily available oxygen delivery device is recommended, in this case B. Note that CPAP and NIV are not routinely used for asthma management except under specialist use, as invasive ventilation is often preferred.

46. D. Type II respiratory failure with a decompensated respiratory acidosis. This gas demonstrates both a type II respiratory failure AND a decompensated respiratory acidosis. The $pO_2$ demonstrates respiratory failure, with a raised $pCO_2$ confirming type II rather than type I respiratory failure. The patient has an acidosis with a pH of 7.28, which in the context of a raised $pCO_2$ is likely to be a respiratory acidosis. Note that the

serum bicarbonate is raised – suggesting that there has been some previous metabolic compensation. The clinical context of an acute exacerbation of COPD tells you that this is likely an acute decompensation of a chronic type II respiratory failure.

47. C. Metabolic acidosis. A low pH with a low $CO_2$ and a low $HCO_3$ demonstrates a metabolic acidosis. The low $pCO_2$ likely demonstrates an incomplete respiratory compensation. Note the relatively low $pO_2$ with 35% oxygen, demonstrating a likely underlying type I respiratory failure, with a high A-a gradient.

48. C. Ventilator-associated pneumonia is a common complication of mechanical ventilation. While B and D can occur in intubated patients, it is a cause of sedative medication not the actual ventilation.

## Chapter 13 The upper respiratory tract

49. C. Croup. The key features are the night time cough, acute history, fevers and barking nature of the cough. The fact that the child is irritable suggests that they are not significantly compromised.

50. A. 0.5 mL of 1:1000 IM adrenaline. Remember that for anaphylaxis, the recommended dose is now always IM not IV (can be given quickly without waiting for access). As it is IM, the more concentrated 1:1000 dose is given, with 0.5 mL given initially. Something worth learning, just in case.

51. A. *Haemophilus influenza* is the commonest cause for an acute epiglottitis. The incidence has therefore reduced given the rise in the HIB vaccine.

## Chapter 14 Asthma

52. E. Weight loss. Unexplained weight loss should prompt further investigation into alternative diagnoses. Intermittent wheeze, chest tightness, cough and breathless are all typical symptoms associated with asthma.

53. A. PEFR 45% predicted. PEFR during a life-threatening asthma exacerbation is <33% or not recordable. A PEFR of 45% predicted would indicate a moderate asthma exacerbation.

54. B. An improvement in $FEV_1$ >12% and 200 mL after bronchodilator administration is consistent with an asthma diagnosis. A FeNO of 50 ppb is positive in adults. Raised eosinophils and nocturnal coughing are common in asthma.

55. D. Prednisolone 40 mg orally for at least 5 days is given when a patient presents with an asthma attack; note that prednisolone 30 mg is given when a COPD patient presents with an exacerbation. As per BTS guidelines,

if an asthmatic patient presents to A&E or hospital with an acute attack, then the GP must be informed within 24 hours of discharge.

## Chapter 15 Chronic obstructive pulmonary disease

56. B. Spirometry. While all the investigations may be appropriate for this patient, post-bronchodilator spirometry is the gold standard for diagnosis with a forced expiratory volume in 1 second to forced vital capacity ratio of <0.7. Chest radiography is useful to exclude other conditions such as lung cancer, infection or interstitial lung disease; echocardiography may be used if cardiac failure is suspected; full blood count may show active infection or polycythaemia and sputum culture is important to assess for active infection.

57. D. Start patient on NIV (bilevel positive airway pressure). The patient has become acidotic and hypercapnic when managed with controlled oxygen therapy and now requires NIV. If after a trial the patient does not respond or cannot tolerate NIV, then she might need referral to intensive care for invasive ventilation. Giving high-flow oxygen or simply reducing the amount of oxygen (as the patient is already hypoxic) is likely to make the situation worse. There is no benefit to additional steroid use if an adequate dose was originally given.

58. C. The influenza vaccination is the most cost-effective treatment in patients with COPD. The COPD value pyramid quantifies the cost-effectiveness of various treatments. After the influenza vaccination, the order of treatments is as follows: smoking cessation, pulmonary rehabilitation, inhalers and telehealth. Of note smoking cessation remains the most important treatment and the one that provides the most patient benefit. This was a tricky question!

## Chapter 16 Disorders of the interstitium

59. C. Asbestos. Asbestos is known to cause asbestosis, pleural plaques, mesothelioma and lung cancer but it is not commonly linked to hypersensitivity pneumonitis.

60. A. An HRCT with bilateral basal honeycomb change. HRCT in IPF typically shows a usual interstitial pneumonia pattern with subpleural peripheral and basal fibrosis and honeycomb change. Consolidation on CT would suggest an alternative process such as infection, as would blood tests suggestive of infection (raised WBC and CRP level). Spirometry in a patient with IPF normally shows a restrictive pattern with a

decreased gas transfer. A chest radiograph showing cardiomegaly and pulmonary oedema suggests cardiac failure, a differential for IPF.

61. D. Coal workers initially get simple pneumoconiosis which tends to usually not have any symptoms associated with the radiographic changes. However, in some cases this progresses to progressive massive fibrosis which results in increased symptoms. Silicosis can also lead to progressive massive fibrosis.

## Chapter 17 Lung cancer

62. C. Liver, bone, brain, adrenals, skin. This is a hard question; reread the chapter and try to remember them.

63. B. A solitary 4-cm left-sided hilar lung tumour with involvement of two ipsilateral hilar lymph nodes but no distal metastases. A mass of 3–5 cm is stage 2. Note the ipsilateral (same side) hilar node involvement giving N1 with no evidence of metastatic disease (M = 0). Answer A demonstrates contralateral node involvement (N = 3) and C is likely metastatic breast cancer. D gives signs of distal metastases (M = 1) while E shows a very small lung lesion which may or may not have clinical significance (more details of features are required).

64. D. Arrange a staging CT. This man appears to have lung cancer; a CT will define the next most suitable investigations. A lateral chest radiograph will add little to the current clinical picture and a cortisol level is not indicated. Tuberculosis or other infection may be a differential diagnosis in this patient, however is less likely and further imaging should be performed first.

65. C. Arrange an urgent CT chest. This patient has superior vena cava obstruction, an oncological emergency. Treatment is with high-dose steroids, radiotherapy or stenting. The presentation does not fit with anaphylaxis or sepsis at this stage, but further active investigation needs to be performed to rule out serious underlying pathology.

66. E. Stopping smoking improves life expectancy even after lung cancer diagnosis. It is never too late to stop! Squamous cell is the commonest lung cancer type in Europe; haemoptysis is seen in around 50% of lung cancer patients. Finger clubbing has many causes including cardiac, abdominal or respiratory. Spinal cord compression occurs because of metastatic disease as a structural complication rather than a paraneoplastic syndrome.

67. B. Hypercalcaemia. The patient's symptoms fit with this and it is a common complication of cancer that can be excluded by a simple blood test.

## Chapter 18 Respiratory infections

68. C. *Streptococcus pneumoniae*.

69. A. *Staphylococcus aureus*. This is a common cause of secondary bacterial infection following influenza. *S. aureus* pneumonia is often rapidly progressive and characteristically causes cavitation on X-ray.

70. B. *Pneumocystis jirovecii*. Pneumocystis is a fungal lung infection that commonly presents with dyspnoea on exertion in immunosuppressed patients. Patients with HIV and a CD4 count $<200 \times 10^6$/L are at risk.

71. D. Ziehl–Neelsen staining is used to identify acid-fast bacilli in TB. Haematoxylin and eosin are common stains used to visualize cell structures more clearly. Congo red is used to identify amyloid.

72. B. Oseltamivir is used in severe cases of influenza, not COVID-19.

## Chapter 19 Bronchiectasis and cystic fibrosis

73. D. Cystic fibrosis is a congenital cause of bronchiectasis. All other options are acquired causes of bronchiectasis.

74. A. High-resolution CT scan to look for typical signs of bronchiectasis such as thickened bronchial walls and the signet ring sign will confirm the diagnosis. A chest radiograph is not diagnostic in bronchiectasis. A sweat test is used to diagnose cystic fibrosis and, as this lady is in her 80s, is not required in this case. Flexible bronchoscopy is useful if unilobar disease owing to obstruction is suspected. Routine blood tests will not diagnose bronchiectasis but may be required if acute infection is suspected.

75. B. The F508del mutation is the most common cystic fibrosis mutation.

## Chapter 20 Pleural disease

76. E. Hypocalcaemia is not a recognized cause of pleural effusion. Organ failure and malignancy (including haematological malignancies) as well as low-albumin states from poor nutrition are all common causes of pleural effusion.

77. A. Bronchial carcinoma. A blood-stained effusion is highly suggestive of pulmonary malignancy, whether bronchial carcinoma or a pleural malignancy.

78. B. Insert a large bore cannula into the midclavicular line of the left second intercostal space. The clinical scenario describes a tension pneumothorax following chest trauma. This is a medical emergency and needle decompression of the pneumothorax should take place before any further investigations such as a chest X-ray or ABG analysis. A chest drain should be inserted

following needle decompression once the patient is stabilized.

79. E. Appearance of pus on pleural aspirate. Aspiration of pus from the pleural cavity is one of the defining features of empyema.

80. C. High-risk characteristics of a pneumothorax are: haemodynamic compromise (tension pneumothorax), significant hypoxia, bilateral pneumothorax, underlying lung disease, ≥50 years of age with significant smoking history or haemothorax.

## Chapter 21 Thromboembolic disease and pulmonary hypertension

81. B. CT pulmonary angiogram. The likely diagnosis in this scenario is pulmonary embolism following a recent deep vein thrombosis. A CT pulmonary angiogram is the gold standard investigation for diagnosis of a pulmonary embolism. Although pulmonary angiography is useful, it has considerably more risks associated with it.

82. B. Oral contraceptive pill. Although a risk factor, the oral contraceptive pill is not on the Wells scoring system for pulmonary embolism clinical probability.

83. B. Rivaroxaban is a direct inhibitor of factor X.

84. B. The most common cause of PH in the United Kingdom is pulmonary artery hypertension. It is accepted that the most common cause in the UK of PH is left heart disease. Pulmonary artery hypertension is rare in the general population.

## Chapter 22 Sleep disorders

85. E. All of the above. Down syndrome creates obstructive anatomy, obesity predisposes to adipose tissue deposition in the neck, acromegaly can cause macroglossia and amyloidosis can lead to deposition into and hypertrophy of soft tissue.

86. A. Continuous positive airway pressure therapy. CPAP is gold standard and first-line treatment in patients with severe OSA. NIV is indicated for patients with hypoventilation which would be accompanied by nocturnal hypoxia.

87. B. He cannot drive, but because he has mild OSA, he does not need to inform the DVLA immediately. He has 3 months to have treatment/modify sleep hygiene and if no better by then, he does need to inform them. This is likely to impact his job, so it is good practice to encourage them to inform their occupational health services.

## Chapter 23 Respiratory manifestations of systemic disease

88. B. A presentation of sarcoidosis combining hilar lymphadenopathy, erythema nodosum, joint symptoms and fever. Lofgren syndrome is a classical presentation of sarcoidosis. The other answers described are A: Churg–Strauss syndrome, C: Miller–Fisher syndrome, D: Caplan syndrome, E: Felty syndrome. Well done if you got them all!

89. E. Ankylosing spondylitis. The key is apical fibrosis. While rheumatoid arthritis is again often associated with lung fibrosis, it typically affects the lung bases. Other causes of apical lung fibrosis include sarcoidosis, pneumoconiosis, silicosis, radiation and tuberculosis.

90. C. Eosinophilic granulomatosis with polyangiitis (formerly known as Churg–Strauss disease) is a small-vessel vasculitis, typically presenting with late-onset asthma. It is characterized by the pathological triad of granulomatous inflammation, eosinophilia (seen on full blood count) and small-vessel vasculitis (purpura may be seen).

# OSCEs and Short Clinical Cases

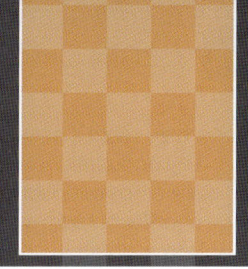

## PLEURAL DISEASE

Vignette: A 76-year-old man presents with breathlessness on exertion and a chest X-ray showing a pleural effusion on the right side.

1. What questions would you ask in the history to help you with the diagnosis?
   - History of breathlessness – duration of breathlessness, change in exercise tolerance (how far could you walk before you got breathless? Now, how far can you walk before you get breathless?), sudden or progressive, Medical Research Council Dyspnoea Scale.
   - Associated symptoms – cough (productive or dry), haemoptysis, chest pain, weight loss, PND, orthopnoea, ankle swelling, calf pain, fevers, night sweats, infective symptoms, risk factors for thromboembolic disease.
   - Systems review – any symptoms suggestive of systemic disease, e.g., connective tissue disorder or undiagnosed malignancy.
   - Other previous medical history – particularly diseases associated with pleural effusions such as cardiac failure, renal failure and rheumatoid arthritis.
   - Current medication history.
   - Occupational exposure – particularly asbestos.
   - Previous tuberculosis exposure.
   - Smoking history – current and previous. Record pack-year history.
   - Performance status.
2. What findings would you expect on physical examination?
   - General inspection – possibly breathless at rest.
   - Stony dull percussion note on the right.
   - Decreased breath sounds on auscultation of the right.
   - Bronchial breathing at the top of the effusion.
3. Your examination confirms the chest radiograph findings. What other investigations would you like to perform?
   - Bloods – clotting, renal function, full blood count including platelets, CRP.
   - Ultrasound right chest with diagnostic pleural aspiration of the right-sided pleural effusion.
   - Computed tomography scan of the chest.

4. Pleural aspiration under ultrasound guidance is performed in clinic. Pleural fluid results show a fluid protein of 34 g/dL and a fluid lactate dehydrogenase (LDH) of 1000. Is this effusion an exudate or a transudate?
   - Exudate.
   - The pleural fluid protein is equivocal (between 25 and 35 g/dL); however, using Light's criteria, this is an exudate, as the LDH is >300.
5. What is the differential diagnosis in this case?
   - The differential diagnosis for an exudative unilateral pleural effusion includes malignancy (pleural, lung, extrathoracic), empyema, parapneumonic effusion, pulmonary embolism, drug-related effusion and an effusion related to connective tissue disorders such as rheumatoid arthritis.

## CRASH COURSE RESPIRATORY OSCE CASES

### OSCE 1 Haemoptysis history

Mr Patel has had a cough for the last 2 months. Yesterday he coughed up some blood. Please take a history from him.

#### Checklist
- Introduce yourself, check patient's details and obtain consent.
- Fully clarify the presenting history. Explore the nature of coughing, the character of sputum produced and the details of the episode of haemoptysis (episodes, volume, colour, associated clots). Is there anything that has brought on these symptoms?
- Explore associated symptoms: shortness of breath, chest pain, palpitations, fevers, weight loss and night sweats.
- Ask about past medical history: Think about other lung conditions or previous infections, conditions causing clotting abnormalities or history of malignancy.
- Take a drug history: Check allergies. Ask about regular medication and correctly identify any anticoagulants or antiplatelet drugs which may exacerbate bleeding.
- Take a social history: Ask about smoking status, including amount per day and duration (calculating

pack-years if possible). Ask about occupation, including any occupational dust exposures. Specifically ask about asbestos exposure. Ask about foreign travel and country of birth, including known TB exposure. Consider home situation and support.

- Explore patient performance status: Ask about exercise tolerance and activity status, including functional state and ability to leave the house.
- Take a family history: Ask about a history of cancer in the family. Consider other hereditary conditions or clotting abnormalities.
- Ask about what the patient thinks this might be and what their concerns are. Address and discuss these where appropriate.
- Summarize your findings and give the opportunity for the patient to ask further questions or add in anything outstanding.

## Questions

1. What are the main causes of haemoptysis?
   - The commonest causes of haemoptysis can be broken down into groups: infective, malignant, autoimmune, vascular and other. Infective causes include bronchitis, pneumonia, pulmonary TB or lung abscess. Malignant causes include primary bronchial carcinomas and metastatic tumours. Autoimmune causes include vasculitis such as Goodpasture's or granulomatosis with polyangiitis. Vascular causes include pulmonary embolism and AV malformations. Other causes include trauma, foreign bodies, systemic coagulopathies or pulmonary endometriosis.
2. What would your next investigations be for this patient?
   - Observations and clinical examination.
   - Bloods – including full blood count, renal and liver functions, inflammatory markers and clotting screen.
   - Sputum examination – send for culture. If the history is suggestive, this could also be sent to assess for acid-fast bacilli and TB culture.
   - ECG – important if PE is part of your differential. Sinus tachycardia is the most common finding, although RV strain and the S1Q3T3 phenomenon can also be seen.
   - Imaging – chest radiography initially. May progress to CT depending on findings.
3. The patient has features in the history suggestive of a possible lung cancer. How would you counsel the patient that this is what you are investigating for?
   - Begin by establishing the patient's own concerns – cancer may be something that they are worried about too. Explain that, while a number of conditions can cause you to cough up blood, one of the conditions that you are concerned about is cancer.

Explain to the patient that you must consider all causes, including malignancy and as a result you feel that it is important to investigate things sooner rather than later. Give time to address the patient's response and tailor your responses accordingly.

4. The patient has features suggestive of active pulmonary TB. How would you manage them?
   - In a hospital setting, you would isolate the patient and ensure they were nursed in a side room with respiratory precautions. Aim to send a minimum of three sputum samples for AFB and TB culture and perform a chest radiograph. Refer to the TB specialist team and consider starting treatment based on senior advice (standard quadruple therapy in the UK currently includes rifampicin, isoniazid, pyrazinamide and ethambutol, although this would be altered if drug-resistant TB was suspected). If TB is confirmed then it is a notifiable disease in the UK and would require public health considerations and contact tracing.

5. The patient has features suggestive of pulmonary embolism. What are the indications for thrombolysis in pulmonary embolism?
   - Massive pulmonary embolism causing haemodynamic instability may require thrombolysis to treat. Indications are: sustained hypotension SBP <90 mmHg, pulselessness, cardiac arrest or profound bradycardia with signs of shock where PE is suspected as the underlying cause.
   - Contraindications to thrombolysis include previous intracranial haemorrhage, ischaemic stroke in the last 3 months (due to the risk of haemorrhage), active bleeding, recent surgery (site depends on timing) or suspected aortic dissection.

## OSCE 2 COPD exacerbation

Mrs Baxter, a lady with known COPD, presents with worsening shortness of breath. Please take a history from her.

## Checklist

- Introduce yourself, check the patient's details and gain consent.
- Clarify the presenting symptoms. Ask about symptom onset and progression of breathlessness, associated features such as cough including change in sputum colour (typically patients have white frothy phlegm with COPD; if becomes yellow or green, then this suggests an infection), wheeze, chest pain, fevers and other associated features. Explore any obvious triggers for this current illness such as infective contacts, new pets or changes of environment.

- Explore the COPD diagnosis. Establish duration of illness, number and frequency of exacerbations and any previous intensive care admissions. Establish current treatments used, adherence and inhaler technique. Consider home oxygen or home nebulizers.
- Take a full past medical history. Include any other lung diseases and conditions predisposing to infection such as diabetes, immunosuppressive conditions or chronic inflammatory states.
- Take a drug history. Always check for allergies. Include inhaler treatments and technique/adherence if not already performed above. Consider prior exacerbation treatments including steroid use and previous antibiotics used.
- Take a social history. Include smoking status and pack-year history. Occupational history, pets and housing status.
- Explore functional status: include distance the patient can walk on flat ground, whether they need walking aids and if they can manage stairs.
- Take a family history, focusing on lung illnesses.
- Explore the patient's ideas and concerns as to what is wrong and what they expect of treatment.
- Summarize the case back to the patient and give them time to ask questions or add in details.

## Questions

1. How do you assess the severity of a COPD exacerbation?
   - Severity is based on clinical assessment. This includes assessing respiratory rate (>30/min), use of accessory muscles and oxygen levels, signs of haemodynamic instability, altered mental status, evidence of hypercarbia or respiratory acidosis and failure of previous community treatment. Mild exacerbations with no adverse features can be managed at home while severe exacerbations require further assessment and hospital admission.
2. What are the next investigation steps for this patient?
   - Assessment includes examination either in an ABCDE assessment format or standard format with observations depending on clinical assessment and features. Blood tests include FBC, UE, LFT and CRP. Arterial blood gas analysis is mandatory for any patient requiring oxygen or showing features of respiratory failure. Sputum culture should be performed. Imaging includes chest radiography to assess for associated pneumonia or pneumothorax.
3. As you perform your investigations, the patient has saturations of 86% on room air and they are placed on nasal oxygen. How would you manage this patient?
   - The patient requires hospital admission for further assessment. Initially, the patient should have target

saturations of >94%. Arterial blood gas assessment is mandatory to look for evidence of hypercapnia and controlled oxygen therapy should thus be used with target saturations of 88%–92% if hypercapnia/raised bicarbonate is present. Treatments include corticosteroid therapy, antibiotics (usually oral unless features of sepsis or severe/resistant infection) and regular nebulized β-agonist and antimuscarinic treatments as initial therapy.
4. Despite your initial treatments, the patient deteriorates further. What are the indications for noninvasive ventilation (NIV) in COPD exacerbation?
   - NIV should be considered in an acute COPD exacerbation where respiratory acidosis (pH <7.35) persists after 1 hour of maximal standard medical therapy. Patients with pH <7.26 are at higher risk of deterioration or treatment failure and should be managed in a high-dependency or intensive care unit where appropriate.
5. What are the contraindications to noninvasive ventilation treatment?
   - Contraindications include noncompliance, inability to protect the airway, facial trauma or burns, recent facial or gastric surgery, impaired GCS and unconscious or respiratory arrest. At the time of consideration for NIV, the escalation status of the patient should be determined, including suitability for invasive ventilation where appropriate.

## OSCE 3 Emergency Station. Anaphylaxis

Mrs Heathcliffe presents to the emergency department with a suspected allergic reaction. Take a brief history and perform a clinical assessment.

## Checklist
- Introduce yourself, gain consent and wash your hands.
- Take a brief focused history of events: ask about allergies, any recent medications, foods or substances taken or other antigens (e.g., bee sting), any known medical history and functional status.
- Assess the patient's airway – if they are able to speak clearly, it is safe to presume patency. Listen for stridor and inspect, providing airway adjuncts where needed.
- Assess the breathing of the patient – look for respiratory rate and accessory muscle use, assess peripheral oxygen saturation and consider arterial gas analysis where appropriate. Auscultate the chest and percuss, listening for evidence of wheeze. Correct with high-flow oxygen through a non–rebreathe mask if deemed suitable.
- Assess the circulation of the patient – assess pulse rate, rhythm and character, peripheral and central perfusion

and capillary refill. Check blood pressure and perform an ECG. Auscultate for heart sounds. Gain IV access with peripheral cannulation. Perform blood tests where appropriate and justify selection.

- Assess for signs of disability. Assess for signs of neurological disability using either the AVPU scale or GCS. Assess for evidence of focal neurological deficit with screening movements and check capillary glucose.
- Assess everything else. Check the legs and abdomen for evidence of other focal pathology.
- Instigate treatments where deemed appropriate at any stage of assessment. Justify any treatment given and include route and dose. If these are not known state that you will look them up prior to administration.
- Reassess the patient after treatments are initiated, starting with A and progressing where appropriate.
- Ask for help. Escalate to a senior colleague when you are no longer comfortable managing the situation.
- Perform a verbal handover of the situation using the SBAR technique to your senior colleague/examiner. Describe the situation, patient background, your key assessment findings and recommendations.

## Questions

1. What is anaphylaxis?
   - Anaphylaxis is a severe and potentially life-threatening reaction to an antigen (e.g., peanuts or a bee sting) to which the body has become hypersensitive. The allergic reaction leads to a systemic reaction caused by a type 1 hypersensitivity IgE-mediated immune response.
2. What are the clinical features of anaphylaxis?
   - Anaphylaxis is characterized by rapidly developing airway, breathing and/or circulatory compromise, usually associated with skin or mucosal changes with an appropriate clinical history. Typical features include flushing, urticarial rash, pruritis, angioedema, throat tightness, shortness of breath, wheezing, dizziness, shock and a sense of impending doom.
3. What are the common causes of anaphylaxis?
   - The commonest causes are insect stings, nuts, other foods, antibiotics, anaesthetic drugs, other drugs and contrast media for radiological scans. Often no identifiable cause is found.
4. The patient has a history and features consistent with anaphylaxis. What treatments should you give?
   - The UK Resuscitation Council recommends for adults the following treatments:
   - 0.5 mL of I M 1:1000 adrenaline as soon as possible. May readminister after 5 minutes if appropriate.
   - Establish/protect airway and administer high-flow oxygen.

- Give a fluid challenge of 500–1000 mL IV crystalloid.
- Give oral nonsedating antihistamines in patients after initial stabilization in patients with persistent skin changes.
- Monitor patient regularly for signs of deterioration.

5. What is the role of mast cell tryptase in anaphylaxis assessment?
   - Mast cell tryptase can be measured to confirm the diagnosis of anaphylactic reaction. Tryptase is part of the mast cell secretory granules, the levels of which sharply increase in anaphylaxis due to mast cell degranulation. Mast cell tryptase peaks around 1 hour after the onset of anaphylactic symptoms and can be measured in a peripheral blood test to confirm diagnosis. Ideally this should be taken three times: as soon as possible after resuscitation, at 1 hour after symptoms and again 24 hours after treatment (to measure baseline level).

## OSCE 4 Asthma history

Miss Jones is a 25 year old with asthma who presents with worsening shortness of breath over the last few weeks. Please take a history from her.

## Checklist

- Introduce yourself, check patient's details and obtain consent.
- Clarify the presenting symptoms. Ask about symptom onset and progression of breathlessness, associated features such as cough including sputum colour, wheeze, chest pain, fevers or night sweats and nasal symptoms. Ask about diurnal variation of symptoms and night symptoms.
- Explore any trigger for this current illness such as infective contacts, new pets or changes of environment.
- Explore relationship of breathlessness to daily activities – any change with work or physical activity.
- Ask about past asthma history – duration of asthma, frequency of exacerbations, previous hospitalizations, previous stays in intensive care. Are symptoms normally controlled with current medication (e.g., waking up in the night due to asthma)? Is she adherent to her usual medications?
- Check if Miss Jones knows her best peak flow measurement. Has she been measuring it recently and if so has it changed?
- Ask about previous medical history – any other medical problems? History of atopy – eczema, allergic rhinitis.
- Take a drug history: Check allergies. Ask about inhaler use and offer to check inhaler technique. Ask about the use of oral steroids – how many courses have been required in the past 12 months? Ask about current and previous medications given for asthma.

- Take a family history: Ask about a history of atopic illness and asthma in the family.
- Take a social history: Ask about smoking status, including amount a day and duration (calculating pack-years if possible). Ask about passive smoke exposure. Ask about occupation, including any occupational dust exposures. Ask about exposures in the home – pets, damp and mould.
- Check the patient has an asthma action plan, that it is up to date and that they are aware of how to use it.
- Ask about what the patient thinks this might be and what their concerns are. Address and discuss these where appropriate.
- Summarize your findings and give the opportunity for the patient to ask further questions or add anything outstanding.

## Questions

1. What symptoms of asthma did this patient present with?
   - Summarize the symptoms of asthma elicited from your history. Asthma is a chronic inflammatory disorder of the airways that causes recurrent episodes of wheeze, chest tightness, breathlessness and cough. It is characterized by variable airflow obstruction. Classically symptoms display diurnal variation and worsen at night.
2. From the history you have taken, what triggers for this patient's worsening symptoms did you identify?
   - It is important to ask about the patient's known asthma triggers and try to identify any precipitating factors for the recent decline in symptoms, for example, a new pet or a recent lower respiratory tract infection.
   - Lifestyle triggers include – smoking, pets, exercise.
   - Environmental triggers include – pollens, exposure to dusts or moulds in the home, cold air, occupational exposures.
   - Physical triggers include – recent infection, stress, menstruation, aspirin.
3. What inhaled medications are commonly used in the treatment of asthma?
   - The main classes of inhaled medications used in asthma are inhaled corticosteroids and bronchodilators. Inhaled corticosteroids, such as budesonide, reduce the formation, release and action of many mediators involved in inflammation. Bronchodilators, such as $\beta_2$-agonists, reduce the resistance to airflow in the respiratory tract.
4. What are the signs of a life-threatening asthma exacerbation?
   - A patient with any one of the following symptoms: PEFR <33%, oxygen saturations <92%, $P_aO_2$ <8kPa, normal $PCO_2$ (4.6–6 kPa), silent chest,

cyanosis, poor respiratory effort, arrhythmia, exhaustion, confusion and coma. Emergency treatment should be initiated immediately with high-flow oxygen, nebulized bronchodilators and oral or intravenous corticosteroids. Senior input and ITU support should be sought immediately.

## OSCE 5 Inhaler Technique

Miss Smith, an 18 year old with recently diagnosed asthma, has come in to your GP surgery today to learn how to use her inhaler correctly. Please explain this to her.

## Checklist

- Introduce yourself, check the patient's details and gain consent.
- Explain what the inhaler device is used for.
- Explain in what circumstances the inhaler should be used – reliever, MART regime.
- Demonstrate the key points on the inhaler including dose count if present.
- Demonstrate and explain how to use the inhaler
  - Prepare the inhaler.
  - Load the dose.
  - Breathe out gently as far as is comfortable.
  - Tightly seal lips around the mouthpiece.
  - Breathe in – quick and deep for dry powdered inhalers, slow and deep for MDIs and soft mist inhalers.
  - Remove inhaler from the mouth and hold breath for as long as comfortable (approximately 10 seconds).
- Assess the patient performing the procedure, give feedback and ask them to repeat the procedure again to refine the technique if necessary.
- Talk to the patient about aftercare – advise to rinse the mouth after using steroid inhalers.
- Explain what a spacer can be used for – demonstrate Volumatic or AeroChamber to patient if present.
- Ask the patient if they have any questions or ongoing concerns.
- Provide information leaflet and check asthma plan if available.
- Thank the patient and wash hands.

## Questions

1. What different types of inhaler devices do you know?
   - Pressurized metered dose inhalers (MDIs) – the medication is stored in a pressurized canister with propellant. The inhaler techniques should include a 'slow and steady' inspiratory breath coordinated with actuation of the device.

- Dry powder inhaler – these release dry powdered medication to the lungs and require a 'fast and deep' inspiratory breath by the patient.
- Soft mist inhaler – these release an aerosolized measured dose of a medication by pressing a button. The inhaler technique is 'slow and steady'.

2. What is the MART regime?
   - MART is single Maintenance And Reliever Therapy. The inhaled therapy used includes both an inhaled corticosteroid and long-acting $\beta_2$-agonist.

3. Do you know any other methods of delivering inhaled medications to a patient?
   - Nebulizers aerosolize liquid medication for inhalation and are driven by either air or oxygen. They are used most frequently in hospital in patients with acute exacerbations of asthma or COPD.

4. What can you tell me about personalized asthma action plans?
   - Personalized asthma action plans inform patients of what to do if their symptoms worsen, how to escalate their treatment and when to seek medical attention. A patient's plan should be reviewed by a specialist asthma nurse during or just after any admission to hospital with asthma.

**Acinus** Airways involved in gaseous exchange, beginning with respiratory bronchioles and ending with the alveoli.

**Alveolar dead space** Air reaching the alveoli that does not partake in gas exchange, for example, because the alveoli are not perfused. This volume is included in physiological dead space.

**Anatomical dead space** Airways that do not partake in gas exchange, that is, from the nose and mouth to and including the terminal bronchioles. This volume is usually about 150 mL and included in physiological dead space.

**Antitussive** A medication that suppresses or relieves coughing (cough suppressant).

**Asthma** An airway disease with symptoms caused by reversible and intermittent airway obstruction. There is underlying inflammation characterized by eosinophilic infiltration. Often associated with other allergic diseases.

**Atelectasis** Collapse of part of the lung.

**Bronchiectasis** Permanent dilatation of the bronchi secondary to chronic infection. It is the end stage of many pulmonary diseases, including cystic fibrosis.

**Bronchitis** See 'Chronic bronchitis'.

**Bronchoalveolar lavage** A diagnostic test performed during bronchoscopy. Saline is squirted down the bronchoscope into the lungs, then sucked back up and the cells collected sent for cytology. The cellular profiles indicate different pathologies.

**Bronchoscopy** A diagnostic technique where a (usually fibreoptic) camera is inserted into the lungs to visualize pathology and take biopsy samples.

**Chronic bronchitis** A disease that is defined clinically by a persistent cough for at least 3 months of the year, for 2 consecutive years. Part of the spectrum of chronic obstructive pulmonary disease.

**Chronic obstructive pulmonary disease (COPD)** A collective term for inflammatory airway diseases (emphysema, chronic bronchitis and others) occurring almost exclusively in smokers, characterized by irreversible and progressive airway obstruction. Inflammation is characterized by neutrophilic infiltration.

**Conducting airways** Airways not involved in gas exchange, that is, airways proximal to respiratory bronchiole.

**Continuous positive airway pressure (CPAP)** A method of noninvasive ventilation whereby air is blown into the airways (positive pressure) for the whole of the respiratory cycle. CPAP is delivered by mask and is a common treatment for obstructive sleep apnoea.

**Corticosteroid (glucocorticosteroid)** A commonly used immunosuppressive drug that acts at a nuclear level to inhibit inflammation.

**Cystic fibrosis** An autosomal-recessive condition causing a defect in the cystic fibrosis transmembrane receptor (CFTR), resulting in abnormally viscous lung secretions. In the lung the mutation predisposes to chronic lung infection and bronchiectasis; it also affects the pancreas and can cause male infertility.

**Emphysema** Defined anatomically as destruction of the alveolar septa resulting in permanent enlargement of the air spaces distal to the terminal bronchiole. Part of the spectrum of chronic obstructive pulmonary disease.

**Haemoptysis** A term to describe the symptom of coughing up blood.

**Hypoxic vasoconstriction** Constriction of pulmonary blood vessels in response to low alveolar oxygen tension. This mechanism acts to prevent a ventilation:perfusion mismatch.

**Interstitial lung disease (ILD)** A diverse group of more than 200 different lung diseases affecting the interstitium (the tissue extending from and including the alveolar epithelium to capillary endothelium).

**Mediastinum** The collective name to describe structures situated in the midline and separating the two lungs. It contains the heart, great vessels, trachea, oesophagus, lymph nodes and phrenic and vagus nerves.

**Mesothelioma** Cancer of the lung pleura, almost always caused by asbestos inhalation.

**Obstructive lung diseases** Diseases which narrow the airways and increase resistance to air flow.

**Physiological dead space** The total amount of air in the lung that does not partake in gas exchange. Includes anatomical dead space and alveolar dead space.

**Pleura** An epithelial lining which covers the external surface of the lungs (visceral pleura) and then is reflected back to line the chest wall (parietal pleura).

**Pleural effusion** Fluid in the pleural space.

**Pneumocytes** The cells lining the alveoli. They are either type I, which are thin and primarily structural, or type II, which are rounded and secrete surfactant.

**Pneumonia** Infection of peripheral lung tissue.

**Pneumothorax** Air in the pleural space; the tension type is a medical emergency.

**Pulmonary embolism** Thrombi lodging in pulmonary vasculature causing ventilation:perfusion mismatches of varying severity. A serious complication of venous thrombosis.

**Pulmonary fibrosis** A restrictive lung disease where lung parenchyma is stiffened by deposition of collagen; the end point of many different lung diseases.

**Respiratory tree** Another name for the airways, particularly referring to their branching pattern. Does not include alveoli.

**Restrictive lung diseases** Diseases which stiffen the lungs so that expansion of the lungs is compromised.

**Sarcoidosis** A multisystem granulomatous disorder of unknown origin that can cause a granulomatous ILD.

**Spirometry** A diagnostic technique used to measure speed of air flow and the volume of air exhaled from the lungs.

**Surfactant** A liquid rich in phospholipids and apoproteins that lines the alveoli to reduce surface tension and defend the host against inhaled pathogens. It is secreted by type II pneumocytes.

**Wheeze** The musical sound heard on expiration, caused by airway narrowing.

# Index

Note: Page numbers followed by *f* indicate figures, *t* indicate tables, and *b* indicate boxes.

249